D1300146

Select Topics in MR Imaging

MAGNETIC RESONANCE IMAGING CLINICS OF NORTH AMERICA

www.mri.theclinics.com

February 2010 • Volume 18 • Number 1

SAUNDERS an imprint of ELSEVIER, Inc.

W.B. SAUNDERS COMPANY
A Division of Elsevier Inc.

1600 John F. Kennedy Boulevard • Suite 1800 • Philadelphia, Pennsylvania 19103-2899

http://www.theclinics.com

MRI CLINICS OF NORTH AMERICA Volume 18, Number 1
February 2010 ISSN 1064-9689, ISBN 13: 978-1-4377-1925-3

Editor: Joanne Husovski
Developmental Editor: Theresa Collier

Magnetic Resonance Imaging Clinics of North America (ISSN 1064-9689) is published quarterly by Elsevier Inc., 360 Park Avenue South, New York, NY 10010-1710. Months of issue are February, May, August, and November. Application to mail at periodicals postage rates is pending at New York, NY and at additional mailing offices. Subscription prices are $309.00 per year (domestic individuals), $455.00 per year (domestic institutions), $150.00 per year (domestic students/residents), $345.00 per year (Canadian individuals), $571.00 per year (Canadian institutions), $448.00 per year (international individuals), $571.00 per year (international institutions), and $217.00 per year (international and Canadian students/residents). International air speed delivery is included in all *Clinics* subscription prices. All prices are subject to change without notice. **POSTMASTER:** Send address changes to *Magnetic Resonance Imaging Clinics*, Elsevier Health Sciences Division, Subscription Customer Service, 3251 Riverport Lane, Maryland Heights, MO 63043. Customer Service (orders, claims, online, change of address): Elsevier Health Sciences Division, Subscription Customer Service, 3251 Riverport Lane, Maryland Heights, MO 63043. Tel:1-800-654-2452 (U.S. and Canada); 314-447-8871 (outside U.S. and Canada). Fax: 314-447-8029. E-mail: journalscustomerservice-usa@elsevier.com (for print support); journalsonlinesupport-usa@elsevier.com (for online support).

Reprints. For copies of 100 or more of articles in this publication, please contact the Commercial Reprints Department, Elsevier Inc., 360 Park Avenue South, New York, NY 10010-1710. Tel.: 212-633-3812; Fax: 212-462-1935; E-mail: reprints@elsevier.com.

Magnetic Resonance Imaging Clinics of North America is covered in the *RSNA Index of Imaging Literature, MEDLINE/PubMed (Index Medicus),* and *EMBASE/Excerpta Medica.*

Printed in the United States of America.

GOAL STATEMENT

The goal of *Magnetic Resonance Imaging Clinics of North America* is to keep practicing physicians up to date with current clinical practice by providing timely articles reviewing the state of the art in patient care.

ACCREDITATION

The *Magnetic Resonance Imaging Clinics of North America* is planned and implemented in accordance with the Essential Areas and Policies of the Accreditation Council for Continuing Medical Education (ACCME) through the joint sponsorship of the University of Virginia School of Medicine and Elsevier. The University of Virginia School of Medicine is accredited by the ACCME to provide continuing medical education for physicians.

The University of Virginia School of Medicine designates this educational activity for a maximum of 15 *AMA PRA Category 1 Credits*™ for each issue, 60 credits per year. Physicians should only claim credit commensurate with the extent of their participation in the activity.

The American Medical Association has determined that physicians not licensed in the US who participate in this CME activity are eligible for a maximum of 15 *AMA PRA Category 1 Credits*™ for each issue, 60 credits per year.

Credit can be earned by reading the text material, taking the CME examination online at http://www.theclinics.com/home/cme, and completing the evaluation. After taking the test, you will be required to review any and all incorrect answers. Following completion of the test and evaluation, your credit will be awarded and you may print your certificate.

FACULTY DISCLOSURE/CONFLICT OF INTEREST

The University of Virginia School of Medicine, as an ACCME accredited provider, endorses and strives to comply with the Accreditation Council for Continuing Medical Education (ACCME) Standards of Commercial Support, Commonwealth of Virginia statutes, University of Virginia policies and procedures, and associated federal and private regulations and guidelines on the need for disclosure and monitoring of proprietary and financial interests that may affect the scientific integrity and balance of content delivered in continuing medical education activities under our auspices.

The University of Virginia School of Medicine requires that all CME activities accredited through this institution be developed independently and be scientifically rigorous, balanced and objective in the presentation/discussion of its content, theories and practices.

All authors/editors participating in an accredited CME activity are expected to disclose to the readers relevant financial relationships with commercial entities occurring within the past 12 months (such as grants or research support, employee, consultant, stock holder, member of speakers bureau, etc.). The University of Virginia School of Medicine will employ appropriate mechanisms to resolve potential conflicts of interest to maintain the standards of fair and balanced education to the reader. Questions about specific strategies can be directed to the Office of Continuing Medical Education, University of Virginia School of Medicine, Charlottesville, Virginia.

The faculty and staff of the University of Virginia Office of Continuing Medical Education have no financial affiliations to disclose.

The authors/editors listed below have identified no professional or financial affiliations for themselves or their spouse/ partner:

Abass Alavi, MD, PhD (Hon), DSc (Hon); Bernd Bittersohl, MD; Peter M. Black, MD, PhD; Eduard de Lange, MD (Test Author); Christian Enzinger, MD; Franz Fazekas, MD; Fiona M. Fennessy, MD, PhD; Joanne Husovski (Acquisitions Editor); Sinchun Hwang, MD; Bobby Kalb, MD; Thomas M. Link, MD; Diego R. Martin, MD, PhD; John M.K. Mislow, MD, PhD; Marie-Louise Montandon, PhD; Elizabeth A. Morris, MD; Paul R. Morrison, MSc; Stefan Ropele, PhD; Ichiro Sakamoto, MD; Khalil Salman, MD; Reinhold Schmidt, MD; Puneet Sharma, PhD; Klaus A. Siebenrock, MD, PhD; Eijun Sueyoshi, MD; Kemal Tuncali, MD; Masataka Uetani, MD; John R. Votaw, PhD; Stefan Werlen, MD; Habib Zaidi, PhD, PD; and Christoph Zilkens, MD.

The authors/editors listed below identified the following professional or financial affiliations for themselves or their spouse/partner:
Alexandra J. Golby, MD is a stockholder for Schering Plough and Johnson & Johnson.
Daniel Havas, MSc is employed by JSW-Lifesciences.
Young-Jo Kim, MD, PhD is an industry funded research/investigator for Siemens Health Care and Bayer Health Care, and is on the Advisory Committee/Board for Siemens Health Care.
Tallal C. Mamisch, MD is a consultant for Siemens Healthcare AG.
Clare M. Tempany, MD is an industry funded research/investigator for NIH and Insightec, Inc, and is a consultant for Insightec, Inc.

Disclosure of Discussion of non-FDA approved uses for pharmaceutical products and/or medical devices
The University of Virginia School of Medicine, as an ACCME provider, requires that all faculty presenters identify and disclose any "off label" uses for pharmaceutical and medical device products. The University of Virginia School of Medicine recommends that each physician fully review all the available data on new products or procedures prior to instituting them with patients.

TO ENROLL

To enroll in the Magnetic Resonance Imaging Clinics of North America Continuing Medical Education program, call customer service at 1-800-654-2452 or visit us online at www.theclinics.com/home/cme. The CME program is available to subscribers for an additional fee of $99.95.

Contributors

CONSULTING EDITORS

VIVIAN S. LEE, MD, PhD, MBA
Professor of Radiology, Physiology, and
Neurosciences; Vice-Dean for Science; and
Senior Vice-President and Chief Scientific
Officer at New York University Langone
Medical Center, New York, New York

LYNNE STEINBACH, MD
Professor of Clinical Radiology and
Orthopaedic Surgery at the University
of California San Francisco in San Francisco,
California

SURESH MUKHERJI, MD
Professor and Chief of Neuroradiology
and Head & Neck Radiology; Professor
of Radiology, Otolaryngology Head Neck
Surgery, Radiation Oncology, Oral Medicine,
and Periodontics at the University of Michigan
Health System in Ann Arbor, Michigan

AUTHORS

ABASS ALAVI, MD, PhD (Hon), DSc (Hon)
Professor of Radiology, Division
of Nuclear Medicine, Hospital of the University
of Pennsylvania, Philadelphia, Pennsylvania

BERND BITTERSOHL, MD
Department of Orthopedic Surgery, University
of Bern, Freiburgstrasse, Switzerland; and
Department of Orthopedic Surgery, University
of Düsseldorf, Duseldorf, Germany

PETER M. BLACK, MD, PhD
Franc D Ingraham Professor, Department
of Neurosurgery, Harvard Medical School,
Brigham and Women's Hospital, Boston,
Massachusetts

CHRISTIAN ENZINGER, MD
Department of Neurology, Medical University
of Graz, Graz, Austria

FRANZ FAZEKAS, MD
Department of Neurology, Medical University
of Graz, Graz, Austria

FIONA M. FENNESSY, MD, PhD
Assistant Professor of Radiology, Harvard
Medical School; and Department of Radiology,
Brigham and Women's Hospital, Boston,
Massachusetts

ALEXANDRA J. GOLBY, MD
Assistant Professor, Department of
Neurosurgery, Harvard Medical School,
Brigham and Women's Hospital, Boston,
Massachusetts

DANIEL HAVAS, MSc
JSW-Research Forschungslabor GmbH,
Graz, Austria

SINCHUN HWANG, MD
Assistant Professor, Weill Medical College of
Cornell University; and Assistant Attending
Radiologist, Department of Radiology,
Memorial Sloan-Kettering Cancer Center,
New York, New York

BOBBY KALB, MD
Department of Radiology, Emory University
School of Medicine, Atlanta, Georgia

YOUNG-JO KIM, MD, PhD
Department of Orthopedic Surgery, Children's
Hospital, Harvard Medical School, Boston,
Massachusetts

THOMAS M. LINK, MD
Professor of Radiology, Department
of Radiology and Biomedical Imaging,
University of California at San Francisco,
San Francisco, California

TALLAL C. MAMISCH, MD
Department of Orthopedic Surgery, University of Bern, Freiburgstrasse, Switzerland; and Department of Radiology, Sonnenhof Clinics, Bern, Switzerland

DIEGO R. MARTIN, MD, PhD
Professor of Radiology and Director of MRI, Department of Radiology, Emory University School of Medicine, Atlanta, Georgia

JOHN M.K. MISLOW, MD, PhD
Department of Neurosurgery, Harvard Medical School, Brigham and Women's Hospital, Children's Hospital Boston, Boston, Massachusetts

MARIE-LOUISE MONTANDON, PhD
Division of Nuclear Medicine, Geneva University Hospital, Geneva, Switzerland

ELIZABETH A. MORRIS, MD
Memorial Sloan-Kettering Cancer Center, New York, New York

PAUL R. MORRISON, MSc
Department of Radiology, Harvard Medical School, Brigham and Women's Hospital, Boston, Massachusetts

STEFAN ROPELE, PhD
Department of Neurology, Medical University of Graz, Graz, Austria

KHALIL SALMAN, MD
Department of Radiology, Emory University School of Medicine, Atlanta, Georgia

REINHOLD SCHMIDT, MD
Department of Neurology, Medical University of Graz, Graz, Austria

PUNEET SHARMA, PhD
Department of Radiology, Emory University School of Medicine, Atlanta, Georgia

ICHIRO SAKAMOTO, MD
Department of Radiology and Radiation Biology, Nagasaki University Graduate School of Biomedical Sciences, Sakamoto, Nagasaki, Japan

EIJUN SUEYOSHI, MD
Department of Radiology and Radiation Biology, Nagasaki University Graduate School of Biomedical Sciences, Sakamoto, Nagasaki, Japan

KLAUS A. SIEBENROCK, MD, PhD
Department of Orthopedic Surgery, University of Bern, Freiburgstrasse, Switzerland

CLARE M. TEMPANY, MD
Professor of Radiology, Harvard Medical School; and Department of Radiology, Brigham and Women's Hospital, Boston, Massachusetts

KEMAL TUNCALI, MD
Instructor in Radiology, Harvard Medical School; and Department of Radiology, Brigham and Women's Hospital, Boston, Massachusetts

JOHN R. VATOW, PhD
Department of Radiology, Emory University School of Medicine, Atlanta, Georgia

MASATAKA UETANI, MD
Department of Radiology and Radiation Biology, Nagasaki University Graduate School of Biomedical Sciences, Sakamoto, Nagasaki, Japan

STEFAN WERLEN, MD
Department of Radiology, Sonnenhof Clinics, Bern, Switzerland

HABIB ZAIDI, PhD, PD
Division of Nuclear Medicine, Geneva University Hospital, Geneva, Switzerland

CHRISTOPH ZILKENS, MD
Department of Orthopedic Surgery, University of Düsseldorf, Duseldorf, Germany; and Department of Orthopedic Surgery, Children's Hospital, Harvard Medical School, Boston, Massachusetts

Contents

Preface   xi

Vivian S. Lee, Lynne Steinbach, and Suresh Mukherji

Origins of Intraoperative MRI   1

John M.K. Mislow, Alexandra J. Golby, and Peter M. Black

> Neurosurgical diagnosis and intervention has evolved through improved neuroimaging, allowing better visualization of anatomy and pathology. This article discusses the various systems that have been designed over the last decade to meet the requirements of neurosurgical patients and opines on the potential future developments in the technology and application of intraoperative MRI. Because the greatest amount of experience with intraoperative MRI comes from its use in brain tumor resection, this article focuses on the origins of intraoperative MRI in relation to this field.

MR Imaging—Guided Interventions in the Genitourinary Tract: An Evolving Concept   11

Fiona M. Fennessy, Kemal Tuncali, Paul R. Morrison, and Clare M. Tempany

> MR imaging-guided interventions are well established in routine patient care in many parts of the world. There are many approaches, depending on magnet design and clinical need, based on MR imaging providing excellent inherent tissue contrast without ionizing radiation risk for patients. MR imaging-guided minimally invasive therapeutic procedures have advantages over conventional surgical procedures. In the genitourinary tract, MR imaging guidance has a role in tumor detection, localization, and staging and can provide accurate image guidance for minimally invasive procedures. The advent of molecular and metabolic imaging and use of higher strength magnets likely will improve diagnostic accuracy and allow targeted therapy to maximize disease control and minimize side effects.

Magnetic Resonance Nephrourography: Current and Developing Techniques   29

Bobby Kalb, John R. Votaw, Khalil Salman, Puneet Sharma, and Diego R. Martin

> MR nephrourography (MRNU) makes it possible to obtain structural and functional data within a single imaging examination without using ionizing radiation. The functional data available with MRNU allows renal physiology to be examined in ways that were not possible previously. Coupled with the exquisite soft-tissue contrast provided by standard MR images, MRNU can provide a comprehensive study that yields critical diagnostic information on structural diseases of the kidneys and collecting system, including congenital and acquired diseases, and also on the full range of the causes of dysfunction in the transplanted kidney.

MR Imaging of the Aorta   43

Ichiro Sakamoto, Eijun Sueyoshi, and Masataka Uetani

> Recent advances in noninvasive imaging methods, such as CT and MR imaging, have replaced most of invasive angiographic procedures in the diagnosis of acquired aortic disease, decreasing the cost and morbidity of diagnosis. This article reviews and illustrates present MR imaging methods for evaluation of the aorta.

Common diseases of the aorta also are discussed with a focus on their unique morphologic and functional features and characteristic MR imaging findings. Knowledge of pathologic conditions of common aortic diseases and proper MR imaging techniques enables accurate and time-efficient aortic evaluation.

Diagnostic Breast MR Imaging: Current Status and Future Directions   57

Elizabeth A. Morris

Breast MRI has become an integral component in breast imaging. Indications have become clearer and better defined. Guidelines and recommendations are evolving and many are recognized and published. Future applications are exciting and may possibly improve our ability to diagnose breast cancer, improving the patient's treatment options and ultimately patient outcome.

Imaging of Lymphoma of the Musculoskeletal System   75

Sinchun Hwang

Imaging plays a crucial role in staging and the assessment of treatment response in patients who have lymphoma of the musculoskeletal system. This article reviews imaging features of lymphoma of bone, muscles, cutaneous, and subcutaneous tissue. At radiography, lymphoma of the bone is most commonly lytic, but the affected bone also can appear deceivingly normal, even when a large tumor is present. At CT, lymphoma of muscle can be homogenous in attenuation, and it may not show contrast enhancement, making tumor detection more difficult. Post-treatment changes often are encountered at MR imaging and positron emission tomography, and when considered in light of the patient's therapy regimen (eg, radiation therapy and granulocyte-colony stimulating factor), they usually can be differentiated from tumor. Post-treatment changes include diffuse FDG uptake in marrow after chemotherapy, indicating rebound of normal marrow, and MR imaging signal abnormalities that may persist for anywhere from a few months to years after treatment.

MR Imaging in Osteoarthritis: Hardware, Coils, and Sequences   95

Thomas M. Link

Whole-organ assessment of a joint with osteoarthritis (OA) requires tailored MR imaging hardware and imaging protocols to diagnose and monitor degenerative disease of the cartilage, menisci, bone marrow, ligaments, and tendons. Image quality benefits from increased field strength, and 3.0-T MR imaging is used increasingly for assessing joints with OA. Dedicated surface coils are required for best visualization of joints affected by OA, and the use of multichannel phased-array coils with parallel imaging improves image quality and/or shortens acquisition times. Sequences that best show morphologic abnormalities of the whole joint include intermediate-weighted fast-spin echo sequences. Also quantitative sequences have been developed to assess cartilage volume and thickness and to analyze cartilage biochemical composition.

MRI of Hip Osteoarthritis and Implications for Surgery   111

Tallal C. Mamisch, Christoph Zilkens, Klaus A. Siebenrock, Bernd Bittersohl, Young-Jo Kim, and Stefan Werlen

Osteoarthritis of the hip joint is caused by a combination of intrinsic factors and extrinsic factors. Different surgical techniques are being performed to delay or halt osteoarthritis. Success of salvage procedures of the hip depends on the existing cartilage and joint damage before surgery; the likelihood of therapy failure rises with advanced osteoarthritis. For imaging of intra-articular hip pathology, MR imaging represents the best technique because of its ability to directly visualize cartilage, superior soft tissue contrast, and the prospect of multidimensional imaging. This article gives an overview on the standard MR imaging techniques used for diagnosis of hip osteoarthritis and their implications for surgery.

MRI in Dementia   121

Reinhold Schmidt, Daniel Havas, Stefan Ropele, Christian Enzinger, and Franz Fazekas

With cognitive disorders increasingly common, clinicians urgently need faster and more accurate tools to classify such disorders and to noninvasively monitor therapeutic interventions. In this review, we provide information on MRI techniques that enable the study of the morphology, neuronal integrity, and metabolism of dementing illnesses. In addition, we explore the usefulness of such techniques as surrogate markers of these diseases.

The Clinical Role of Fusion Imaging Using PET, CT, and MR Imaging   133

Habib Zaidi, Marie-Louise Montandon, and Abass Alavi

Multimodality image registration and fusion have a key role in routine diagnosis, staging, restaging, and the assessment of response to treatment, surgery, and radiotherapy planning of malignant disease. The complementarity between anatomic (CT and MR imaging) and molecular (SPECT and PET) imaging modalities is well established and the role of fusion imaging widely recognized as a central piece of the general tree of clinical decision making. Moreover, dual modality imaging technologies including SPECT/CT, PET/CT, and, in the future, PET/MR imaging, now represent the leading component of contemporary health care institutions. This article discusses recent advances in clinical multimodality imaging, the role of correlative fusion imaging in a clinical setting, and future opportunities and challenges facing the adoption of multimodality imaging.

Index   151

Magnetic Resonance Imaging Clinics of North America

FORTHCOMING ISSUES

Breast MR Imaging
Linda Moy, MD and
Cecilia Mercado, MD,
Guest Editors

MR Imaging of the Neonate
Claudia Hillenbrand, PhD
and Thierry Huisman, MD,
Guest Editors

Normal Variants and Pitfalls in Musculoskeletal MR Imaging
William Morrison, MD
and Adam Zoga, MD,
Guest Editors

RELATED INTEREST

Breast Pathology
Laura Collins, MD
Surgical Pathology Clinics, June 2009

THE CLINICS ARE NOW AVAILABLE ONLINE!

Access your subscription at:
www.theclinics.com

Welcome to Magnetic Resonance Imaging Consulting Editors

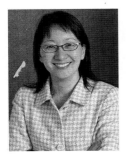
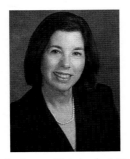
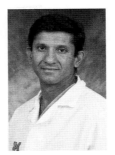

Vivian S. Lee, MD, PhD, MBA   Dr. Lynne Steinbach, MD   Dr. Suresh Mukherji, MD

Welcome to three *MRI Clinics* consulting editors for 2010 and 2011. They are Vivian S. Lee, MD, PhD, MBA; Lynne Steinbach, MD; and Suresh Mukherji, MD.

Dr. Lee is Professor of Radiology, Physiology, and Neurosciences; Vice-Dean for Science; and Senior Vice-President and Chief Scientific Officer at New York University Langone Medical Center, New York, New York.

Dr. Steinbach is Professor of Clinical Radiology and Orthopaedic Surgery at the University of California San Francisco in San Francisco, California.

Dr. Mukherji is Professor and Chief of Neuroradiology and Head & Neck Radiology; Professor of Radiology, Otolaryngology Head Neck Surgery, Radiation Oncology, Oral Medicine, and Periodontics at the University of Michigan Health System in Ann Arbor, Michigan.

These editors bring their combined skills in imaging and their respective specialty focus to this series. We are proud and pleased to have this stellar team join the *MRI Clinics*. Forthcoming are clinically relevant topics in magnetic resonance imaging of value and importance to imaging professionals of all experience levels.

Magn Reson Imaging Clin N Am 18 (2010) xi
doi:10.1016/j.mric.2009.10.001

mri.theclinics.com

Origins of Intraoperative MRI

John M.K. Mislow, MD, PhD, Alexandra J. Golby, MD*,
Peter M. Black, MD, PhD

KEYWORDS

- Intraoperative • MRI • Functional
- Neurosurgery • Brain • Tumor • Epilepsy

Successful neurosurgical procedures hinge on the accurate targeting of regions of interest. Resection of brain tumors is enhanced by the surgeon's ability to accurately define margins. Epileptic foci are identified by coregistration of functional and anatomic information, and stereotactic targets must be pinpointed with submillimetric accuracy for surgical efficacy. Specialized neuronavigational tools have been developed over the last 20 years to assist surgeons in these endeavors; the development of MRI-guided navigation systems represents a significant improvement in the surgical treatment of various intracranial lesions. The ability for most intraoperative image guidance systems to remain faithful to the anatomy once the cranium has been opened remains problematic, however. "Brain shift," the term applied to the dynamic change that intracranial anatomy undergoes after craniotomy, burr hole placement, drainage of cerebrospinal fluid, or resection of a lesion, compromises the localization of neural structures in space relative to where they were when preoperative images were acquired (**Fig. 1**).[1–8] Gliomas also pose a particular challenge to surgeons because many of these tumors (particularly low-grade gliomas) do not possess distinct capsules. As a result, even well-trained human eyes are incapable of discerning where the border of the lesion ends and viable brain begins. This uncertainty leads to two problems: (1) inadequate resection secondary to the surgeon stopping at what appears to be grossly abnormal tissue (so as to avoid neurologic damage) and (2) neurologic damage caused by aggressive surgery in which resection ends only when clearly normal brain tissue is visualized.

Only intraoperatively acquired images can provide neurosurgeons with the information needed to perform real-time, image-guided surgery. Uncertainty is reduced significantly when the surgeon places an instrument at the edge of what is believed to be the resection cavity, and a small nodule of tumor is immediately identified by intraoperative imaging. Avoidance and preservation of eloquent cortex such as motor, speech, and visual areas depend on precise identification of these regions during the procedure. The boundary between tumor and viable neural tissue is often difficult to see with the naked eye, so the superimposition of functional MRI, diffusion tensor imaging, and awake cortical mapping images eliminates a surgeon's uncertainty in determining tumor boundary and shifting brain structures. This leads to surgeons achieving maximal lesion resection while minimizing untoward neurologic sequelae. Maximal lesion resection is a principal goal in tumor resection because abundant evidence indicates that a more complete resection directly impacts the survival time of patients with low- and high-grade gliomas.[9–18]

ORIGINS OF INTRAOPERATIVE MRI: 0.5T OPEN-CONFIGURATION PROTOTYPE

The origin of iMRI for neurosurgery was the Magnetic Resonance Therapy (MRT) Unit at

This article originally appeared in the *Neurosurgery Clinics*: April 2009 Volume 20, Issue 2. This article was supported by the following NIH grants: NCRR, U41-RR019703 (AJG); NCI P01CA067165-11 NINDS, K08-NS048063-02 (AJG); and The Brain Science Foundation (AJG).
Department of Neurosurgery, Harvard Medical School, Brigham and Women's Hospital, 75 Francis Street, Boston, MA 02115, USA
* Corresponding author.
E-mail address: agolby@partners.org (A.J. Golby).

Magn Reson Imaging Clin N Am 18 (2010) 1–10
doi:10.1016/j.mric.2009.09.001
1064-9689/09/$ – see front matter © 2010 Elsevier Inc. All rights reserved.

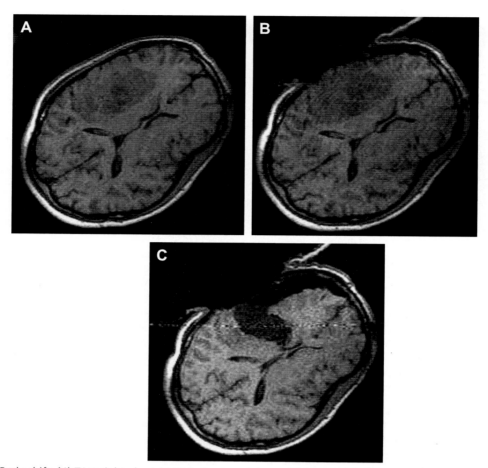

Fig. 1. Brain shift. (*A*) T1-weighted axial MRI before craniotomy. (*B*) Same axial plane MRI after craniotomy performed. (*C*) MRI after lesion resection. Note the significant shift of intracranial contents after craniotomy, cerebrospinal fluid drainage, and lesion resection.

Brigham and Women's Hospital (BWH) in Boston, Massachusetts. It began as a collaborative project among four groups: Ferenc Jolesz of the Department of Radiology at BWH, engineers at General Electric Medical Systems (Milwaukee, Wisconsin), the neurosurgical service at BWH with Dr. Peter Black as head, and the department of otorhinolaryngology with Marvin Fried as director. Throughout the late 1980s, these physicians and scientists collaborated in the development of an open-configuration MRI scanner that allowed surgery to be performed with concurrent intraoperative image guidance. At the time of inception, the closed-configuration of conventional MRI systems precluded direct access to the patient; therefore, fundamental changes in magnet and coil design and display methods were necessary to fully realize the concept of iMRI. This concept was a radical departure from MR physics of the time, with the magnetic field highest in the space between the double donut.

Early interventional procedures in an open MRI system were performed in a low-field imager by Gronemeyer and colleagues.[19,20] This system provided access to patients through a horizontal gap in its magnet. Access was significantly limited, however, and open surgeries that required full access to patients were impractical. Based on this information, after discussing several alternative designs, a "double donut" magnet system that would allow free access to patients within the magnetic field was chosen by BWH for development.[21] The initial research and development phase came to fruition in 1994 with the completion and installation of a prototype midfield intraoperative MRI system (GE 0.5-T Signa SP) unit at the BWH (**Fig. 2**).[22–24]

Direct access to patients was achieved by the construction of two vertically oriented superconducting magnets with coils in separate but communicating cryocoolers. This design results in a vertical gap between the coils through which

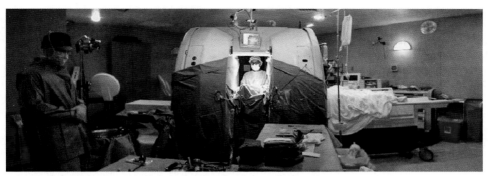

Fig. 2. The MRT unit at BWH. The General Electric Signa 0.5-T iMRI is an open-configuration "double donut" system that allows the surgeon to operate between each superconductive magnet coil (pictured).

patients can be fully accessed during image acquisition. Niobium tin, which has a maximum superconducting transition at higher temperatures than the more common niobium titanium, allows for sufficient cooling of the coils and thermal shield with cryocooler assembly, which eliminates the need for liquid helium coolant. This design resulted in a significantly increased area of patient access: the modified magnet provides a spherical imaging volume 30 cm in diameter and a 56-cm wide area of patient access, allowing surgeons and first assistants to be positioned on either side of patients.[21] In addition to the wide patient access area, the configuration of the "double-donut" magnet allows the position of patients within the imager to be flexible; the table can be inserted into the magnet along two orthogonal axes ("end docked" and "side docked"), which allows convenient access to different areas of anatomy. Because of the open configuration of the MRT, surgeons can perform various percutaneous, interventional, endoscopic, or open surgical procedures while standing or sitting and simultaneously viewing intraoperatively obtained MRI displayed on monitors placed in the gap of the magnet.

Many challenges needed to be met during the original implementation of iMRI, including the development of MRI-compatible equipment, instruments, and various tools along with the integration of the intraoperative display of images, the audiovisual communication among the team members, and the interactive manipulation of image data.

The initial phase of the iMRI project was slowed down by the unavailability of MR-compatible surgical instruments. In many cases, extensive changes were required to adapt instruments and equipment to the unique electromagnetic environment.[25–28] Many ferromagnetic surgical instruments were replaced by titanium, providing the

essential capabilities required for craniotomies without becoming a ballistic hazard. Several metallic instruments that were not ferromagnetic still caused a substantial artifact when placed near a target within the imaging field of view and could not be used. An early problem was the headholder, which had to be firm, nonferromagnetic, and flexible. It was possible to create a headholder similar to the Mayfield device made of high performance plastic, but it took many months. The next challenge was the power drill; for more than a year, the only procedures that could be done were biopsies because there was no way to turn a craniotomy flap. The Midas Rex Corporation (Medtronic, Minniapolis, Minnesota) finally was able to create a nonferromagnetic drill. The operating microscope was the third major device to be created; it was possible to create a plastic microscope with nonferromagnetic joints that, although simple, was adequate. Finally, we were able to develop a bipolar coagulator whose current would not interfere with the magnetic field. Each of these technologic developments took 6 to 12 months to complete, but gradually it was possible to do surgery in the intraoperative GE Signa system just as readily as in a routine operating room. Anesthesia and patient monitoring systems that did not emit any electronic noise and could function during a scan were developed and installed within the MRT suite[29]; fortunately, they had been created for performing pediatric MR imaging under anesthesia.

The development of imaging during surgery led to the "Surgical Planning Laboratory" at BWH. The occurrence of surgically induced volumetric deformations known as brain shift has been well established. There were no detailed analyses, however, of the changes that occur during surgery. As a result, Gering and colleagues[30] at BWH developed a volumetric display software (3D Slicer; www.slicer.org) that allowed quantitative analysis of the degree and direction of brain shift (**Fig. 3**). For 25 patients, multiple intraoperative volumetric image acquisitions were extensively evaluated. It was found that brain shift is a continuous dynamic process that evolves differently in distinct brain regions. The authors concluded that only serial imaging or continuous data acquisition can provide consistently accurate image guidance.[30,31] Further refinements in tracking intraoperative brain deformation were performed in a pilot study by Archip and colleagues in 2008.[32]

The combination of the 0.5-T iMRI and three-dimensional slicer transformed the MRT into an exceptionally effective tool for neurosurgeons. Since the first craniotomy for brain tumor resection in 1996, more than 1000 craniotomies for intracranial tumor resection have taken place in the MRT (40% low-grade gliomas, 50% high-grade gliomas, and 10% other intracranial lesions such as metastases, meningiomas, and vascular malformations).[33,34] In most patients with brain tumor operated on in the MRT, resection rates of 80% or more were achieved.[10] This percentage reinforces the value of iMRI in extension of lifespan of patients, because patients with subtotal tumor resection are at a higher risk of recurrence and death compared with patients with gross total tumor removal.

EXPANDING THE SCOPE OF OPEN-CONFIGURATION INTRAOPERATIVE MRI

The BWH MRT was the original iMRI system but it was by no means the last. Because of the specialized nature of the equipment, the entire MRT suite needed to be custom-made to accommodate the scanner. Room shielding, coolant, and power consumption were only a few of the expensive and high-maintenance aspects of the MRT. iMRI had proven itself to be a powerful tool in the hands of neurosurgeons attempting to achieve maximal tumor resection while preserving neurologic function, but how could institutions and practitioners take advantage of this technology without embarking on the expense of a major remodeling of their operative suite?

There were several answers, all driven by neurosurgeons. A major center was Erlangen, where Rudolph Fahlbusch helped to develop multiple concepts of Siemens for intraoperative imaging. This system moved from a side-opening low field to a system in which a table rotated into and out of a 1.5-T closed-bore magnet. Fahlbusch showed that for pituitary tumors and low-grade gliomas this system had a major advantage over other systems. A second answer was driven by the Israeli surgeon Moshe Hadani and his group.[35] Initially introduced in 2001 by Hadani and collagues,[35] the PoleStar (Medtronic Navigation, Louisville, Colorado) N-10 iMRI offered an open-configuration, portable 0.12-T magnet that required only modest remodeling of the operative suite. The device was stored in what amounted to a small garage within the operating theater. The N-10's compact size and low magnetic footprint allowed units to be integrated into multiple institutions' conventional operating rooms. Despite a slightly increased time for induction of anesthesia and intubation, the units made a significant and

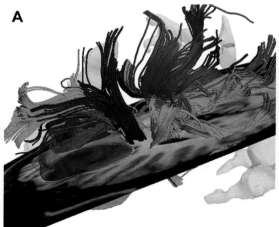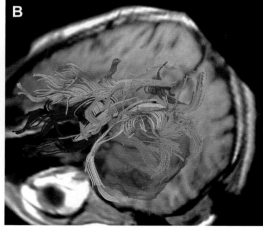

Fig. 3. Intraoperative colocalization using iMRI images and 3-D Slicer software. (*A*) Tumor, functional MRI, and diffusion tensor imaging are colocalized with standard MRI. (*B*) After craniotomy is performed, 3-D Slicer compensates for brain shift, allowing surgeons to visualize not only shift of gross neuroanatomy but also functional regions and white matter tracts.

positive impact on the safety and completeness of tumor resection in adult and pediatric intracranial procedures.[36–41] PoleStar recently introduced a higher-field (0.15-T) N-20 (**Fig. 4**), and initial evaluations confirm that the accuracy, versatility, and quality of this new-generation iMRI scanner are at least as good as the N-10. Clearly further clinical analysis of the accuracy on clinical cases using the N-20 is needed to confirm that these results will bear out in surgical reality.[36,37,42]

Other open-configuration iMRIs have since been developed. A 0.3-T horizontal iMRI by Hitachi at the University of Cincinnati[43,44] is a customized diagnostic iMRI, but the draping configuration does not lend itself to the sterile nature of neurosurgical interventions.

ORIGINS OF CLOSED-CONFIGURATION INTRAOPERATIVE MRI

A significant shortfall of the BWH MRT was the relatively low field offered by such a specialized system: the 0.5-T field did not yield image resolution comparable to contemporary diagnostic 1.5-T and 3-T MRI scanners. Initially, the basis of the

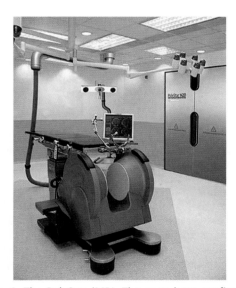

Fig. 4. The PoleStar iMRI. The open-bore configuration PoleStar N-20, despite its low-field 0.15-T magnet, has allowed many institutions to take advantage of iMRI without completely remodeling their operative suite to accommodate a larger, high-field stationary iMRI. The Polestar is compact enough to be stored in a shielded room (pictured on the right side of the figure) when not in use. If a smaller room cannot be dedicated to storage, an in-suite "hangar" can be set up to shield the magnet when not in use. (*Courtesy of* Medtronic Navigation, Louisville, CO; with permission.)

double-donut design was that sacrifice of high-field imaging was acceptable if the patient did not have to be moved. This paradigm of imaging on demand proved to be efficient and effective over more than a decade. The field moved toward a paradigm of "in and out" imaging, however, primarily to enable the use of more off-the-shelf scanners. Surgical teams have developed protocols for moving patients in and out of the scanner that are relatively rapid and efficient. Methods to maintain patient registration data throughout the procedure were developed using an integrated overhead navigation camera or fixed markers on patients.[45,46] As a result of these findings, it was felt that the next iteration that should evolve from the original open-configuration MRT would be developed from a high-field, closed-bore system. Consequently, several static closed-bore 1.5-T and 3-T systems have been installed in a growing number of institutions.[46,47] They are essentially hybrid systems that can be used for imaging or surgery.

The IMRIS system was developed by a neurosurgeon, Dr Garnette Sutherland of Calgary, Alberta, Canada. This system offers a unique intraoperative rail-mounted system in which the scanner is brought to patients (**Fig. 5**). By enabling the MR system to move to patients, the system allows for improved surgical work-flow and enhanced patient safety in the surgical environment. The 70-cm bore 1.5-T magnet is able to move from room to room via a ceiling-mounted rail system, which allows the system to be shared between two operating rooms. A magnet room that is separated from the operating room via sliding radiofrequency- and sound-shielded doors allows the magnet to be used for diagnostic studies when not used in the surgical theater. The suite is designed around the IMRIS magnet and features an MR-compatible operating room table, application-specific 8-channel intraoperative radiofrequency coils, and head fixation devices specifically designed to fit with the IMRIS operating room table and radiofrequency coils. Nine systems have been installed worldwide, with more than 1000 surgeries performed with these systems. Twelve additional systems are currently in stages of installation. The next generation IMRIS suites will feature a 3-T magnet with capacity for biplanar angiography within the magnet room.

FUTURE HORIZONS OF INTRAOPERATIVE MRI
Intraoperative MRI Robotics

In the iMRI suite, manual manipulation of instruments limits the precision and repeatability of

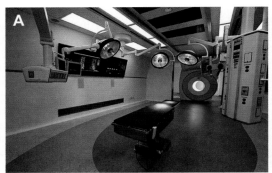
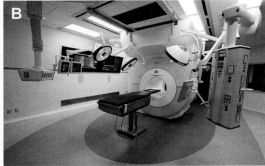
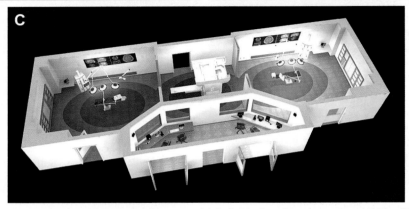

Fig. 5. The IMRIS iMRI. The IMRIS iMRI suite features a high-field, closed-bore magnet. (*A*) The IMRIS magnet in its storage room, shielding doors opened to show its relation to the operative suite when not in use. (*B*) The magnet has moved on its ceiling-mounted rails to its position over the region of the patient's head. The 1.5-T magnet can be brought from its park position in the storage room to a fully operational position within the operating room in less than 90 seconds, allowing for efficient scanning while still remaining unobtrusive. (*C*) An example of the IMRIS magnet serving two separate operating rooms. (The magnet can swivel 180° in the storage room to orient the working end toward the appropriate operating room.) (*Courtesy of* IMRIS, Inc, Winnipeg, Manitoba, Canada.)

placement, particularly when surgeons have their attention divided between multiple surgical team members, image displays, and the surgical field. As closed-bore systems predominate, the ability to manipulate tools remotely becomes increasingly important. For this reason, several groups have considered the use of instrument manipulation via robotics.[48,49] In the late 1990s, Chinzei and colleagues[50] developed one of the first MRI-compatible robotic manipulators, and the resulting positioning device was integrated into the MRT to form an MRI-guided interventional system.[51–53] Despite its revolutionary concept, this robot is designed exclusively for the original open-bore 0.5-T MRT, so its use is limited to few facilities. An MRI-compatible surgical robot suited for the new generation of closed-bore iMRI systems may offer more applicability and versatility in the neurosurgical community at large.

To enhance a surgeon's ability within the closed-bore iMRI environment, Sutherland and colleagues[54] developed an MRI-compatible neurosurgical robot, the NeuroArm (**Fig. 6**). The robot is compact enough to function within the confines of the 70-cm bore MRI, is entirely MRI compatible, and features haptic feedback. The latter feature is a significant step in the progression of neurosurgical assistive technologies, because real-time tactile feedback is known to reduce error and increase efficiency.[49,55] Haptic data may be recorded in a real case and replayed off-line. This feature represents a powerful educational tool for neurosurgeons-in-training, allowing them to develop an understanding of tactile experience of manipulating delicate neural tissue.

FUTURE INTRAOPERATIVE MRI SUITES

Since the first biopsy was performed in the BWH MRT in 1995, researchers, engineers, and surgeons have been collaborating on developing the next-generation iMRI. In 2009, the National

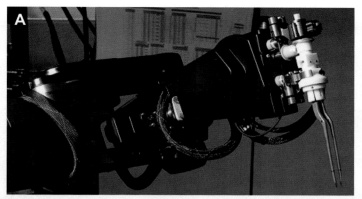
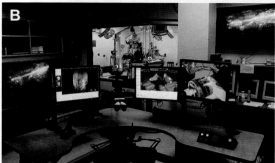
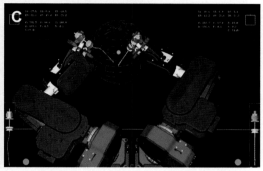

Fig. 6. The NeuroArm MRI-compatible neurosurgical robot. (*A*) Detailed picture of one of the NeuroArm's two operative limbs, with bipolar cautery attachment. (*B*) Command center for NeuroArm robot, where surgeon is seated and driving the movements of the robot through haptic-feedback controllers. (*C*) Real-time virtual reality display of the robot's position is delivered to the surgeon. Other virtual reality displays feature colocalization of MRI, functional MRI, and diffusion tensor imaging. (*Courtesy of* NeuroArm, Calgary, Alberta, Canada.)

Center for Image Guided Therapy at BWH will open the Advanced Multimodality Image Guided Operating (AMIGO) suite, a multimodality image-guided operating suite dedicated to intraoperative guidance (**Fig. 7**).[56] The suite will allow neurosurgeons to use 3-T MRI scans, positron emission tomographic (PET)/CT scans, ultrasound, radiographic fluoroscopy, and microscopy to update preoperative plans. The seamless unification of multiple intraoperative images promises the effective delivery of superior care for a wide range of medical conditions.

The AMIGO will be a three-room, 5700-sq-ft interventional suite with an operating room and, on opposing sides of it, a GE (Waukesha, Wisconsin) Discovery STE 64-slice PET-CT scanner and a GE 3-T 750 DVMR scanner. Staff will move patients under general anesthesia via a specialized surgical table through the operating room, PET suite, and MR suite using the table's wheels or between the patient beds of the PET and MR suite on a mobile transfer tabletop. The seamless nature of patient transfer helps to address the concern over patient safety prompted by previous generations of static closed-bore iMRI systems. Other imaging devices will include ultrasound, radiographic fluoroscopes, and surgical navigation equipment. All components are designed to function in an integral manner.

As a state-of-the-art suite, the AMIGO is designed for the implementation and further development and refinement of multimodal imaging in diagnosis and therapy, such as enabling biopsies and the removal of any unwanted tissue to occur with enhanced accuracy during the same treatment session. Within the AMIGO, imaging modalities will be used in conventional and novel ways. For example, in addition to being used as it customarily is, ultrasound will be tested under research protocols within the AMIGO for its potential to monitor brain shift in real-time during neurosurgery.[56] The new understandings and techniques emerging from within the AMIGO will enable clinicians to better understand areas of interest; plan, monitor, or change treatment; navigate through a procedure or operation; and know how, where, and when to best apply a novel therapy.

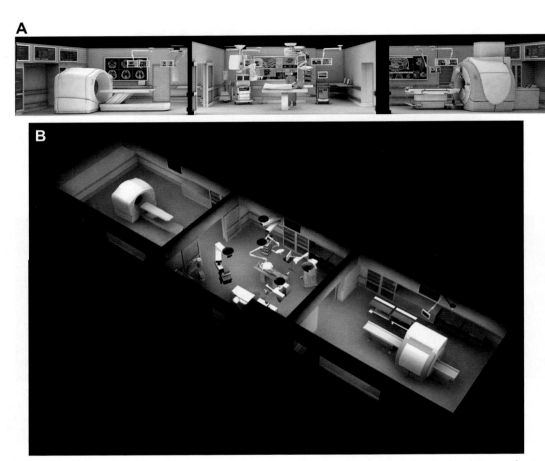

Fig. 7. The Advanced Multimodality Image Guided Operative (AMIGO) suite at the National Center for Image Guided Therapy, BWH and the Harvard Medical School. In AMIGO, real-time anatomic imaging modalities such as radiography and ultrasound are combined with the cross-sectional digital imaging systems of PET-CT and MRI. (*A, B*) Cross-sectional and oblique views of the three-room suite composed of a PET-CT (*left room*), state-of-the-art operating room, and 3.0-T MRI (*right room*). (*Courtesy of* GE Healthcare, Wauwatosa, WI; with permission.)

SUMMARY

In this article, we present a comprehensive framework describing the motivation, development, and evolution of contemporary iMRI in neurosurgery. We describe several key iMRI systems that have developed over the last 15 years, several of which have been evaluated in clinical cases at BWH and others that remain in developmental stages. Although the origins of iMRI can be traced to open-bore MRI at the BWH MRT, the framework for future growth and refinement will be applicable in closed-MRI systems and multimodal operating rooms that are currently on the cusp of operational capacity. Image-guided surgical navigation systems and robotics will be invaluable for applications in closed, high-field MRI magnets, particularly for applications in which real-time imaging is critical. Because targeting with submillimetric precision is required for functional neurosurgical procedures such as deep brain stimulation, gene therapy, and cell transplantation therapeutic strategies, iMRI suites will be of great importance for the future success of functional neurosurgery as a field.

The iMRI suite is a hybrid, combining elements of an interventional radiology unit, an MRI facility, and operating room. In this setting, the respective role and communication among team members (eg, surgeons, radiologists, MR technologists, nurses, anesthesiologists, computer scientists, and engineers) is of paramount importance. In the increasingly technologically driven field of medicine and science, the human factor remains the most critical.

ACKNOWLEDGMENTS

The authors dedicate this in memory of John M.K. Mislow our dear friend and esteemed colleague.

REFERENCES

1. Tronnier VM, Wirtz CR, Knauth M, et al. Intraoperative diagnostic and interventional magnetic resonance imaging in neurosurgery. Neurosurgery 1997;40(5):891–900.

2. Wirtz CR, Tronnier VM, Bonsanto MM, et al. Image-guided neurosurgery with intraoperative MRI: update of frameless stereotaxy and radicality control. Stereotact Funct Neurosurg 1997;68(1–4 Pt 1):39–43.

3. Maurer CR Jr, Hill DL, Martin AJ, et al. Investigation of intraoperative brain deformation using a 1.5-T interventional MR system: preliminary results. IEEE Trans Med Imaging 1998;17(5):817–25.

4. Nimsky C, Ganslandt O, Hastreiter P, et al. Intraoperative compensation for brain shift. Surg Neurol 2001; 56(6):357–64 [discussion: 64–5].

5. Ferrant M, Nabavi A, Macq B, et al. Serial registration of intraoperative MR images of the brain. Med Image Anal 2002;6(4):337–59.

6. Soza G, Grosso R, Labsik U, et al. Fast and adaptive finite element approach for modeling brain shift. Comput Aided Surg 2003;8(5):241–6.

7. Hastreiter P, Rezk-Salama C, Soza G, et al. Strategies for brain shift evaluation. Med Image Anal 2004;8(4):447–64.

8. Clatz O, Delingette H, Talos IF, et al. Robust nonrigid registration to capture brain shift from intraoperative MRI. IEEE Trans Med Imaging 2005;24(11):1417–27.

9. Berger MS, Deliganis AV, Dobbins J, et al. The effect of extent of resection on recurrence in patients with low grade cerebral hemisphere gliomas. Cancer 1994;74(6):1784–91.

10. Claus EB, Horlacher A, Hsu L, et al. Survival rates in patients with low-grade glioma after intraoperative magnetic resonance image guidance. Cancer 2005;103(6):1227–33.

11. Keles GE, Anderson B, Berger MS. The effect of extent of resection on time to tumor progression and survival in patients with glioblastoma multiforme of the cerebral hemisphere. Surg Neurol 1999;52(4): 371–9.

12. Lacroix M, Abi-Said D, Fourney DR, et al. A multivariate analysis of 416 patients with glioblastoma multiforme: prognosis, extent of resection, and survival. J Neurosurg 2001;95(2):190–8.

13. Berger MS, Rostomily RC. Low grade gliomas: functional mapping resection strategies, extent of resection, and outcome. J Neurooncol 1997;34(1): 85–101.

14. Fernandez-Hidalgo OA, Vanaclocha V, Vieitez JM, et al. High-dose BCNU and autologous progenitor cell transplantation given with intra-arterial cisplatinum and simultaneous radiotherapy in the treatment of high-grade gliomas: benefit for selected patients. Bone Marrow Transplant 1996;18(1):143–9.

15. Johannesen TB, Langmark F, Lote K. Progress in long-term survival in adult patients with supratentorial low-grade gliomas: a population-based study of 993 patients in whom tumors were diagnosed between 1970 and 1993. J Neurosurg 2003;99(5): 854–62.

16. McGirt MJ, Chaichana KL, Gathinji M, et al. Independent association of extent of resection with survival in patients with malignant brain astrocytoma. J Neurosurg 2008;110:156–62.

17. Sakata K, Hareyama M, Komae T, et al. Supratentorial astrocytomas and oligodendrogliomas treated in the MRI era. Jpn J Clin Oncol 2001;31(6):240–5.

18. Wirtz CR, Knauth M, Staubert A, et al. Clinical evaluation and follow-up results for intraoperative magnetic resonance imaging in neurosurgery. Neurosurgery 2000;46(5):1112–20 [discussion: 20–2].

19. Gronemeyer D, Seibel R, Erbel R, et al. Equipment configuration and procedures: preferences for interventional microtherapy. J Digit Imaging 1996;9(2): 81–96.

20. Gronemeyer DH, Seibel RM, Schmidt A, et al. Two- and three-dimensional imaging for interventional MRI and CT guidance. Stud Health Technol Inform 1996;29:62–76.

21. Schenck JF, Jolesz FA, Roemer PB, et al. Superconducting open-configuration MR imaging system for image-guided therapy. Radiology 1995;195(3): 805–14.

22. Alexander E 3rd, Moriarty TM, Kikinis R, et al. The present and future role of intraoperative MRI in neurosurgical procedures. Stereotact Funct Neurosurg 1997;68(1–4 Pt 1):10–7.

23. Alexander E 3rd, Moriarty TM, Kikinis R, et al. Innovations in minimalism: intraoperative MRI. Clin Neurosurg 1996;43:338–52.

24. Moriarty TM, Kikinis R, Jolesz FA, et al. Magnetic resonance imaging therapy: intraoperative MR imaging. Neurosurg Clin N Am 1996;7(2):323–31.

25. Kanal E. An overview of electromagnetic safety considerations associated with magnetic resonance imaging. Ann N Y Acad Sci 1992;649:204–24.

26. Kanal E, Borgstede JP, Barkovich AJ, et al. American College of Radiology White Paper on MR Safety: 2004 update and revisions. AJR Am J Roentgenol 2004;182(5):1111–4.

27. Kanal E, Borgstede JP, Barkovich AJ, et al. American College of Radiology White Paper on MR Safety. AJR Am J Roentgenol 2002;178(6):1335–47.

28. Kettenbach J, Kacher DF, Kanan AR, et al. Intraoperative and interventional MRI: recommendations for

a safe environment. Minim Invasive Ther Allied Technol 2006;15(2):53–64.

29. Black PM, Moriarty T, Alexander E 3rd, et al. Development and implementation of intraoperative magnetic resonance imaging and its neurosurgical applications. Neurosurgery 1997;41(4):831–42 [discussion: 42–5].

30. Gering DT, Nabavi A, Kikinis R, et al. An integrated visualization system for surgical planning and guidance using image fusion and an open MR. J Magn Reson Imaging 2001;13(6):967–75.

31. Nabavi A, Black PM, Gering DT, et al. Serial intraoperative magnetic resonance imaging of brain shift. Neurosurgery 2001;48(4):787–97 [discussion: 97–8].

32. Archip N, Clatz O, Whalen S, et al. Compensation of geometric distortion effects on intraoperative magnetic resonance imaging for enhanced visualization in image-guided neurosurgery. Neurosurgery 2008;62(3 Suppl 1):209–15 [discussion: 15–6].

33. Oh DS, Black PM. A low-field intraoperative MRI system for glioma surgery: is it worthwhile? Neurosurg Clin N Am 2005;16(1):135–41.

34. Jolesz FA, Talos IF, Schwartz RB, et al. Intraoperative magnetic resonance imaging and magnetic resonance imaging-guided therapy for brain tumors. Neuroimaging Clin N Am 2002;12(4):665–83.

35. Hadani M, Spiegelman R, Feldman Z, et al. Novel, compact, intraoperative magnetic resonance imaging-guided system for conventional neurosurgical operating rooms. Neurosurgery 2001;48(4):799–807 [discussion: 9].

36. Gerlach R, du Mesnil de Rochemont R, Gasser T, et al. Feasibility of Polestar N20, an ultra-low-field intraoperative magnetic resonance imaging system in resection control of pituitary macroadenomas: lessons learned from the first 40 cases. Neurosurgery 2008;63(2):272–84 [discussion: 84–5].

37. Ntoukas V, Krishnan R, Seifert V. The new generation Polestar N20 for conventional neurosurgical operating rooms: a preliminary report. Neurosurgery 2008;62(3 Suppl 1):82–9 [discussion: 89–90].

38. Samdani AF, Schulder M, Catrambone JE, et al. Use of a compact intraoperative low-field magnetic imager in pediatric neurosurgery. Childs Nerv Syst 2005;21(2):108–13 [discussion: 14].

39. Levivier M, Wikler D, De Witte O, et al. PoleStar N-10 low-field compact intraoperative magnetic resonance imaging system with mobile radiofrequency shielding. Neurosurgery 2003;53(4):1001–6 [discussion: 7].

40. Schulder M, Sernas TJ, Carmel PW. Cranial surgery and navigation with a compact intraoperative MRI system. Acta Neurochir Suppl 2003;85:79–86.

41. Kanner AA, Vogelbaum MA, Mayberg MR, et al. Intracranial navigation by using low-field intraoperative magnetic resonance imaging: preliminary experience. J Neurosurg 2002;97(5):1115–24.

42. Salas S, Brimacombe M, Schulder M. Stereotactic accuracy of a compact intraoperative MRI system. Stereotact Funct Neurosurg 2007;85(2–3):69–74.

43. Bohinski RJ, Kokkino AK, Warnick RE, et al. Glioma resection in a shared-resource magnetic resonance operating room after optimal image-guided frameless stereotactic resection. Neurosurgery 2001;48(4):731–42 [discussion: 42–4].

44. Nimsky C, Ganslandt O, Fahlbusch R. 1.5 T: intraoperative imaging beyond standard anatomic imaging. Neurosurg Clin N Am 2005;16(1):185–200, vii.

45. Lipson AC, Gargollo PC, Black PM. Intraoperative magnetic resonance imaging: considerations for the operating room of the future. J Clin Neurosci 2001;8(4):305–10.

46. Hushek SG, Martin AJ, Steckner M, et al. MR systems for MRI-guided interventions. J Magn Reson Imaging 2008;27(2):253–66.

47. Hall WA, Truwit CL. Intraoperative MR-guided neurosurgery. J Magn Reson Imaging 2008;27(2):368–75.

48. Louw DF, Fielding T, McBeth PB, et al. Surgical robotics: a review and neurosurgical prototype development. Neurosurgery 2004;54(3):525–36 [discussion: 36–7].

49. McBeth PB, Louw DF, Rizun PR, et al. Robotics in neurosurgery. Am J Surg 2004;188(4A Suppl):68S–75S.

50. Chinzei K, Miller K. Towards MRI guided surgical manipulator. Med Sci Monit 2001;7(1):153–63.

51. Hata N, Tokuda J, Hurwitz S, et al. MRI-compatible manipulator with remote-center-of-motion control. J Magn Reson Imaging 2008;27(5):1130–8.

52. Dimaio SP, Archip N, Hata N, et al. Image-guided neurosurgery at Brigham and Women's Hospital. IEEE Eng Med Biol Mag 2006;25(5):67–73.

53. DiMaio SP, Pieper S, Chinzei K, et al. Robot-assisted needle placement in open-MRI: system architecture, integration and validation. Stud Health Technol Inform 2006;119:126–31.

54. Sutherland GR, Latour I, Greer AD. Integrating an image-guided robot with intraoperative MRI: a review of the design and construction of neuroArm. IEEE Eng Med Biol Mag 2008;27(3):59–65.

55. Rizun PR, McBeth PB, Louw DF, et al. Robot-assisted neurosurgery. Semin Laparosc Surg 2004;11(2):99–106.

56. Advanced Multimodality Image Guided Operating (AMIGO) Suite. 2008. Available at: http://www.ncigt.org/pages/AMIGO. Accessed November 2, 2008.

MR Imaging–Guided Interventions in the Genitourinary Tract: An Evolving Concept

Fiona M. Fennessy, MD, PhD*, Kemal Tuncali, MD,
Paul R. Morrison, MSc, Clare M. Tempany, MD

KEYWORDS

- Uterine fibroids
- Magnetic resonance guided focused ultrasound surgery (MRgFUS) • Genitourinary tract • Prostate cancer
- Radiofrequency ablation • Brachytherapy

MR imaging–guided interventions are a well-established form of routine patient care in many centers around the world. There are many different approaches, depending on magnet design and clinical need. The rationale behind this is based initially on MR imaging providing excellent inherent tissue contrast, without ionizing radiation risk for patients. MR imaging–guided minimally invasive therapeutic procedures have major advantages over conventional surgical procedures. In the genitourinary tract, MR imaging guidance can play a role in tumor detection, localization, and staging and can provide accurate image guidance for minimally invasive procedures for the confirmation of pathology, tumor treatment, and treatment monitoring. Depending on the body part accessed, a customizable magnet bore configuration and magnetic resonance (MR)-compatible devices can be made available. The advent of molecular and metabolic imaging and the use of higher strength magnets likely will improve diagnostic accuracy and allow patient-specific targeted therapy, designed to maximize disease control and minimize side effects.

GENITAL TRACT: FEMALE

One of the most unique and exciting MR-guided interventional procedures in the female pelvis is MR-guided focused ultrasound surgery (MRgFUS). In addition, MR is used to guide other interventions and therapies, such as biopsies and gynecologic tumor treatments. The latter have been done in several centers, guiding the placement of radiation catheters for delivery of high-dose radiation in cervical or endometrial cancer.[1]

MAGNETIC RESONANCE–GUIDED FOCUSED ULTRASOUND SURGERY FOR TREATING UTERINE FIBROIDS

Uterine fibroids are the most common female pelvic tumor, occurring in approximately 25% of women.[2] Although many patients remain asymptomatic, others suffer from symptoms, such as pelvic pain, menorrhagia, dysmenorrhagia, dyspareunia, urinary frequency, and infertility. Ultrasound (US) usually is the first diagnostic imaging modality of choice for fibroids, demonstrating a well-defined, usually hypoechoic mass. Providing good inherent tissue contrast, MR imaging is the optimal modality for fibroid detection, accurate localization, and volumetrics.

A wide spectrum of treatment options for uterine fibroids exists, ranging from expectant waiting to medical management to myomectomy to hysterectomy. Women, however, increasingly are seeking

This article originally appeared in *Radiologic Clinics of North America* 2008;46(1):149–66.
This work was supported in part by National Institutes of Health grant U41RR019703.
Department of Radiology, Harvard Medical School/Brigham and Women's Hospital, 75 Francis Street, Boston, MA 02115, USA
* Corresponding author.
E-mail address: ffennessy@partners.org (F.M. Fennessy).

less invasive treatment options, perhaps motivated by fertility preservation and the possibility of reduced postprocedure recovery time. A good example of a less invasive choice is uterine artery embolization, a procedure that has demonstrated significant growth and interest since its introduction in 1995.[3] Only MRgFUS, however, is completely noninvasive. Approved by the United States Food and Drug Administration (FDA) in October 2004, much of the worldwide experience with MRgFUS has been with treatment of uterine fibroids, with more than 3500 patients treated to date.

Fundamentals of Magnetic Resonance–Guided Focused Ultrasound Surgery

The potential surgical application of focused ultrasound surgery (FUS) was first demonstrated in 1942.[4] Since then, it has been evaluated extensively in animal [5,6] and human[7] brains and in the kidney, prostate, liver, bladder,[8–11] and eye[12] within clinical trials. Clinical acceptance, however, was hampered because of the difficulty in controlling the focal spot position, defining the beam target precisely, and coping with the lack of feedback about thermal damage.

MR imaging can satisfy the requirements of FUS, having excellent anatomic resolution and high sensitivity for tumor visualization, thereby offering accurate planning of the tissue to be targeted. By exploiting the temperature dependence of the water proton resonant frequency,[13] MR-based temperature mapping is possible. This allows for targeting of the beam during subthreshold US exposures [14] and online estimation of the ablated volume.[15,16] Phase imaging is used to estimate the temperature-dependent proton resonant-frequency shift using a fast spoiled gradient-re-called-echo sequence (SPGR).[17] Therefore, obtaining temperature-sensitive MR images before, during, and after each sonication can monitor tissue temperature elevations, including any slight elevations in normal adjacent surrounding tissue, thereby preventing damage.

Magnetic Resonance–Guided Focused Ultrasound Surgery Equipment for Fibroid Treatment

Sonications are performed using an MR-compatible focused US system that is built into a table that docks with a compatible MR scanner. The system consists of a focused piezoelectric phased-array transducer (208 elements, frequency 0.96–1.14 MHz) that is located within the specially designed table surrounded by a water tank. A thin plastic membrane covers the water tank and allows the US beam to propagate into the tissue.

Patients lie in a prone position in the magnet, with the anterior abdominal wall positioned over the water tank. The location of the focal spot is controlled electronically by the transducer array that controls the volume of coagulation necrosis.

Patient Selection for Magnetic Resonance–Guided Focused Ultrasound Surgery of Uterine Fibroids

The FDA has approved this procedure for premenopausal women who have symptomatic uterine fibroids and who have no desire for future pregnancy. This treatment is not indicated for pregnant women, postmenopausal women, or those who have contraindications to contrast-enhanced MR imaging. If multiple fibroids are present, clinical symptomatology and accessibility to the target fibroids are reviewed and a target fibroid is selected. The anterior abdominal wall is evaluated for extensive scarring. Those women who have such scarring are excluded from treatment because of the risk for skin burns.[18]

Treatment Planning

Immediately before treatment, T2-weighted fast spin-echo images in three orthogonal planes are obtained to plan the beam path to the targeted lesion. The MR images are analyzed to evaluate the area to be treated for possible obstructions. Although patients who have extensive anterior abdominal wall scarring in the beam path generally are excluded at screening, it may be possible, however, to treat women who have abdominal wall scarring that is not extensive by angling the beam path, ensuring that the scar is not traversed (Fig. 1). Filling of the urinary bladder by Foley catheter clamping also may help in moving the uterus and selected fibroid into a position away from the abdominal wall scar. Coursing bowel loops lying anterior to the uterus at the level of the uterine fibroid also may cause treatment-planning difficulties. Placement of a gel spacing device may allow the bowel loops to be displaced out of the treatment field, thereby enlarging the acoustic window and allowing for greater treatment volume (Fig. 2).

Clinical Trials in the Treatment of Uterine Fibroids with Magnetic Resonance–Guided Focused Ultrasound Surgery

Multicenter clinical trials investigating the use of MRgFUS in the treatment of uterine fibroids, which subsequently resulted in device labeling by the FDA, were performed at five medical centers across the United States in addition to centers in the United Kingdom, Germany, and Israel. Follow-up of many patients is ongoing.

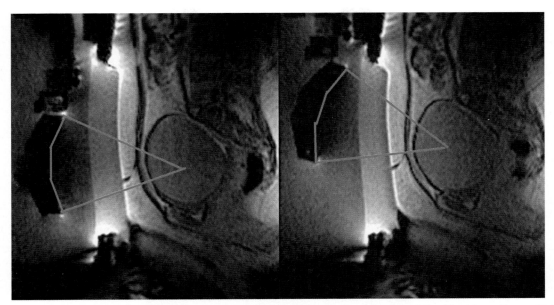

Fig. 1. Linear scar through the subcutaneous tissue lies between the transducer and the fibroid, on the sagittal localizer image on the *left*. The sagittal localizer image on the *right* is obtained after tilting the transducer superiorly, without moving the patient, allowing treatment planning that will not course through the anterior abdominal subcutaneous tissue scar. (*Reproduced from* Fennessy FM, Tempany CM. A review of magnetic resonance imaging-guided focused ultrasound surgery of uterine fibroids. Top Magn Reson Imaging 2006;17(3):173–9; with permission.)

Enrollment for phase I/II began in 1999 to assess the safety and feasibility of MRgFUS in the treatment of fibroids. Eligible patients underwent MRgFUS followed by hysterectomy, and subsequent pathologic examination of the uterus and fibroid showed that MRgFUS did result in hemorrhagic necrosis in the area of nonperfusion on the post-treatment MR.[19,20]

Phase III of the clinical trial involved treatment of larger volumes of fibroids in women who had symptomatic uterine fibroids who otherwise would have opted for hysterectomy (**Fig. 3**). To date, the longest-term follow-up—in 359 patients—is up to 24 months.[21] These patients reported durable symptom relief. Those who had a greater nonperfused treatment volume fared better, with fewer of

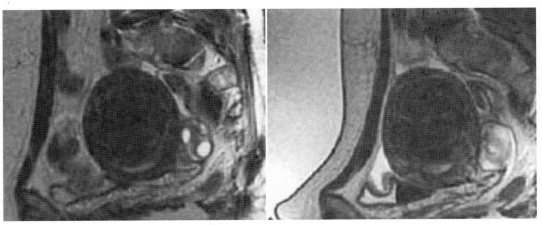

Fig. 2. The sagittal localizer image on the *left* demonstrates bowel loops coursing between the anterior abdominal wall and the uterine fibroid. After placement of a spacer device (sagittal localizer image on the *right*) under the anterior abdominal wall, the bowel loops are displaced, allowing for treatment through a larger acoustic window. (*Reproduced from* Fennessy FM, Tempany CM. A review of magnetic resonance imaging-guided focused ultrasound surgery of uterine fibroids. Top Magn Reson Imaging 2006;17(3):173–9; with permission.)

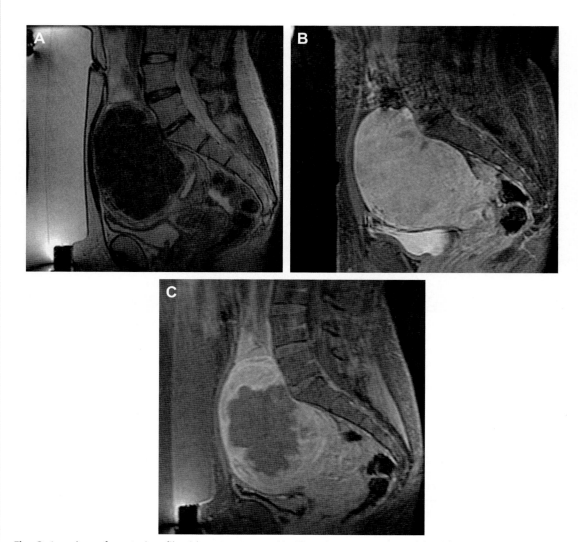

Fig. 3. Imaging of a uterine fibroid pretreatment (*A, B*) and post-treatment (*C*) with MRgFUS. Sagittal T2-weighted image (*A*), obtained with the patient in the prone position overlying the US transducer, demonstrates a large solitary uterine fibroid of low-signal intensity. Sagittal SPGR post gadolinium (*B*) demonstrates homogenous enhancement of the fibroid. After treatment, sagittal SPGR post gadolinium (*C*) demonstrates a new large nonperfused area within the fibroid, consistent with treatment-induced necrosis.

these patients undergoing additional fibroid treatment. These findings concur with those of Fennessy and colleagues,[22] where greater clinical outcome was found in those treated with a modified treatment protocol that allowed for greater nonperfused fibroid volumes post treatment.

CRYOTHERAPY FOR UTERINE FIBROIDS

MR-guided cryotherapy is a minimally invasive procedure. It involves a percutaneous approach in an interventional setting with multiple (1 to 5) needle-like 17-G cryotherapy probes. Each probe

creates a tear-drop shaped volume of frozen tissue about its tip (approximately 2.5-mm diameter); the simultaneous use of multiple probes gives a larger volume of treated tissue in the same time frame as treating with a single probe. The freeze is provided by pressurized argon gas that circulates within the probe. Typical treatments involve a cycling of the gas that delivers a freeze-thaw-freeze to destroy tissue, with each stage of the cycle 10 to 15 minutes in duration. MR imaging–guided cryotherapy has been evolving through experiment and clinical use during the past 20 years to target a range of tumors in various organ systems.[23] Compared with US that has shadow artifacts, visibility of the ice ball for monitoring is not as limited.

There are several promising reports of MR imaging–guided cryotherapy to treat symptomatic patients who have uterine fibroids.[24–27] During cryotherapy, the ice appeared as a signal void in the image as a result of the short MR relaxation time of the solid ice, giving a clear demarcation between frozen and unfrozen tissue. Though all reported relief from deleterious symptoms, short-term clinical outcome, however, is reported in only 8 of 9 treated patients, who demonstrated on average, 65% volume reduction in uterine size.[25]

One of these studies [26] was performed transvaginally, with the investigators proposing that such an approach had the advantage of providing direct access, especially for submucosal tumors. Procedures usually are performed with epidural anesthesia in a horizontally open MR imaging scanner with multiple 2- to 3-mm cryotherapy probes (**Fig. 4**). Gradient-echo and T2-weighted spin-echo sequences were used to guide probe placement and monitor the treatment cycle of freeze-thaw-freeze (**Fig. 5**).

Percutaneous ablation of fibroids is a nascent procedure and not practiced widely. This method of ablation has found a place in treating other parts of the body but not necessarily treating uterine fibroids, possibly because of the recent emergence of other minimally invasive procedures, such as uterine artery embolization, or noninvasive procedures, such as MRgFUS.

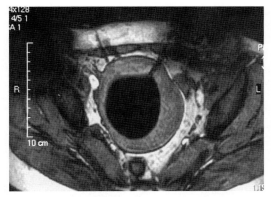

Fig. 5. Axial T2-weighted spin-echo sequence demonstrating a probe in the left anterolateral aspect of a uterine fibroid. The diffuse low-signal intensity in the fibroid represents the ice-ball. (*Courtesy of* Yusuke Sakuhara, MD, Department of Radiology, Hokkaido University Hospital, Sapporo, Japan.)

GENITAL TRACT: MALE

The leading cause of cancer death in men over 50, prostate cancer, affects one man in six in his lifetime. The American Cancer Society estimates that in 2007 in the United States, 218,890 new cases of prostate cancer will be diagnosed, and approximately 27,050 men will die of the disease.[28] There is only a 33% 5-year survival rate in men who have metastatic disease,[29] making early tumor detection and localized treatment a necessity.

MR IMAGING–GUIDED PROSTATE BIOPSY

Early diagnosis and cancer localization within the prostate gland usually are found through digital examination and serum prostate-specific antigen (PSA) measurement, followed by transrectal ultrasound (TRUS)-guided biopsy. Image-guided prostate biopsy with ultrasound (US) has become a universally accepted tool,[30] but because of a low sensitivity and specificity for tumor detection,[31] interest continues in the development of a more accurate technique. In addition, for men who have increasing PSA levels and repeatedly negative TRUS-guided prostate biopsies (the concern being that a sampling error may result in a false-negative biopsy), for those in whom a transrectal biopsy is not possible, or for those who are reluctant to undergo transrectal biopsy because of its recognized complications, such as infection, hematuria, hematospermia, and rectal bleeding,[32–34] an alternative approach may be necessary.

MR imaging can outline prostate architecture and substructure. Although the specificity for

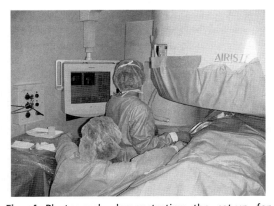

Fig. 4. Photograph demonstrating the set-up for percutaneous MR imaging–guided cryotherapy for uterine fibroids in an open horizontal 0.3-T AIRIS II (Hitachi, Tokyo, Japan) scanner. (*Courtesy of* Yusuke Sakuhara, MD, Department of Radiology, Hokkaido University Hospital, Sapporo, Japan.)

diagnosis may be limited, MR imaging can demonstrate suspicious nodules in the peripheral zone, the most common site for prostate cancer. On T2-weighted images, tumor is demonstrated most commonly by focal or diffuse regions of decreased signal intensity relative to the high-signal-intensity normal peripheral zone. MR imaging is used most routinely for staging men who have known cancer. The reported accuracy of prostate cancer detection and staging on MR images varies widely, with reports of accuracy ranging from 54% to 93%, likely because of differences in techniques and interobserver variability.[35–38]

Its role in detection and characterization, particularly in the initial diagnosis of high-risk patients or those who have previous negative biopsy findings but persistently high PSA levels, is increasing as techniques such as MR spectroscopy imaging (MRSI) and dynamic contrast enhancement become more widely available. The ultimate role and application in clinical practice, however, remain controversial.[35] MR imaging contributes significant incremental value to TRUS-guided biopsy and digital rectal examination in cancer detection and localization in the prostate.[39] It offers an excellent second-line alternative to those who have failed to obtain a diagnosis with conventional methods.

MR Imaging–Guided Prostate Biopsy: Technique

Two basic strategies have been explored for MR imaging–guided prostate biopsy. The first is coregistration of previously acquired diagnostic MR images to TRUS images, localizing suspected tumor lesions on MR and correlating these locations to the US.[40] The second strategy is stereotactic needle interventions within diagnostic MR scanners using careful patient positioning. By implementing surgical navigation software originally developed for neurosurgery[41,42] and adapting the technical capabilities of MR imaging–guided prostate brachytherapy in an open configuration magnet,[43] biopsy of suspected tumor foci in the peripheral zone is made possible (Fig. 6).[44] In addition, the feasibility of transrectal needle access to prostate tumors has been assessed in a closed-bore 1.5-T magnet[45–48] in a small number of patients, which potentially could provide for additional functional and spectroscopic imaging in comparison with a 0.5-T scanner. The procedure requires the use of a specialized device that consists of a needle guide and support system. The same guidance also has been used recently in a 3-T system.[49]

Larger studies of clinical usefulness, however, are necessary. With progress in biologic imaging of the prostate gland, it is likely that MR imaging guidance will play an increasing role in the diagnosis and treatment of prostate cancer.

MR Imaging–Guided Prostate Biopsy: The Future

The move toward targeted interventions, for diagnosis and treatment, underscores the need for precise image-guided needle placement. Based on a patient's anatomy and lesion detection in pretreatment MR imaging, a graphic planning interface that allows desired needle trajectories to be specified, through MR-compatible robotic assistance, recently has been described.[50] Avoiding the limitations of a fixed-needle template is a positive move forward for tissue sampling and treatment. As the field of prostate imaging moves to higher strength magnets, namely 3 T, the biopsy devices are reconfigured to allow sampling in a closed-bore environment. A recent study of prostate biopsy using 3-T MR imaging guidance described it as a promising tool for detecting and sampling cancerous regions in patients who have known prostate cancer[49]; however, the role (even at 3 T) of MR imaging–guided prostate biopsy as a screening tool in patients who have elevated PSA levels and recent previous negative biopsy remains to be determined.

MR IMAGING–GUIDED BRACHYTHERAPY FOR PROSTATE CANCER

Established options for the management of localized prostate cancer include one or a combination of the following: radical prostatectomy, external beam radiation therapy, brachytherapy, or watchful waiting. In radiation therapy, the goal is to achieve the prescribed dose throughout the prostate gland while minimizing toxicity to adjacent structures and minimizing morbidity from the procedure. Prostate brachytherapy is one of the more popular radiation methods in the prostate and involves the percutaneous placement of I-125 radiation seeds into the gland under image guidance. This is done most commonly with TRUS. It also can be done with MR guidance and the goal in both procedures is to optimize seed placement and allow maximal dose to the prostate peripheral zone tumor and minimal dose to the urethra and rectum.

Imaging-guided radiation therapy, therefore, allows directed tumor treatment, decreasing the chances of disease spreading outside the gland, while healthy prostate tissue and its neighboring structures are not overdosed. This is extremely

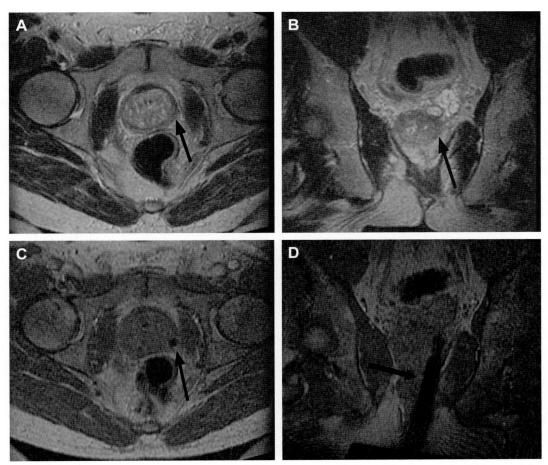

Fig. 6. Imaging before and during MR imaging–guided prostate biopsy. Axial (*A*) and coronal (*B*) T2-weighted spin-echo sequence outline areas to be biopsied. In this example, an area in the left midgland is demonstrated (*arrow*), reformatted to the same spatial location as the corresponding real-time axial (*C*) and coronal images (*D*) taken during needle insertion. The biopsy needle is seen in cross section as a circle of low-signal intensity (*arrow*) on the axial gradient-echo real-time image (*C*) and as a longitudinal area of low-signal intensity (*arrow*) on the coronal gradient-echo real-time image (*D*).

important for structures such as the urethra, in which over-radiation may cause stricture and fistualization that can be avoided with good image guidance.[51,52] Radiation dose fall-off is sharp at the rectal wall and at the urethra. Unlike external beam radiotherapy, there is no entrance or exit dose. Brachytherapy, therefore, has the potential to achieve superior tumor control with decreased morbidity and side effects. It is not, however, without its own set of complications, such as rectal irritation and ulceration, incontinence, and impotence resulting from inadvertent delivery of radiation dosing to the rectum, bladder, and urethra.

Patient Selection

Low-risk prostate cancer patients who have a high probability of organ-confined disease are screened appropriately with an endorectal coil MR for potential treatment with brachytherapy monotherapy. Most centers include patients who have stage T1-T2a (according to the American Joint Committee on Cancer/International Union Against Cancer 1997 staging), PSA level of 10 ng/mL or less, and a Gleason score of 6 or lower. The few contraindications to the procedure include prior transurethral resection of the prostate or morbid obesity (equipment cannot sustain the weight).

Procedure

MR-guided prostate brachytherapy using open configuration 0.5-T and 1.5-T scanners are described.[43,45] Using the open 0.5-T magnet, patients are placed supine between the two magnets in the lithotomy position under general anesthesia. A Foley catheter is inserted, the skin is prepared and draped in a sterile fashion, and a template for needle guidance is placed against the perineum. A rectal obturator then is placed and T2-weighted images are acquired in the axial, coronal, and sagittal planes and used to outline the urethra, peripheral zone, and anterior rectal wall. Surgical simulation software outlines these areas, and the targeted volume is calculated using designated planning software.[53] Seed number and depth of catheter insertion are calculated.

While gradient-echo MR images are obtained in real time,[44] seed-loaded catheters then are positioned in the prostate gland (**Fig. 7**). The images are compared to their intended locations, according to the radiation therapist plan. Dose-volume histograms of the urethra, anterior rectal wall, and target volume are obtained before final deployment of seeds. Six weeks after the procedure, CT imaging (to identify the seeds accurately) and MR imaging (for prostate anatomic correlation) are fused to calculate the final dose distribution to the gland and surrounding tissues.

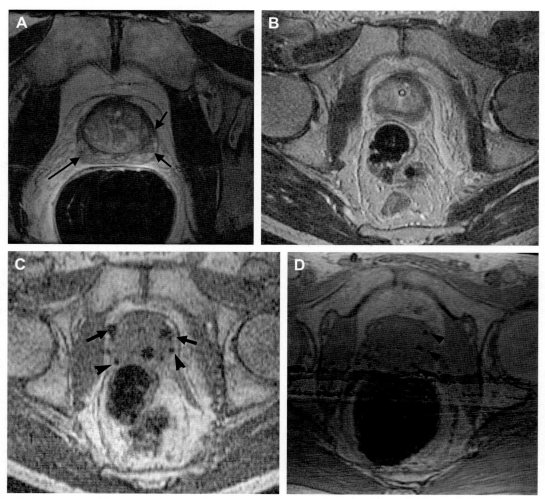

Fig. 7. Pre-, intra-, and postoperative MR imaging–guided brachytherapy in prostate cancer. Preoperative 1.5-T (*A*) axial T2-weighted spin-echo image through the prostate base, demonstrating low signal intensity in the peripheral zone (*arrows*), previously demonstrated to be tumor. Intraoperative 0.5-T (*B*) axial T2-weighted spin-echo T2 weighted spin-echo image through the same area. Intraoperative axial gradient-echo MR images (*C*) obtained in real time during needle and seed placement in the prostate base. The larger round areas represent the needles (*arrows*), before deployment, and the small round areas represent the deployed seeds (*arrowheads*). A postoperative axial SPGR (*D*) through the prostate base demonstrates multiple round areas of low signal in the peripheral zone (*arrowheads*), consistent with deployed seeds.

Although open-bore magnets offer good patient accessibility and allow satisfactory prostate tumor and anatomic depiction, higher-quality MR intervention images in a closed 1.5-T system also have been investigated.[45] This system uses a customized perineal template, an endorectal imaging coil, and a lockable positioning arm. Patients are placed in the left lateral decubitus position. Although patient accessibility with this technique may be limited because of the closed-bore configuration and the 60-cm diameter bore, the investigators found that dependence on deformable registration between image sets (high-field 1.5-T diagnostic images and low-field–strength interventional images) was reduced.

Outcomes

Short-term toxicity after MR-guided brachytherapy is rare, with no gastrointestinal or sexual dysfunction reported during the first month after treatment.[54] Within 24 hours of removal of the Foley catheter, acute urinary retention was reported in 12% of men, which was self-limited to within 1 to 3 weeks of treatment. Prostatic volume and transitional zone volume, determined by MR imaging, and number of brachy therapy seeds placed were found to be significant predictors of acute urinary retention.

The long-term genitourinary and rectal toxicity was compared between those who received MR-guided brachytherapy alone and those who received combined MR-guided brachytherapy and external beam radiation therapy.[55] The 4-year estimates of rectal bleeding requiring coagulation for patients who underwent MR-guided brachytherapy compared with patients who received combined-modality therapy were 8% versus 30%. The 4-year estimate of freedom from radiation cystitis was 100% versus 95% for patients who received MR-guided brachytherapy alone and patients who received combined-modality therapy, respectively. In a separate study evaluating the long-term toxicity in patients who received MR-guided brachytherapy as a salvage procedure for radiation therapy failure,[56] the 4-year estimate of grade 3 or 4 gastrointestinal or genitourinary toxicity was reported at 30% of all patients, with 13% requiring an intervention, such as a colostomy or urostomy for fistula repair.

Supplemental external beam radiotherapy, in addition to brachytherapy seed implantation, has been given to patients who have intermediate- to high-risk prostate cancer (according to the D'Amico risk stratification for prostate cancer).[57] This combination of radiation therapy has demonstrated good long-term results,[58,59] resulting in a 15-year biochemical relapse-free survival equal to 80.3% for intermediate-risk disease and 67.2% for high-risk disease.

Brachytherapy: The Future

The current manual method of needle placement, using a fixed-needle template guide, constrains needle orientation. The manual method also makes use of manual computation and transcription of needle coordinates that are prone to human error. The future points toward a system that incorporates an interactive planning interface with MR-compatible robotic assistance. Such a device, which serves as a dynamic guide for precise needle placement, has been developed.[60] Likely the future direction for percutaneous MR imaging–guided prostatic interventions, this MR-compatible robotic device has been integrated with a software planning interface, allowing physicians to specify desired needle trajectories based on MR imaging anatomy.

FOCUSED ULTRASOUND SURGERY IN THE PROSTATE

As discussed previously regarding the female genital tract, there is growing interest in MRgFUS because of its many potential applications as a minimally invasive therapy. US-guided FUS (USgFUS) has been used predominantly in Europe for the treatment of prostate cancer. Limitations include difficulty in treating the anterior prostate or small-volume prostates, and lack of long-term follow-up.

Literature describing the results of USgFUS for prostate cancer suggests that USgFUS treatment is a valuable option for well-differentiated and moderately differentiated tumors and for local recurrence after external-beam radiation therapy.[61–63] USgFUS treatment is whole-gland therapy, without selective tumor-directed targeted treatment, that should allow for minimal disruption of normal function. USgFUS arguably is limited by the lack of direct temperature and thermal dose measurements during thermocoagulation. Without the latter, the energy delivery cannot be controlled or monitored nor can the thermal dose be measured accurately.

To address these challenges, MR imaging–compatible prostate applications have been developed for hyperthermia,[64] and phased-array applicators for thermal ablation.[65] Insightec (Haifa, Israel) has developed a MRgFUS system for prostate treatment (**Fig. 8**). A major potential advantage of MR imaging guidance is its ability to map functional changes in prostate tissue, with the possibility of 3-D tumor mapping before

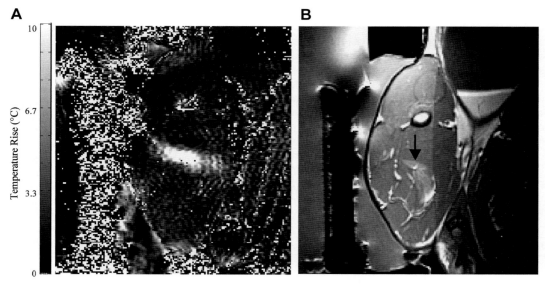

Fig. 8. (*A*) MR imaging–based temperature image during a sonication (130 W for 30 seconds) into rabbit thigh muscle during a test of an MR imaging–compatible transrectal phased array applicator for MRgFUS of prostate. (*B*) The thermal lesion (*arrow*) seen in T2-weighted imaging. The bright region to the right of the lesion is a tissue fascia layer. (*From* Sokka SD, Hynynen K. The feasibility of MRI-guided whole prostate ablation with a linear aperiodic intracavitary ultrasound phased array. Phys Med Biol 2000;45:3373–83; with permission.)

and during treatment. Overall, noninvasive thermal ablation using MR imaging guidance should improve prostate treatment significantly and its application should increase in the near future.

MR IMAGING–GUIDED CATHETER-BASED ULTRASOUND THERMAL THERAPY OF THE PROSTATE

In a similar mode, catheter-based US devices (in interstitial and transurethral configurations) have been evaluated in canine prostate models in vivo and found to produce spatially selective regions of thermal destruction in the prostate.[66–68] Transurethral US devices with tubular transducers have been developed, which can coagulate sectors of the prostate using pre-shaped angular patterns.[69,70] Devices with finer spatial control using planar[71,72] or curvilinear transducers[73] can be rotated slowly using a computer-controlled, MR-compatible stepper motor while under MR imaging guidance and feedback (**Fig. 9**). The feasibility of MR imaging–guided interstitial US thermal therapy of the prostate has been evaluated in an in vivo canine prostate model.[66] MR imaging–compatible, multielement interstitial US applicators were used. The applicators were inserted transperineally into the prostate with the energy

directed ventrally away from the rectum. This study demonstrated a large volume of ablated tissue within the prostate and, importantly, demonstrated contiguous zones of thermal coagulation. At least in an animal model and using MR guidance, transurethral and interstitial treatment strategies have, therefore, demonstrated significant potential for thermal ablation of localized prostate cancer.

URINARY TRACT

Renal cell carcinoma (RCC) is the sixth leading cause of cancer death,[74] and its incidence in the United States is rising.[75] Partial nephrectomy, a nephron-sparing surgical method, has replaced radical nephrectomy for the treatment of small RCC. Less invasive methods also have emerged that can be performed laparoscopically (partial nephrectomy and cryosurgery) or percutaneously (radiofrequency ablation [RFA] and cryoablation). Image-guided percutaneous ablations have the potential to replace others as the least invasive and least costly[76] of all nephron-sparing treatments clinically available, particularly in patients who are poor surgical candidates because of comorbid disease and patients who have renal insufficiency, solitary kidney, or multiple RCC.

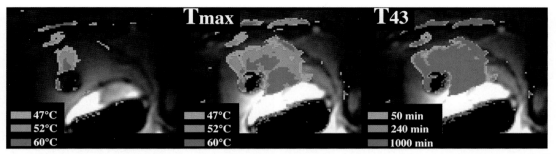

Fig. 9. MR imaging–guided catheter-based US thermal therapy of the prostate: real-time temperature image (*left*), maximum temperature image (*middle*), and thermal dose (*right*) of the prostate during catheter-based US thermal therapy. The transurethral catheter, with a rotating curvilinear transducer array, is depicted as the round low-signal intensity structure within the prostate gland.[69] (*Courtesy of* Kim Butts Pauly, PhD, Viola Rieke, MD, and Graham Sommer, PhD, Stanford University School of Medicine, Stanford, CA; and Chris Diederich, PhD, UCSF, San Francisco, CA.)

MR IMAGING–GUIDED RADIOFREQUENCY ABLATION IN THE KIDNEY

RFA is a focal thermal tumor therapy method in which tissue is heated by an electric current. The current is present with a high density surrounding a percutaneously placed electrode that is driven by an electrical generator. The circuit is completed by the placement of grounding pads on a patient. The electrode is placed interstitially and intended to be activated to create a volume of coagulative necrosis in place of the tumor.

Many reports of successful treatment of renal tumors with percutaneous RFA have been published.[77–85] Real-time monitoring of RFA, however, is not possible with CT or US because the thermal ablation zone is not visible with these imaging modalities. RFA can be monitored with MR imaging.[86,87]

But with limitations. Radiofrequency energy has to be interrupted during MR imaging because of the significant interference it causes otherwise. Furthermore, the temperature-sensitive, very short repetition time/echo time gradient-echo sequences typically are not suitable for detailed visualization of retroperitoneal anatomy.

Specific to MR imaging–guided RFA in the kidney, the first report was an in vivo study in porcine kidney.[88] The procedures were performed in a 0.2-T open magnet and demonstrated the suitability of MR imaging for guiding needle placement and the benefit of its inherent soft-tissue sensitivity where the electrode could be placed and the thermal lesion observed. Clinical studies of MR imaging–guided RFA in the kidney subsequently reported the safety and efficacy of the procedure[87,89] in tumors less than 4 cm in diameter. No recurrences at 25 months' post procedure were reported.

Overall, RFA is a feasible therapeutic modality for kidney lesions, under MR imaging, CT, or US guidance.[90] Although RFA is performed more routinely under CT guidance, many practices turn to MR imaging for the assessment and long-term follow-up of treated patients.[91–93]

MR IMAGING–GUIDED PERCUTANEOUS CRYOTHERAPY OF RENAL TUMORS

Cryoablation, a focal thermal tumor therapy method which uses extreme cold to establish coagulative necrosis, has several advantages over RFA. While RFA may require the need to perform multiple overlapping ablations of larger tumors, with percutaneous cryoablation, larger tumors can be treated simultaneously with the placement of multiple applicators.[94,95] Evidence suggests that renal tumors more likely are treated in one session with cryoablation compared to RFA.[96] Lower doses of medications are required for intravenous conscious sedation suggesting that percutaneous cryoablation of renal tumors is associated with less intraprocedural pain than with percutaneous RFA.[97]

US monitoring of cryoablation is limited by an inability to image the entire ice ball because of acoustic shadowing from the edge closest to the US probe.[98] Cryoablation of renal tumors can be monitored with CT because the ice ball is readily apparent as a hypoattenuating structure in the renal parenchyma.[94,95,98–103] There are two main limitations with CT, however. One is that the portion of the ice ball in the perinephric fat, a hyperattenuating region, provides only a modest contrast-to-noise ratio[104,105] compared to surrounding fat, and the ablation zone edge is not demarcated clearly in fatty tissue (**Fig. 10**A). This limits its use for real-time monitoring of the effect of ablation on adjacent critical structures, such as bowel, ureter, pancreas, and adrenal gland. Another is that the streak artifact created

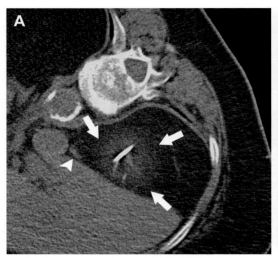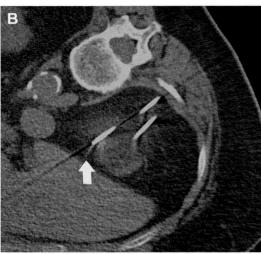

Fig. 10. CT–guided percutaneous cryotherapy of renal yumors. A 77-year-old woman who had RCC of the right kidney upper pole. Unenhanced transverse CT images obtained during percutaneous cryoablation performed in the right lateral decubitus position show that (*A*) low contrast-to-noise ratio and poor edge definition of ice ball (*arrows*) in the perinephric fat renders assessment for overlap of ablation zone with adjacent adrenal gland (*arrowhead*) difficult, and (*B*) streak artifact from applicator interferes with visualization of portion of the ice ball (*arrow*).

by the applicators with CT imaging can interfere with ice ball visibility (**Fig. 10B**).

Since the initial clinical reports of MR imaging–guided percutaneous cryoablation of renal tumors[98,100] in 2001, several investigators have shown the feasibility and safety of the procedure,[106–112] all demonstrating the advantages of MR imaging monitoring during percutaneous cryoablation procedures.

MR imaging depicts the ice ball as a signal void region with high contrast-to-noise ratio compared to surrounding tissues, with sharp edge definition in multiple planes and with minimal applicator artifact (**Fig. 11**). Ice ball volume on intraprocedural MR imaging correlates well with volume of cryonecrosis on postprocedural MR imaging.[113] Because the ice ball is well depicted on all pulse sequences, the ablation can be monitored using pulse sequences that display tumor or adjacent critical structures best.[111] If images demonstrate incomplete coverage of tumor, additional applicators may be placed to improve coverage.[111,112] Alternatively, if the ice ball edge approaches adjacent critical structures, the freezing can be stopped.[111] Applicators can be controlled individually. Additional maneuvers to reduce risk for injury to surrounding bowel, such as water instillation described for CT-guided ablations,[114] also can be performed during MR imaging–guided cryoablations.[111] A noninvasive method of external manual displacement of bowel during MR imaging–guided cryoablation of renal tumors also

is described—a maneuver unique to cryoablation procedures performed in an open-configuration interventional MR imaging unit.[115]

Limitations of MR imaging–guided cryoablation include the high cost of MR imaging units and its limited availability, generally long procedure times, smaller gantry sizes compared to CT scanners, and inability to detect ST-T segment changes of cardiac ischemia on an EKG in the magnetic environment during procedures.

In summary, image-guided percutaneous ablative therapies have the potential to replace conventional surgical treatment of small RCC. Compared with other image-guided ablative therapies, with its vast advantages and minimal limitations, MR imaging–guided percutaneous cryoablation is well poised to play an important role in the management of renal tumors.

THE FUTURE

Recent developments in MR imaging paralleling those in computer-assisted surgery have set up an ideal environment for MR-compatible robotic systems and manipulators. Materials used in mechatronic devices inside the magnet ideally should have a magnetic susceptibility similar to that of human tissue and be electrical insulators to avoid image distortion. Although image quality is reduced because of reduction in static field strength, interventional open-bore magnets have fewer spatial constraints. Alternatively, closed

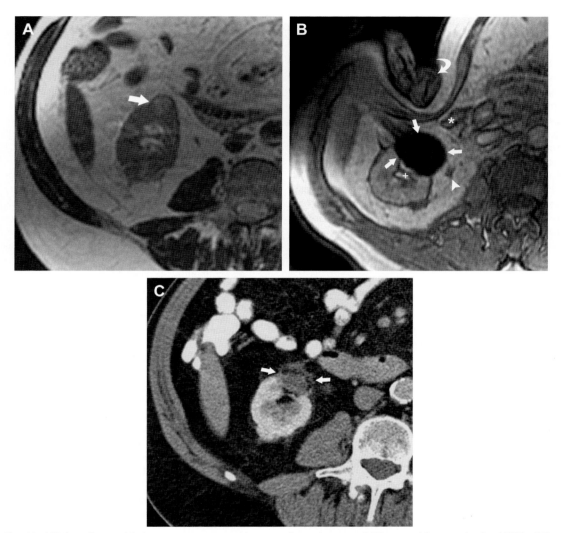

Fig. 11. MR imaging–guided percutaneous cryotherapy of renal tumor. A 70-year-old man who had RCC of the right kidney lower pole treated with MR imaging–guided percutaneous cryoablation. (*A*) Transverse T2-weighted fast recovery fast spin–echo sequence image obtained before treatment in 1.5-T MR image shows a small exophytic renal mass in the lower pole of the right kidney anteriorly (*arrow*). (*B*) Intraprocedural transverse gradient-echo image obtained in 0.5-T open configuration interventional MR imaging shows that sharp edge definition of signal void ice ball (*arrows*) contributes to monitoring of tumor coverage and assessment of proximity to adjacent ureter (*arrowhead*), renal collecting system (+), and colon (*), which is being displaced by an interventionalist's hand (*curved arrow*). (*C*) An 18-month follow-up contrast-enhanced transverse CT image shows no enhancement in the involuted ablation zone (*arrows*).

MR scanners can impose severe constraints on procedural manipulations, despite their imaging advantage of higher field strengths. New wide- and short-bore 1.5-T magnets (Espree, Siemens, Erlangen, Germany) will expand the use of interventional MR imaging. Emerging use of 3-T magnets for interventions will bring about improved monitoring of thermal therapies. Much research is underway evaluating material selection, position detection sensors, different actuation models and techniques, and design strategies.[116] Once the engineering hurdle is overcome, systems must undergo clinical validation before introduction into the commercial realm.

SUMMARY

MR imaging has become part of routine care in many places around the world, for tumor detection, localization, and staging. In the genitourinary tract, MR imaging guidance is playing an increasing role in minimally invasive procedures for confirmation of tumor pathology and for tumor treatment and treatment monitoring. It offers inherent ability for tumor detection and biopsy guidance and, currently, MR-guided ablative therapies are an increasing and real alternative to more invasive surgical options. As the capabilities of MR imaging expand and newer imaging modalities become more accessible (PET imaging, for example), the need for nonrigid registration of multiple modalities will be necessary. A combination of functional imaging and high-resolution tumor detail in the genitourinary tract, in a patient-specific treatment environment, should increase demand and the use of semi-invasive or noninvasive technology. Clearly, the pressure is on to provide MR-compatible devices and methodology that easily integrate with imaging and are supportive of patients' clinical needs.

REFERENCES

1. Stewart AJ, Viswanathan AN. Current controversies in high-dose-rate versus low-dose-rate brachytherapy for cervical cancer. Cancer 2006;107(5):908–15.
2. Stewart EA. Uterine fibroids. Lancet 2001;357:293–8.
3. Ravina J, Herbreteau D, Ciraru-Vigneron N, et al. Arterial embolisation to treat uterine myomata. Lancet 1995;346:671–2.
4. Lynn JG, Zwemer RL, Chick AJ, et al. A new method for the generation and use of focused ultrasound in experimental biology. J Gen Physiol 1942;26:179–93.
5. Fry WJ, Barnard JW, Fry FJ. Ultrasonically produced localized selective lesions in the central nervous system. Am J Phys Med 1955;34:413–23.
6. Lele PP. A simple method for production of trackless focal lesions with focused ultrasound: physical factors. J Physiol 1962;160:494–512.
7. Heimburger RF. Ultrasound augmentation of central nervous system tumor therapy. Indiana Med 1995;78:469–76.
8. Gelet A, Chapelon JY, Bouvier R, et al. Local control of prostate cancer by transrectal high intensity focused ultrasound therapy: preliminary results. J Urol 1999;161:156–62.
9. Paterson RF, Barret E, Siqueira TM Jr, et al. Laparoscopic partial kidney ablation with high intensity focused ultrasound. J Urol 2003;169(1):347–51.
10. Yang R, Sanghvi NT, Rescorla FJ, et al. Extracorporeal liver ablation using sonography-guided high-intensity focused ultrasound. Invest Radiol 1992;27(10):796–803.
11. Watkin NA, Morris SB, Rivens IH, et al. A feasibility study for the non-invasive treatment of superficial bladder tumours with focused ultrasound. Br J Urol 1996;78(5):715–21.
12. Lizzi FL, Deng CX, Lee P, et al. A comparison of ultrasonic beams for thermal treatment of ocular tumors. Eur J Ultrasound 1999;9(1):71–8.
13. Ishihara Y, Calderon A, Watanabe H, et al. A precise and fast temperature mapping using water proton chemical shift. Magn Reson Med 1995;34(6):814–23.
14. Hynynen K, Vykhodtseva NI, Chung AH, et al. Thermal effects of focused ultrasound on the brain: determination with MR imaging. Radiology 1997;204(1):247–53.
15. Chung AH, Jolesz FA, Hynynen K. Thermal dosimetry of a focused ultrasound beam in vivo by magnetic resonance imaging. Med Phys 1999;26(9):2017–26.
16. McDannold N, Tempany CM, Fennessy FM, et al. Uterine leiomyomas: MR imaging-based thermometry and thermal dosimetry during focused ultrasound thermal ablation. Radiology 2006;240(1):263–72.
17. Chung AH, Hynynen K, Colucci V, et al. Optimization of spoiled gradient-echo phase imaging for in vivo localization of focused ultrasound beam. Magn Reson Med 1996;36(5):745–52.
18. Leon-Villapalos J, Kaniorou-Larai M, Dziewulski P. Full thickness abdominal burn following magnetic resonance guided focused ultrasound therapy. Burns 2005;31(8):1054–5.
19. Tempany CM, Stewart EA, McDannold N, et al. MR imaging-guided focused ultrasound surgery of uterine leiomyomas: a feasibility study. Radiology 2003;226(3):897–905.
20. Stewart EA, Gedroyc WM, Tempany CM, et al. Focused ultrasound treatment of uterine fibroid tumors: safety and feasibility of a noninvasive thermoablative technique. Am J Obstet Gynecol 2003;189(1):48–54.
21. Stewart EA, Gostout B, Rabinovici J, et al. Sustained relief of leiomyoma symptoms by using focused ultrasound surgery. Obstet Gynecol 2007;110(2 Pt 1):279–87.
22. Fennessy FM, Tempany C, McDannold N, et al. Uterine leiomyomas: MR imaging-guided focused ultrasound surgery–results of different treatment protocols. Radiology 2007;243(3):885–93.
23. Morrison PR, Silverman SG, Tuncali K, et al. MRI guided cryotherapy. J Magn Reson Imaging 2008;27(2):410–20.
24. Sewell PE, Arriola RM, Robinette L, et al. Real-time I-MR-imaging-guided cryoablation of uterine fibroids. J Vasc Interv Radiol 2001;12(7):891–3.
25. Cowan BD, Sewell PE, Howard JC, et al. Interventional magnetic resonance imaging cryotherapy of uterine fibroid tumors: preliminary observation. Am J Obstet Gynecol 2002;186(6):1183–7.
26. Dohi M, Harada J, Mogami T, et al. MR-guided transvaginal cryotherapy of uterine fibroids with

a horizontal open MRI system: initial experience. Radiat Med 2004;22(6):391–7.

27. Sakuhara Y, Shimizu T, Kodama Y, et al. Magnetic resonance-guided percutaneous cryoablation of uterine fibroids: early clinical experiences. Cardiovasc Intervent Radiol 2006;29(4): 552–8.

28. American Cancer Society. Cancer facts and figures 2007. Publication no. 500807. Atlanta (GA): American Cancer Society; 2006.

29. American Cancer Society. Cancer facts and figures. Publication no. 500807. Atlanta (GA): American Cancer Society; 2008.

30. Lee F, Gray JM, McLeary RD, et al. Prostatic evaluation by transrectal sonography: criteria for diagnosis of early carcinoma. Radiology 1986;158: 91–5.

31. Terris MK. Sensitivity and specificity of sextant biopsies in the detection of prostate cancer; preliminary report. Urology 1999;54:486–9.

32. Aus G, Hermansson CG, Hugosson J, et al. Transrectal ultrasound examination of the prostate: complications and acceptance by patients. Br J Urol 1993;71:457–9.

33. Collins GN, Lloyd SN, Hehir M, et al. Multiple transrectal ultrasound-guided prostatic biopsies: true morbidity and patient acceptance. Br J Urol 1993; 71:460–3.

34. Rodriguez LV, Terris MK. Risks and complications of transrectal ultrasound guided prostate needle biopsy: a prospective review of the literature. J Urol 1998;160:2115–20.

35. Rifkin MD, Zerhouni EA, Gatsonis CA, et al. Comparison of magnetic resonance imaging and ultrasonography in staging early prostate cancer: results of a multi-institutional cooperative trial. N Engl J Med 1990;323:621–6.

36. Schnall MD, Pollack HM. Magnetic resonance imaging of the prostate gland. Urol Radiol 1990; 12(2):109–14.

37. Cornud F, Flam T, Chauveinc L, et al. Extraprostatic spread of clinically localized prostate cancer: factors predictive of pT3 tumor and of positive endorectal MR imaging examination results. Radiology 2002;224(1):203–10.

38. Outwater EK, Petersen RO, Siegelman ES, et al. Prostate carcinoma: assessment of diagnostic criteria for capsular penetration on endorectal coil MR images. Radiology 1994;193(2):333–9.

39. Mullerad M, Hricak H, Kuroiwa K, et al. Comparison of endorectal magnetic resonance imaging, guided prostate biopsy and digital rectal examination in the preoperative anatomical localization of prostate cancer. J Urol 2005;174:2158–63.

40. Perrotti M, Han KR, Epstein RE, et al. Prospective evaluation of endorectal magnetic resonance imaging to detect tumor foci in men with prior negative prostatic biopsy: a pilot study. J Urol 1999;162:1314–7.

41. Hata N, Morrison PR, Kettenbach J, et al. Computer-assisted intra-operative MRI monitoring of interstitial laser therapy in the brain: a case report. SPIE J Biomed Optics 1998;3:302–11.

42. Gering D, Nabavi A, Kikinis R, et al. An integrated visualization system for surgical planning and guidance using image fusion and interventional imaging. Medical Image Computing and Computer-Assisted Intervention (MICCAI), Cambridge, England September 22, 1999.

43. D'Amico AV, Cormack R, Tempany CM, et al. Real-time magnetic resonance image-guided interstitial brachytherapy in the treatment of select patients with clinically localized prostate cancer. Int J Radiat Oncol Biol Phys 1998;42:507–15.

44. Hata N, Jinzaki M, Kacher D, et al. MR imaging-guided prostate biopsy with surgical navigation software; device validation and feasibility. Radiology 2001;220:263–8.

45. Susil RC, Camphausen K, Choyke P, et al. System for prostate brachytherapy and biopsy in a standard 1.5 T MRI scanner. Magn Reson Med 2004; 52(3):683–7.

46. Susil RC, Menard C, Kreiger A, et al. Transrectal prostate biopsy and fiducial marker placement in a standard 1.5T magnetic resonance imaging scanner. J Urol 2006;175(1):113–20.

47. Beyersdorff D, Winkel A, Hamm B, et al. MR imaging-guided prostate biopsy with a closed MR unit at 1.5 T: initial results. Radiology 2005;234(2): 576–81.

48. Kreiger A, Susil RC, Menard C, et al. Design of a novel MRI compatible manipulator for image guided prostate interventions. IEEE Trans Biomed Eng 2005;52(2):306–13.

49. Singh AK, Kreiger A, Lattouf JB. Patient selection determines the prostate cancer yield of dynamic contrast-enhanced magnetic resonance imaging-guided transrectal biopsies in a closed 3-Tesla scanner. BJU Int 2008;101(12):181–5.

50. DiMaio SP, Pieper S, Chinzei K, et al. Robot-assisted needle placement in open MRI: system architecture, integration and validation. Comput Aided Surg 2007;12(1):15–24.

51. Lee WR, Hall MC, McQuellon RP, et al. A prospective quality-of-life study in men with clinically localized prostate carcinoma treated with radical prostatectomy, external beam radiotherapy, or interstitial brachytherapy. Int J Radiat Oncol Biol Phys 2001;51(3):614–23.

52. Zelefsky MJ, Yamada Y, Marion C, et al. Improved conformality and decreased toxicity with intraoperative computer-optimized transperineal ultrasound-guided prostate brachytherapy. Int J Radiat Oncol Biol Phys 2003;55(4):956–63.

53. Kooy HM, Cormack RA, Mathiowitz RV, et al. A software system for interventional magnetic resonance image-guided prostate brachytherapy. Comput Aided Surg 2000;5(6):401–13.

54. D'Amico AV, Cormack R, Kumar S, et al. Real-time magnetic resonance imaging-guided brachytherapy in the treatment of selected patients with clinically localized prostate cancer. J Endourol 2000; 14:367–70.

55. Albert M, Tempany CM, Schultz, et al. Late genitourinary and gastrointestinal toxicity after magnetic resonance image-guided prostate brachytherapy with or without neoadjuvant external beam radiation therapy. Cancer 2003;98(5):949–54.

56. Nguyen PL, Chen MH, D'Amico AV, et al. Magnetic resonance image-guided salvage brachytherapy after radiation in select men who initially presented with favorable-risk prostate cancer: a prospective phase 2 study. Cancer 2007;110(7):1485–92.

57. D'Amico AV, Moul J, Carroll PR, et al. Cancer-specific mortality after surgery or radiation for patients with clinically localized prostate cancer managed during the prostate-specific antigen era. J Clin Oncol 2003;21(11):2163–72.

58. Sylvester JE, Grimm PD, Blasko JC, et al. 5-Year biochemical relapse free survival in clinical Stage T1-T3 prostate cancer following combined external beam radiotherapy and brachytherapy; Seattle experience. Int J Radiat Oncol Biol Phys 2007; 67(1):57–64.

59. Lawton CA, DeSilvo M, Lee WR, et al. Results of a phase II trial of transrectal ultrasound-guided permanent radioactive implantation of the prostate for definitive management of localized adenocarcinoma of the prostate (radiation therapy oncology group 98-05). Int J Radiat Oncol Biol Phys 2007; 67(1):39–47.

60. Chinzei K, Miller K. Towards MRI guided surgical manipulator. Med Sci Monit 2001;7:153–63.

61. Poissonier L, Chapelon JY, Rouviere O, et al. Control of prostate cancer by transrectal HIFU in 227 patients. Eur Urol 2007;51(2):381–7.

62. Uchida T, Ohkusa H, Nagata Y, et al. Treatment of localized prostate cancer using high-intensity focused ultrasound. BJU Int 2006;97(1):56–61.

63. Ficarra V, Antoniolli SZ, Novara G, et al. Short-term outcome after high-intensity focused ultrasound in the treatment of patients with high-risk prostate cancer. BJU Int 2006;98(6):1193–8.

64. Smith NB, Buchanan MT, Hynynen K. Transrectal ultrasound applicator for prostate heating monitored using MRI thermometry. Int J Radiat Oncol Biol Phys 1999;43(1):217–25.

65. Sokka SD, Hynynen KH. The feasibility of MRI-guided whole prostate ablation with a linear aperiodic intracavitary ultrasound and phased array. Phys Med Biol 2000;45(11):3378–83.

66. Nau WH, Diederich CJ, Ross AB, et al. MRI-guided interstitial ultrasound thermal therapy of the prostate: a feasibility study in the canine model. Med Phys 2005;32(3):733–43.

67. Pauly KB, Diedrich CJ, Rieke V, et al. Magnetic resonance-guided high-intensity ultrasound ablation of the prostate. Top Magn Reson Imaging 2006;17(3):195–207.

68. Diederich CJ, Nau WH, Ross AB, et al. Catheter-based ultrasound applicators for selective thermal ablation: progress towards MRI-guided applications in prostate. Int J Hyperthermia 2004;20(7): 739–56.

69. Diederich CJ, Stafford RJ, Nau WH, et al. Transurethral ultrasound applicators with directional heating patterns for prostate thermal therapy: in vivo evaluation using magnetic resonance thermometry. Med Phys 2004;31(2):405–13.

70. Hazle JD, Diederich CJ, Kangasniemi M, et al. MRI-guided thermal therapy of transplanted tumors in the canine prostate using a directional transurethral ultrasound applicator. J Magn Reson Imaging 2002;15(4):409–17.

71. Chopra R, Burtnyk M, Haider MA, et al. Method for MRI-guided conformal thermal therapy of prostate with planar transurethral ultrasound heating applicators. Phys Med Biol 2005;50(21):4957–75.

72. Ross AB, Diederich CJ, Nau WH, et al. Highly directional transurethral ultrasound applicators with rotational control for MRI guided prostatic thermal therapy. Phys Med Biol 2004;49(1): 189–204.

73. Ross AB, Diederich CJ, Nau WH, et al. Curvilinear transurethral ultrasound applicator for selective prostate thermal therapy. Med Phys 2005;32(6):1555–65.

74. Godley PA, Ataga KI. Renal cell carcinoma. Curr Opin Oncol 2000;12:260–4.

75. Chow WH, Devesa SS, Warren JL, et al. Rising incidence of renal cell cancer in the United States. JAMA 1999;281:1628–31.

76. Link RE, Permpongkosol S, Gupta A, et al. Cost analysis of open, laparoscopic, and percutaneous treatment options for nephron-sparing surgery. J Endourol 2006;20:782–9.

77. Gervais DA, McGovern FJ, Wood BJ, et al. Radiofrequency ablation of renal cell carcinoma: early clinical experience. Radiology 2000;217:665–72.

78. Ogan K, Jacomides L, Dolmatch BL, et al. Percutaneous radiofrequency ablation of renal tumors: technique, limitations, and morbidity. Urology 2002;60:954–8.

79. Farrell MA, Charboneau WJ, DiMarco DS, et al. Imaging-guided radiofrequency ablation of solid renal tumors. AJR 2003;180:1509–13.

80. Mayo-Smith WW, Dupuy DE, Parikh PM, et al. Imaging-guided percutaneous radiofrequency ablation of solid renal masses: technique and

outcomes of 38 treatment sessions in 32 consecutive patients. AJR 2003;180:1503–8.

81. Roy-Choudhury SH, Cast JE, Cooksey G, et al. Early experience with percutaneous radiofrequency ablation of small solid renal masses. AJR 2003;180:1055–61.

82. Su LM, Jarrett TW, Chan DYS, et al. Percutaneous computed tomography-guided radiofrequency ablation of renal masses in high surgical risk patients: preliminary results. Urology 2003;61:26–33.

83. Zagoria RJ, Hawkins AD, Clark PE, et al. Percutaneous CT-guided radiofrequency ablation of renal neoplasms: factors influencing success. AJR 2004;183:201–7.

84. Gervais DA, McGovern FJ, Arellano RS, et al. Radiofrequency ablation of renal cell carcinoma: part 1, indications, results, and role in patient management over 6-year period and ablation of 100 tumors. AJR 2005;185:64–71.

85. Varkarakis IM, Allaf ME, Inagaki T, et al. Percutaneous radiofrequency ablation of renal masses: results at a 2-year mean followup. J Urol 2005;174:456–60.

86. Lewin JS, Connell CF, Duerk JL, et al. Interactive MRI-guided radiofrequency interstitial thermal ablation of abdominal tumors: clinical trial for evaluation of safety and feasibility. JMRI 1998;8:40–7.

87. Lewin JS, Nour SG, Connell CF, et al. Phase II clinical trial of interactive MR imaging-guided interstitial radiofrequency thermal ablation of primary kidney tumors: initial experience. Radiology 2004; 232(3):835–45.

88. Merkle EM, Shonk JR, Duerk JL, et al. MR-guided RF thermal ablation of the kidney in a porcine model. AJR Am J Roentgenol 1999;173(3):645–51.

89. Boss A, Clasen S, Kuczyk M, et al. Magnetic resonance-guided percutaneous radiofrequency ablation of renal cell carcinomas: a pilot clinical study. Invest Radiol 2005;40(9):583–90.

90. Boss A, Clasen S, Kuczyk M, et al. Image-guided radiofrequency ablation of renal cell carcinoma. Eur Radiol 2007;17(3):725–33.

91. Merkle EM, Nour SG, Lewin JS. MR imaging follow-up after percutaneous radiofrequency ablation of renal cell carcinoma: findings in 18 patients during first 6 months. Radiology 2005;235(3):1065–71.

92. Memarsadeghi M, Schmook T, Remzi M, et al. Percutaneous radiofrequency ablation of renal tumors: midterm results in 16 patients. Eur J Radiol 2006;59(2):183–9.

93. Kawamoto S, Permpongkosol S, Bluemke DA, et al. Sequential changes after radiofrequency ablation and cryoablation of renal neoplasms: role of CT and MR imaging. Radiographics 2007;27(2):343–55.

94. Atwell TD, Farrell MA, Callstrom MR, et al. Percutaneous cryoablation of 40 solid renal tumors with US guidance and CT monitoring: initial experience. Radiology 2007;243:276–83.

95. Atwell TD, Farrell MA, Callstrom MR, et al. Percutaneous cryoablation of large renal masses: technical feasibility and short-term outcome. AJR 2007;188: 1195–200.

96. Matina SF, Ahrarb K, Cadedduc JA, et al. Residual and recurrent disease following renal energy ablative therapy: a multi-institutional study. J Urol 2006; 176:1973–7.

97. Allaf ME, Varkarakis IM, Bhayani SB, et al. Pain control requirements for percutaneous ablation of renal tumors: cryoablation versus radiofrequency ablation—initial observations. Radiology 2005; 237:366–70.

98. Tacke J, Speetzen R, Heschel I, et al. Imaging of interstitial cryotherapy—an in vitro comparison of ultrasound, computed tomography, and magnetic resonance imaging. Cryobiology 1999;38:250–9.

99. Saliken J, McKinnon J, Gray R. CT for monitoring cryotherapy. AJR 1996;166:853–5.

100. Sandison GA, Loye MP, Rewcastle JC, et al. X-ray CT monitoring of iceball growth and thermal distribution during cryosurgery. Phys Med Biol 1998; 43:3309–24.

101. Gupta A, Allaf ME, Kavoussi LR, et al. Computerized tomography guided percutaneous renal cryoablation with the patient under conscious sedation: initial clinical experience. J Urol 2006;175:447–53.

102. Permpongkosol S, Link RE, Kavoussi LR, et al. Percutaneous computerized tomography guided cryoablation for localized renal cell carcinoma: factors influencing success. J Urol 2006;176:1963–8.

103. Littrup PJ, Ahmed A, Aoun HD, et al. CT-guided percutaneous cryotherapy of renal masses. J Vasc Interv Radiol 2007;18:383–92.

104. Harada J, Dohi M, Mogami T, et al. Initial experience of percutaneous renal cryosurgery under the guidance of a horizontal open MRI system. Radiat Med 2001;19:291–6.

105. Shingleton WB, Sewell J, Patrick E. Percutaneous renal tumor cryoablation with magnetic resonance imaging guidance. J Urol 2001;165:773–6.

106. Shingleton WB, Sewell PE. Percutaneous renal cryoablation of renal tumors in patients with von Hippel-Lindau disease. J Urol 2002;167:1268–70.

107. Shingleton WB, Sewell PE. Percutaneous cryoablation of renal cell carcinoma in a transplanted kidney. BJU International 2002;90:137–8.

108. Sewell PE, Howard JC, Shingleton WB, et al. Interventional magnetic resonance image-guided percutaneous cryoablation of renal tumors. South Med J 2003;96:708–10.

109. Shingleton WB, Sewell PE. Cryoablation of renal tumours in patients with solitary kidneys. BJU International 2003;92:237–9.

110. Kodama Y, Abo D, Sakuhara Y, et al. MR-guided percutaneous cryoablation for bilateral multiple renal cell carcinoma. Radiat Med 2005;23:303–7.

111. Silverman SG, Tuncali K, vanSonnenberg E, et al. Renal tumors: MR imaging guided percutaneous cryotherapy–initial experience in 23 patients. Radiology 2005;236:716–24.

112. Miki K, Shimomura T, Yamada H, et al. Percutaneous cryoablation of renal cell carcinoma guided by horizontal open magnetic resonance imaging. Int J Urol 2006;13:880–4.

113. Silverman SG, Tuncali K, Adams DF, et al. MR imaging-guided percutaneous cryotherapy of liver tumors: initial experience. Radiology 2000;217:657–64.

114. Farrell MA, Charboneau JW, Callstrom MR, et al. Paranephric water instillation: a technique to prevent bowel injury during percutaneous renal radiofrequency ablation. AJR 2003;181:1315–7.

115. Tuncali K, Morrison PR, Tatli S, et al. MRI-guided percutaneous cryoablation of renal tumors: use of external manual displacement of adjacent bowel loops. Eur J Radiol 2006;59:198–202.

116. Elhawary H, Zivanovic A, Davies B, et al. A review of magnetic resonance imaging compatible manipulators in surgery. Proc Inst Mech Eng [H] 2006;220(3):413–24.

Magnetic Resonance Nephrourography: Current and Developing Techniques

Bobby Kalb, MD, John R. Votaw, PhD, Khalil Salman, MD, Puneet Sharma, PhD, Diego R. Martin, MD, PhD*

KEYWORDS

• MRI • Liver • Nephrourography

The MR imaging techniques used for liver are well suited for renal analysis. A useful imaging protocol includes a combination of (1) breath-hold T2-weighted single-shot echo-train coronal and axial images, with at least one plane performed with fat suppression; (2) T1-weighted gradient echo (GRE) precontrast axial and coronal fat-suppressed images; and (3) T1-weighted gadolinium-enhanced arterial capillary– and delayed-phase images. T1-weighted imaging using newer three-dimensional (3D) GRE sequences (eg, 3D volumetric interpolated breath-hold examination [VIBE], T1-weighted fast acquisition multiple excitation [FAME], or 3D T1-weighted high resolution isotropic volume examination [THRIVE]), combined with gadolinium enhancement, has improved spatial resolution for resolving masses and vascular anatomy. T2-like imaging using breath-hold balanced echo true free-induction with steady-state precession (TFISP) imaging may provide additional information for urographic evaluation of the collecting system, with urine having high signal on such images. Additionally, acquisition of pre- and postcontrast 3D GRE images performed with identical field of view, resolution, and slice parameters allows the precontrast images to be used as a subtraction mask. The resultant image shows only areas of increased signal caused by gadolinium enhancement. This technique may be useful for determining vascularity and tumor within a high-signal protein- or blood-containing renal lesion.

NORMAL KIDNEY

The advantages of MR multiplanar imaging are exploited by combining axial and coronal imaging, allowing optimal visualization of the renal pelvis and poles (**Fig. 1**). The use of dynamic gadolinium-enhanced T1 imaging combined with rapid acquisition may be referred to as "functional MR nephrourography" (MRNU).

MR NEPHROUROGRAPHY—STRUCTURE

In the past, obtaining both structural and functional data of the kidneys has not been possible without compromise involving one or both of these areas. With increasingly rapid image acquisition, however, MRNU offers the ability to capture simultaneously exquisite anatomic detail and physiologic data in parameters that have not been previously possible, even with traditional nuclear medicine techniques.

To obtain structural and functional renal data simultaneously, several imaging sequences are

This article originally appeared in the *Radiologic Clinics* of North America 2008;46(1):11–24.

Bobby Kalb was supported in part by a Bracco Clinical Translational Body MRI Training Award.

Department of Radiology, Emory University School of Medicine, Building A, Suite AT622, Atlanta, GA 30322, USA

* Corresponding address.

E-mail address: dmartin@emory.edu (D.R. Martin).

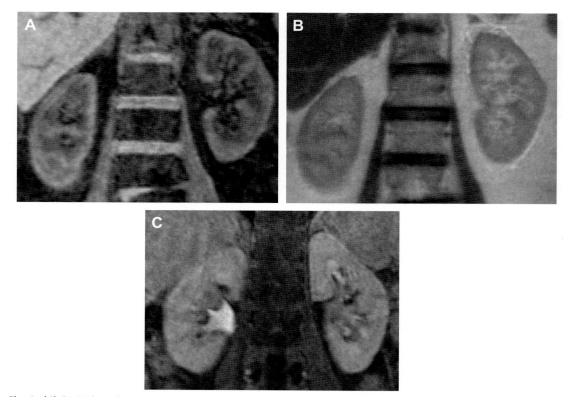

Fig. 1. (*A*) On T1 imaging, normal cortico-medullary differentiation (CMD) is seen with the cortex slightly brighter than skeletal muscle and the medulla relatively dark. Inherent CMD usually is best shown on T1 fat-suppressed images. (*B*) On T2 imaging, CMD is reversed relative to T1 imaging, with brighter-signal medulla, and lower-signal cortex. Gadolinium enhancement in the arterial-capillary phase (20-second delay) shows enhancement of the cortex. (*C*) Delayed gadolinium-enhanced interstitial-phase images show filling in of the medulla and subsequent excretion of contrast into the renal pelvis.

needed. T2-weighted images offer excellent morphologic evaluation of the kidneys and collecting system. The intrinsic signal characteristics of T2-bright urine contrast well with isointense urothelium, allowing the identification of filling defects within the collecting system. Distension of the urinary system with the administration of furosemide has been shown to be helpful,[1] although many clinically significant abnormalities of the collecting system, especially the bladder, often can be identified even with minimal distension because of the intrinsic contrast resolution on T2-weighted sequences. The relative contribution of T2-weighted images may be increased in patients who have significantly impaired renal function, because the visibility of the collecting system does not depend completely on the excretion of contrast material, a requirement of gadolinium-chelate–enhanced imaging.

In addition, with the use of relatively motion-insensitive T2-weighted half-Fourier acquisition single-shot turbo spin-echo (HASTE) sequences, high-quality images of the kidneys can be obtained even in free-breathing patients. Pulse sequences that use steady-state magnetization, such as TFISP, also can demonstrate the morphology of the collecting system in the absence of excretion. Like T2-weighted HASTE sequences, TFISP has excellent in-plane motion insensitivity and may display collecting system morphology in a nondistended system better than single-shot T2-weghted images, although this advantage should be balanced against a drop in contrast resolution compared with T2-weighted sequences. A disadvantage of two-dimensional (2D) T2-weighted images is the inability to reconstruct the images in a volume format. Volume-acquired 3D T2-weighted images, however, may be acquired to generate a maximum-intensity projection (MIP) dataset that can demonstrate collecting system morphology in a rotating manner from multiple-projection reconstructions, similar to the MIP reconstructions often used in vascular imaging.[2] Multiple projection reconstructions provide a powerful anatomic overview of the collecting system helpful for referring clinical services. Disadvantages of the 3D technique are a significant increase in data acquisition time compared with single-slice T2-weighted HASTE and loss of the motion insensitivity inherent in the 2D technique. Respiratory gating with a 2D navigation system can be used but at the expense of further increases in the total acquisition time for all the slices.

3D GRE contrast-enhanced T1-weighted sequences are another mainstay of MR nephrourography. Although T2-weighted images provide excellent contrast resolution and morphologic data, postcontrast 3D GRE images can provide functional data in addition to complementary views of tissue contrast. Precontrast T1-weighted images are ideal for displaying hemorrhage and proteinaceous debris. Dynamic contrast-enhanced images at varying time points allow the identification of neoplastic processes involving either the renal parenchyma or the urothelium. For example, early contrast-enhanced images clearly demonstrate enhancement of the urothelium against a background of dark urine before the excretion of gadolinium. This inherent contrast differential allows identification of enhancing tumors within the renal pelvis, ureters, or bladder, even in the setting of poorly functioning kidneys with diminished excretion. Tumor visibility is enhanced with the routine use of fat suppression, causing the surrounding retroperitoneal fat to become dark. This technique has the effect of allowing enhancing tissues to fill the available gray-scale values, allowing easier depiction of urothelial neoplastic processes (**Fig. 2**). Use of a 3D volume acquisition with thin partitions allows the initial coronal data to be reformatted into additional imaging planes as desired to enhance lesion detection further. Disadvantages to the 3D T1-weighted technique include sensitivity to motion, which can degrade images significantly in a free-breathing patient. Additional techniques to shorten the acquisition time (eg, increased parallel processing acceleration) can reduce these detrimental effects but at the cost of a decreased signal-to-noise ratio. Contrast enhancement of the collecting system is dependent on renal excretion, which may be reduced markedly with severe renal disease. This problem is not unique to MR imaging, however, and is encountered in both nuclear renal scintigraphy and CT urography. Thus MR imaging provides still another advantage by having alternative contrast strategies using T2-weighted imaging to visualize the collecting system even when the kidney's excretory function may be severely impaired.

In addition to morphologic imaging, 3D GRE images are the critical sequences necessary for the quantitative evaluation of renal function with MR imaging. Advances in parallel processing and in undersampling and underfilling of k-space have reduced imaging times so that a coronal volume of images through the kidneys can be acquired in 0.9 seconds with these techniques. Repeated T1-weighted GRE acquisitions through the kidneys every second during the administration of intravenous gadolinium allows the calculation of differential glomerular filtration rate (GFR) and renal blood flow (RBF) for each kidney.

MR NEPHROUROGRAPHY—FUNCTION

The clinical management of patients who have kidney diseases is somewhat limited by the lack of readily available noninvasive methods to test and follow renal function, to diagnose causes of renal dysfunction, or to monitor treatment response. Among the most commonly used tests for evaluation of renal function are measurement of serum creatinine level, endogenous creatinine clearance, and urinalysis for measurement of proteinuria. These indirect measures of renal GFR and loss of filtration integrity are insensitive and nonspecific and do not supply information that would differentiate the right kidney from the left.[3] Accurate 24-hour urine collections are challenging generally, and it is particularly difficult to ensure accuracy in younger patients.

There remains a clinical need for a sensitive and noninvasive in vivo imaging method that can be performed quickly and safely to provide regionally specific functional information about the kidney and to facilitate repeated evaluation, especially when there is a need for monitoring the progression of disease or the response to a treatment. Although nuclear medicine methods such as renal scintigraphy[4,5] have been used for determining renal function, these techniques suffer from low spatial resolution and do not provide detailed analysis of both structure and function. Furthermore, Technetium-99m mercaptoacetyltriglycine (MAG-3), commonly used in nuclear renal imaging, is an agent actively excreted by the renal tubules, and the rate of excretion does not measure the GFR. The use of radioactive tracers, particularly in monitoring applications where the study will be repeated, raises the concern of radiation risk.[6,7] This concern is particularly important when dealing with younger or pregnant patients. Dynamic CT imaging has been used,[8] but it also involves undesirable risks from ionizing radiation. In the setting of acute renal disease, or in patients who have risk factors such as diabetes mellitus, CT may be dangerous because it uses potentially nephrotoxic iodinated contrast agents.[9]

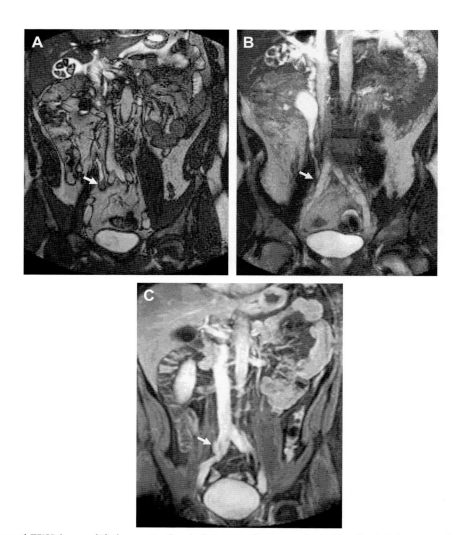

Fig. 2. Coronal TFISP image (*A*) demonstrating isointense soft tissue within the distal right ureter (*arrow*) contrasted against high-signal urine, again seen with (*B*) a MIP reconstruction of the TFISP images. (*C*) This filling defect corresponds exactly to a focal area of enhancement (*arrow*) demonstrated on the coronal 3D GRE sequence, confirming the presence of tumor and not stone or clot, neither of which would demonstrate enhancement. Surgical pathology returned a diagnosis of transitional cell carcinoma.

Advantages of MR imaging include the ability to achieve scans with higher temporal resolution than obtained with CT and nuclear scans and with higher spatial resolution than obtained with nuclear scans, without the exposure to ionizing radiation that occurs with CT and nuclear scans. Important measures of renal function can be related to RBF and GFR. From these parameters the filtration fraction can be determined. Recently, the potential of gadolinium-enhanced dynamic MR imaging, or MRNU, of the kidney has emerged as having the capacity to measure GFR.[10–14] This method uses rapid "snapshots" of the kidney at different time points following administration of a gadolinium-chelate paramagnetic contrast agent, combining

mathematical modeling of tracer kinetics to determine RBF[10] and GFR.[13,15] There has been development and evolving validation of gadolinium-chelate perfusion MR imaging techniques for the evaluation of GFR, relying on its behavior as a filtered agent without active excretion or uptake from the renal tubules.

Several methods have been developed for estimating the GFR from dynamic nuclear medicine data, but all are hampered by the poor counting statistics of such dynamic studies and the problem of accounting for the extrarenal component of the signal. Recently, several groups have applied the methods developed for nuclear medicine to dynamic MR imaging data acquired in conjunction with an injection of the contrast agent gadolinium-diethylenetriamine pentaacetic acid. In applying these techniques to MR imaging data, several issues must be addressed. First, although nuclear medicine measures the activity, and hence the concentration, of the contrast agent directly, in MR imaging the contrast agents change signal by altering the relaxation times of the tissue, producing a linear relationship with the concentration over only a limited range of concentrations. Second, the exact relationship between the signal and concentration depends on the flip angle used, and because the flip angle varies across the slice in 2D studies, time-consuming corrections are required for 2D data, making these unsuitable for routine clinical applications. Third, to obtain an adequate signal-to-noise ratio, it generally is necessary to use surface array coils for the reception of the signal, which in turn can lead to local variations in signal intensity that complicate the analysis of the data. One approach that the present authors have advocated [10] addresses these problems by using a slow injection of contrast over 10 seconds to limit the arterial concentration, by using a 3D technique and discarding the outer slices to ensure a uniform flip angle, and by using the precontrast signal to correct for spatial variations in the signal intensity.

Calculation of the individual RBF and GFR from gadolinium-enhanced MRNU can be coupled with measurement of the individual kidney volumes (cortex plus medulla). This technique makes it possible to determine RBF and GFR in proportion to a unit measure of kidney volume that can be expressed, for example, as RBF or GFR per milliliter of kidney. This value may provide an additional functional parameter for monitoring renal dysfunction and response to interventions, which previously was not possible in the clinical setting (**Fig. 3**). Potential applications range across the full spectrum of renal diseases.

IMAGING TECHNIQUES
Gadolinium-enhanced Renal Perfusion-distribution Imaging

Both 2D and 3D GRE techniques have been proposed to capture the critical period when the infused gadolinium arrives in the renal artery. The principle that has been adopted is that the blood flow to the kidney can be determined in the first few seconds as the gadolinium contrast agent perfuses the renal parenchyma; the GFR then can be measured by measuring the total amount of gadolinium agent within the entire kidney parenchyma as a function of time with the data collected up to the point of urinary excretion. The strength of

2D techniques is that a turbo-flash sequence can be implemented providing a fast acquisition method that is relatively insensitive to motion, as has been used to evaluate cardiac perfusion. A limitation of this approach is that volumetric determination of total kidney signal and volume is less accurate. Using 3D GRE provides volumetric data for more accurate evaluation of total kidney signal and volume. A challenge has been to acquire 3D GRE with a sufficiently short acquisition time to provide the necessary temporal resolution demanded from the kinetic modeling. Volumetric GRE also is more motion sensitive. The present authors have approached this problem by using 3D GRE with a high degree of acceleration to achieve the necessary short acquisition time and to reduce motion sensitivity. Use of surface coils with parallel processing inherently corrects for coil element sensitivity profile and helps overcome the problem of positional changes in signal intensities within the field of view.

The authors have adopted a technique to achieve a long infusion period combined with a minimal gadolinium concentration. The objectives are to produce a more uniform arterial gadolinium concentration over the period of data collection and to maintain the gadolinium concentration at the lowest detectable level, to minimize susceptibility effects. They administer the gadolinium agent using a dual-syringe power injector at a dose of 0.1 mmol/kg diluted into a total volume of 60 mL with normal saline and injected at a rate of 0.6 mL/s. Renal perfusion imaging is performed during the first pass using a coronal 3D GRE technique with fat saturation and centric-radial k-space acquisition using a 430-mm^2 field of view, 96 matrix (60% scan percentage, reconstructed to 256), recovery time/echo time/flip angle of 3.7/1.7ms/30°, 30 slices at a 2.8-mm slice thickness, 120 k-lines/segment, and a sensitivity encoding factor of 3. These parameters result in an acquisition time of 0.9 seconds per dynamic scan. The resultant images have an acceptable signal-to-noise ratio and provide adequate spatial resolution. A benefit of this highly accelerated acquisition time is that the imaging may be performed during normal breathing with negligible motion-related image deterioration.

IMAGE ANALYSIS

Proposals for modeling the kinetics have ranged from the simple two-compartment analysis, based on the Patlak-Rutland model,[13,16,17] to more complex models that range to seven compartments.[15] The authors have adopted a model that takes into consideration the blood, interstitial,

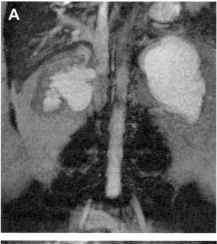

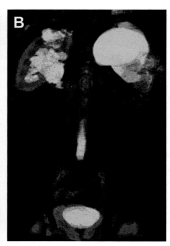

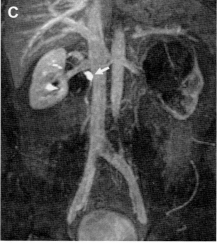

D

	RIGHT	LEFT
Vol (ml)	159.6	45.7
RBF (ml/s)	6.3	1.0
RBF (ml/min)	379.5	62.2
RBF/Vol (min-1)	2.38	1.36
GFR/Vol (min-1)	0.37	0.13
Fitration Fraction	0.16	0.1
GFR (ml/min)	59 (91%)	6 (9%)
-Total=65 ml/min		

Fig. 3. A 52-year-old man who presented with unexplained bilateral hydronephrosis based on ultrasound examination. (*A*) Coronal TFISP MIP shows what appears to be bilateral hydronephrosis affecting the pelvis and calyces, moderate on the right and severe on the left side. (*B*) Colorization of the coronal MIP image is possible using readily available commercial image postprocessing software. In this case, it incrementally accentuates the severely dilated collecting system of the left kidney, including interconnecting dilated calyces and pelvis. (*C*) The right kidney calyces are mildly blunted. Coronal post-gadolinium contrast-enhanced 3D GRE MIP shows no detectable excretion of contrast after 10 minutes. There is excretion from the right kidney and filling of the bladder. This image shows that the major calyces and the pelvis are compressed and thinned, and the proximal ureter (*arrow*) is draped over the medial border of the fluid filled structure shown on the coronal TFISP images. These findings are in keeping with large peripelvic cysts. (*D*) The summary of quantitative information derived from the gadolinium-enhanced MRNU shows that the function of the right kidney is within expected limits, but the left kidney is markedly impaired, with the loss of approximately two thirds of the left renal parenchyma volume as compared with the right kidney. This study shows that the MRNU provides a unique array of structural and functional information that is important for an accurate diagnosis and for optimized management.

and filtered tubular compartments in keeping with a three-compartment model. They believe that a three-compartment model provides sufficient sophistication to account for the major regions of gadolinium distribution and have been able to validate their belief empirically by showing excellent fit between the measured and the predicted values in a variety of disease states.

The relative signal from within each kidney is calculated to determine the signal contribution from the contrast agent perfusion. The bulk kidney signal represents the total amount of gadolinium agent present in the kidney per unit time. The three dynamic signal-intensity time courses (aorta, right kidney, and left kidney) are evaluated. They have modeled three compartments (blood, extracellular space, and glomerular filtration), as described

later. An assumption required for the analysis discussed here is that the measured increased signal within an image voxel, either within the feeding artery or within the kidney parenchyma, is proportional to the amount of gadolinium within the respective voxel. They have performed phantom studies to show that maintaining the low gadolinium administration rate maintains the blood concentration within a range that retains a mostly linear relationship between the gadolinium concentration and the increase in signal intensity over background.[10]

Each total perfused kidney volume (cortex and medulla) can be segmented using a semiautomatic algorithm based on user-defined intensity thresholds (**Fig. 4**), morphologic erosion/dilation, and region growing steps.[10,18] Renal pelvis, pelvic

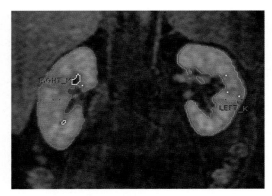

Fig. 4. Representative coronal 3D GRE contrast-enhanced image showing manually placed segmentation of right (*green*) and left (*red*) kidney. The last image just before appearance of contrast spillage into the pelvic collecting system is used for this process to ensure inclusion of the entire renal parenchyma.

vessels, and adjacent soft tissues are excluded from the renal segments. Additionally, a dynamic signal-intensity mask is created in the descending aorta to serve as the input function. These segmented binary masks of the kidneys and aorta are applied to the images at each time point and are adjusted for position changes related to respiration. Positional correction to account for respiration can be performed manually or by motion-tracking software. The authors have found that for images acquired during restful breathing in regions of interest around the kidney, and particularly in transplanted kidneys where motion is inherently negligible, motion-corrected results often are not significantly different from the uncorrected results.

The output from the perfusion masks is a time course of signal intensity in the aorta and each kidney. Summing the number of pixels in the kidney mask and multiplying by the voxel size provides the perfused kidney volume, V.

The mean signal intensity for the renal volumes is calculated for each 0.9-second scan. Relative signal values are determined by the formula $(S_t - S_0) / S_0$, where S_t is the signal at time t and S_0 is the mean pre-contrast signal, calculated from the mean of at least three unenhanced precontrast images. The relative signal is used both to isolate the signal contribution from the contrast agent perfusion and to help eliminate residual signal variations that may result from imperfect coil spatial sensitivity corrections or other field inhomogeneities.

CALCULATION OF SINGLE-KIDNEY RENAL BLOOD FLOW

Fick's first law of diffusion states that the rate of uptake of gadolinium within the kidney is equal to

the blood flow through the organ times the arterial-venous difference in the concentration of the tracer (gadolinium signal in this application). In this approach, data collection must focus on the kidney images acquired before venous drainage of gadolinium from the kidney. Hence, the RBF may be determined from Eq. 1:

$$C_T(t)V = F \int_0^t C_a(s - t_d)\,ds \qquad \textbf{Eq. 1}$$

where C_T is the measured gadolinium tissue concentration in the whole kidney, V is the kidney volume, F is the blood flow into the kidney, C_a is the measured gadolinium concentration in the artery supplying the kidney, and t_d is the time difference between when the gadolinium is measured in the artery and the kidney. It is recognized that in application, V is the volume of the kidney region of interest, and C_T is the average pixel intensity inside this region. Thus VC_T is proportional to the total amount of gadolinium in the kidney. This approach has been described in detail.[10]

CALCULATION OF SINGLE-KIDNEY GLOMERULAR FILTRATION RATE
Gadolinium Systemic Model, Analysis of Arterial Curve

Assuming the equilibration of gadolinium is fast relative to the clearance, then clearance of gadolinium through the kidney can be considered a first-order concentration-driven process (**Fig. 5**). Under these conditions, gadolinium clears exponentially from the system with a characteristic half-life related to the GFR. Hence, gadolinium concentration at the measurement point after injection of a very short bolus at the input point is expected to have the general shape known as the point spread function:

$$y_g(t) = \begin{cases} a_1 e^{-p_1(t-t_c)^2} & t \le t_c \\ \left(a_1 - a_2\right)e^{-p_2(t-t_c)^2} + a_2 e^{-p_3(t-t_c)} & t > t_c \end{cases}$$

where the a represents amplitude, p the rate constant, and t_c is the time of the peak. The amount of dispersion is characterized by the width of the peak at half of its height (full width half maximum, FWHM). Equation parameters are determined by minimizing the error-weighted chi-square function using Powell's method. The error was assumed to be fractional (ie, 12% of the value) and was determined by fitting a single exponential to the tail of the aorta curve and taking the standard deviation about the fit value. The tail (long after the injection has stopped) of the aorta curve is affected by the clearance rate of gadolinium

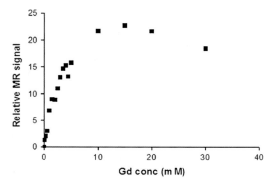

Fig. 5. The MR signal response of the 3D GRE perfusion sequence as a function of gadolinium concentration (Gd conc), as determined with an array of gadolinium-doped plasma phantoms. Signal intensities were measured after the fifth dynamic scan to ensure the system was in steady state, as expected with in vivo conditions. There is an apparent region of linearity between MR signal intensity and gadolinium concentration below approximately 3.5 mM, allowing the simple use of physiologic models, such as the two-compartment model, for describing changes in tracer concentrations. Beyond the linearity threshold, the relationship between signal and gadolinium concentration is no longer predictable, and the kinetic model cannot be used. This phenomenon occurs primarily because of T1 and T2* effects of the imaged species, in addition to effects of sequence parameters such as the flip angle.

from the blood and is well described by a single exponential function.

Gadolinium Kidney Model, Analysis of Kidney Curve

The general shape of the curve of gadolinium concentration in the kidney over time was modeled with three phases. The first phase is a rapid increase in concentration occurring after gadolinium enters the kidney but before any gadolinium appears in the renal vein. This process is proportional to the amount of blood flowing into the kidney. The second phase lasts until the end of the infusion. During this phase, the gadolinium concentrations in the blood and extracellular space are in quasi-equilibrium, with the blood concentration being greater. Both concentrations increase because the constant infusion is adding gadolinium to the system faster than it is being cleared via the kidney. The third phase begins at the end of infusion and lasts until gadolinium appears in the ureter (the end of the study). After a short transient in this phase, there is a greater concentration in the blood, and gadolinium continues to accumulate in the kidney (**Fig. 6**). A

mathematical model of gadolinium in the renal system has been elaborated.[19]

Briefly, the gadolinium concentration throughout the kidney at time t is modeled with the following time-dependent coupled equations:

$$\frac{\partial C_a(x,t)}{\partial t} = -\frac{F}{A}\frac{\partial C_a(x,t)}{\partial x}$$
$$- K_1 C_a(x,t) + \frac{k_2 V_e}{LA}C_e(x,t)$$

$$\frac{\partial C_e(x,t)}{\partial t} = K_1\frac{LA}{V_e}C_a(x,t) - (k_2+k_3)C_e(x,t)$$

$$\frac{\partial C_t(x,t)}{\partial t} = k_3\frac{V_e}{V_t}C_e(x,t)$$

V_e and V_t represent the total volumes of the interstitial and tubular portions of the kidney. All concentrations are zero at time $t = 0$. The input condition, $C_a(0,t)$, is the measured curve from the descending aorta (after a suitable shift for the transit time between the descending aorta and kidney measurements). These equations were solved numerically by finite differencing using a two-step Lax-Wendroff method. As a quality-control step, the accuracy of the solution is verified by dividing the time step size (dt) in half and checking that the solution does not change. Because the MR imaging signal is a global kidney signal, the calculated values must be summed over the entire kidney. Hence, the measured data are identified to be

$$MRI(t) = \int_0^L (LAC_a(x,t)+V_e C_e(x,t)$$

$$+ V_t C_t(x,t))dx \qquad \textbf{Eq. 2}$$

The parameters of interest, F, k_1, k_2, k_3, are adjusted using Powell's algorithm until the model estimate (Eq. 2) matches the measured value in the region of interest as closely as possible (least squares difference). Then blood flow into the kidney, F, is obtained. The GFR is the amount of blood that flows into the kidney multiplied by fraction of the blood that enters the tubules (Fk3).

Measurement accuracy

Measurement of RBF using the MRNU technique has been compared with phase-contrast imaging, and the results show no significant differences between the methods.[20]

Different methods have been used to compare MRNU-derived GFR measurements against different standards of reference, including GFR determined by scintigraphic [18] and iothalamate [21] clearance methods. The authors also have

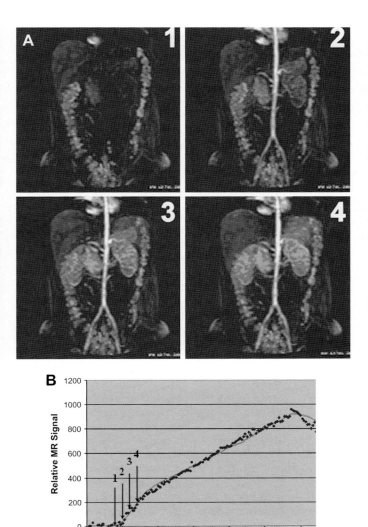

Fig. 6. (*A*) Selected dynamic coronal MIP series of contrast enhanced 3D GRE 0.9-second scans with a 430-mm² field of view, 96 matrix (reconstructed to 256), recovery time/echo time/flip angle of 3.7/1.7ms/30°, 30 slices at 2.8-mm slice thickness, acquired in a freely breathing subject just before the arrival of contrast in the aorta and kidneys (*1*), followed by sample points (*2–4*) within the first 7 seconds from the time contrast has arrived showing progressive enhancement of the kidneys. (*B*) The relative MR signal from the left kidney from each 0.9-second scan is shown as an individual point in relation to the time of acquisition. The points indicated by numbered *arrows* (*1–4*) indicate the acquisition time and measured renal signal of the corresponding MIP image shown in panel A. The solid line represents the curve calculated using Eq. 2. The first 10 seconds of data fit Eq. 1 and were used to calculate "F," a parameter in Eq. 2 (see text). The first few seconds of data are acquired from the time contrast arrives within the kidney until the time contrast exits the kidney in the renal vein. The degree of calculated curve fit to the measured data serves as indirect support for the assumptions made in the kinetic modeling.

compared their MRNU technique with the inulin clearance method. Although not used routinely because of its expense and complexity, inulin clearance generally is accepted as the reference standard for measuring GFR,. The authors' findings show high correlation with GFR measured concurrently by the inulin clearance technique (**Fig. 7**). In this example, five patients who had normal to moderately impaired renal function were studied first by MRNU and immediately afterwards by the inulin technique.

CLINICAL APPLICATIONS
Congenital Anomalies and Obstruction

There has been considerable clinical experience in the use of MRNU in the analysis of congenital anomalies of the urinary tract. Congenital

anomalies of the urinary tract are common in young children, with a frequency of between 1:650 and 1:1000, and are one of the major causes of renal insufficiency and renal failure. An initial diagnosis commonly is made on an antenatal ultrasound scan, but the complete postnatal evaluation requires both anatomic and functional information. Currently ultrasound is used to provide somewhat limited anatomic information, and a nuclear medicine test is used to obtain functional information. Combined MR anatomic and functional imaging may have a marked impact on the management of pediatric patients.[2]

The differential renal function as measured by dynamic renal scintigraphy (DRS) is based on the integration of the tracer curve over a range of time points at which the tracer is assumed to be located predominantly in the parenchyma. The

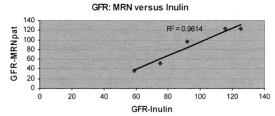

Fig. 7. Correlation plot between GFR measured concurrently by inulin and by MRNU technique in five patients. The GFR ranged from normal to moderately impaired by chronic renal disease. The inulin study results in a total GFR for both kidneys. The MRNU GFR results are shown as the sum of individually calculated GFR measurements for each kidney. The correlation shows good linear least squares fit. There is an apparent persistent offset with the MRNU technique showing a lower GFR value for each patient. The reason for this apparent bias remains the focus of continued investigation.

spatial resolution of DRS studies is limited; fixed time limits are used because the exact location of the tracer cannot be confirmed by visual inspection of the images. Because DRS measurements are based on projection images of the whole kidney, they measure the activity in the whole kidney but inadvertently may include the collecting system or adjacent soft tissues, such as spleen or liver. The MRNU approach provides high-resolution 3D volumes and avoids the limitations of the scintigraphic methods (**Fig. 8**). The methodology presented here makes a clear distinction between functioning and nonfunctioning tissue and accounts for the effects of cortical scarring or unusual morphology, such as seen in the polycystic or dysplastic kidneys often encountered in the pediatric population.

The ability to determine GFR as a function of renal volume provides additional potential application. Currently, GFR in children is indexed most often with body surface area.[22,23] Using functional MRNU, it is possible that normalizing GFR and RBF to the volume of renal parenchyma may provide more precise comparisons of the renal function of an obstructed kidney over time or between pediatric patients. It is hoped that this approach may yield a better understanding of patients at risk for progressive loss of renal function who may benefit from interventions and help determine the benefits of therapies.

The Transplanted Kidney

Repeated diagnostic imaging of a transplanted kidney often is needed to evaluate complications and to determine optimal intervention.

Complications may be categorized as prerenal (vascular complications), renal (intrinsic parenchymal disease), and postrenal (obstruction). Currently, differentiation between different categories and disease entities requires a combination of multiple imaging modalities to evaluate both structure and function, using CT, ultrasound, nuclear scintigraphy, and MR imaging to varying degrees. MRNU may offer a comprehensive analysis that provides a higher diagnostic yield than has been possible previously.

Prerenal causes of transplant dysfunction can be discerned with MR angiography techniques that already are widely in use. Intrinsic parenchymal disease is a diagnostic challenge with purely anatomic imaging, although it may be suggested by increased cortical T2 signal and loss of corticomedullary differentiation. Serial evaluation of GFR and RBF, however, can provide quantitative evaluation of transplant function, providing an earlier clue to acute or chronic rejection and potentially reducing the need for biopsy, which introduces its own complications. Postrenal causes of transplant dysfunction primarily involve obstruction of the collecting system (**Fig. 9**) and of venous outflow. The collecting system may be evaluated morphologically in excellent anatomic detail, even in the absence of contrast excretion (with the use of T2-weighted images), allowing identification of an anatomic site of narrowing. Dynamic acquisition of images allows more precise evaluation of the contrast transit time into the collecting system than possible with nuclear medicine. Evaluation of the transplant renal vein usually is a trivial matter when employing 3D postcontrast VIBE or THRIVE sequences.

LIMITATIONS

Although MRNU is a robust technique offering a large amount of clinically useful data, there are a few limitations. The most significant is the relatively poor sensitivity of MR imaging of calcium,[24] resulting from a combination of decreased proton density and increased T2 relaxation rates.[25] Large stones may be identified as hypointense filling defects within the collecting system on T2-weighted images, but smaller stones usually are invisible with MR imaging. The contribution of small stones to impaired renal function is uncertain, and the presence of small stones in a donor kidney is not a contraindication to renal transplantation.[26] If stone disease is a primary consideration in evaluation of the genitourinary system, low-dose unenhanced CT remains the modality of choice.

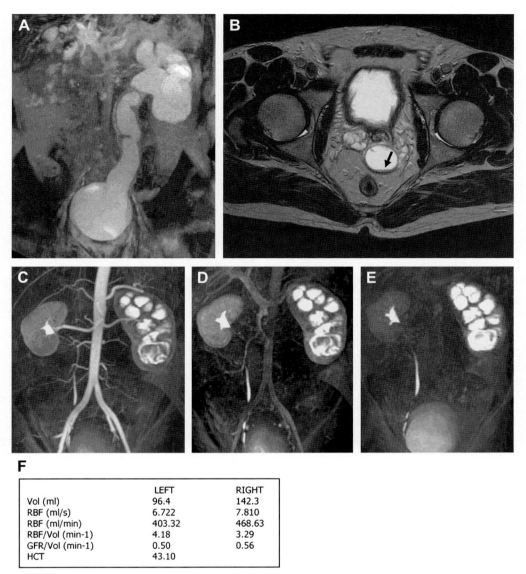

	LEFT	RIGHT
Vol (ml)	96.4	142.3
RBF (ml/s)	6.722	7.810
RBF (ml/min)	403.32	468.63
RBF/Vol (min-1)	4.18	3.29
GFR/Vol (min-1)	0.50	0.56
HCT	43.10	

Fig. 8. A 38-year-old man with ectopic insertion of the left ureter resulting in obstruction. (*A*) Coronal TFISP MIP shows severe left-side hydronephrosis and hydroureter to the level of the bladder. (*B*) Axial T2 fast spin-echo image at the level of the bladder shows that the severely distended distal ureter ectopically passes posterior to the seminal vesicle, where it narrows abruptly to a thin channel. Note the sedimentation (*arrow*) collecting along the dependent wall of the left ureter. Panels *C, D,* and–*E* show progressively delayed post-gadolinium coronal 3D GRE images. The collecting system is severely distended, the kidney size is enlarged overall, but the parenchyma and particularly the medullary component of the kidney appear thinned. (*F*) The summary of the quantitative analysis from the MRNU study. A concurrent MAG-3 nuclear study measured a differential function of 46% on the left and 54% on the right. The MRNU shows that the differential GFR is greater than that measured on MAG-3 and shows that the overall GFR is mildly impaired (stage 2 disease). This finding is in keeping with the mildly elevated creatinine level persistently measuring between 1.5 and 1.8 mg/dL during the time of these scans. The MAG-3 scan lacks the spatial resolution to evaluate the degree of loss in parenchyma in the left kidney and blurs together adjacent soft tissues such as the spleen. In the setting of obstruction, the kidney and the collecting system cannot be separated anatomically, and the capacitance of the severely dilated pelvis makes interpretation of clearance results challenging. The MR examination provides a comprehensive evaluation that includes determination of the cause of the obstruction. In the setting of urinary obstruction, therapeutic intervention depends on understanding both the cause of the disease and the degree of residual function of the affected kidney to evaluate the potential value of therapy. In this patient, the quantitative GFR for each kidney cannot be determined by the MAG-3 examination alone. The MRNU results suggest that this patient is dependent on both kidneys to achieve an acceptable combined GFR and that any improvements in left renal function may have significant impact.

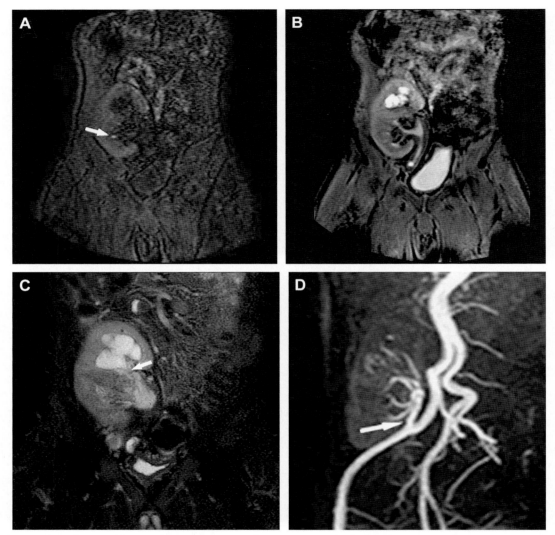

Fig. 9. Selected coronal images from an MRNU study in a patient who had undergone renal transplantation and who had impaired renal function initially misdiagnosed as caused by ureteric obstruction at the ureterovesical junction. Imaging was performed with 3D GRE over a 3-minute period during administration of low-dose gadolinium infusion. Images were acquired every 6 seconds. (*A*) A selected slice, reconstructed at 2-mm thickness, acquired 2.5 minutes from the time contrast first appeared in the renal artery, shows the first appearance of contrast at the tip of a lower pole papilla (*arrow*), representing a renal transit time at the upper limit of normal. (*B*) The upper-pole transit time was impaired at 5 minutes, and the upper-pole calyces fill later and show marked dilation 7 minutes after first arrival of contrast. (*C*) On a 9-minute image, the lower-pole calyces have normal configuration, and the upper-pole major calyx demonstrates stenosis (*arrow*). (*D*) Angiographic phase images can be viewed using MIP images and on an oblique coronal view show a normal renal transplant artery anastomosis (*arrow*). This complex case was delineated on MRNU after multiple attempts with ultrasound, scintigraphy, and biopsy failed to yield a comprehensive picture of the abnormalities.

Another limitation to consider is the recent association between certain gadolinium agents, in the setting of renal failure and the systemic condition of nephrogenic systemic fibrosis (NSF).[27,28] First described by Cowper and colleagues,[20] NSF is a systemic disease presenting initially as thickening and hardening of the skin, possibly leading to permanent disability. Most cases have been associated with the use of gadodiamide,[2] a linear-structure gadolinium agent that is more than 1 million times less stable than the most stable macrocyclic chelate in clinical use. Several case studies have reported the deposition of gadolinium within the soft tissues of patients who have NSF, and the disease may be secondary to deposition of toxic dissociated gadolinium within the soft tissues of patients who have renal failure.[2] The causes of NSF are multifactorial, but the common requirements for disease include severe renal disease (at least stage 4; GFR <30 mL/min) and use of gadodiamide. Furthermore, there is a dose relationship between the gadolinium agent and NSF,[29,30] and the dose may be cumulative over multiple prior doses. Even in the presence of these factors, the rates of NSF are on the order of 2% to as high as 5%.[29,31,32] The authors believe that the risk of NSF may be minimized by the use of more stable gadolinium chelates and by a reduction in the cumulative lifetime dose in patients who have renal failure. These measures should allow the continued judicious use of contrast-enhanced MR imaging in this patient population. For each patient, the risk and benefits must be considered. For patients who have normal to moderately impaired renal function (stage 3; GFR of 30–59 mL/min), the clinical risk for NSF seems to be immeasurably small. Similarly, the risk of NSF with the use of usual doses of the more stable agents has remained immeasurably small, even in high-risk patients who have severe renal insufficiency (stage 4 or 5) or who are receiving dialysis.

SUMMARY

MRNU is a powerful tool that makes it possible to obtain both structural and functional data within a single imaging examination that does not use ionization radiation, a significant benefit, especially in younger patients. The functional data available with MRNU allow renal physiology to be examined in ways that were not possible previously, including measurements of individual renal GFR and RBF and simultaneous measurement of individual renal perfused and functional volumes. Coupled with the exquisite soft tissue contrast provided by the standard MR images, MRNU can provide a comprehensive study that yields critical diagnostic information on structural diseases of the kidneys and collecting system, including congenital and acquired diseases, and also the full range of the causes of dysfunction in the transplanted kidney.

REFERENCES

1. Ergen FB, Hussain HK, Carlos RC, et al. 3D excretory MR urography: improved image quality with intravenous saline and diuretic administration. J Magn Reson Imaging 2007;25(4):783–9.

2. Grattan-Smith JD, Jones RA. MR urography in children. Pediatr Radiol 2006;36(11):1119–32 [quiz: 1228–9].

3. Lacour B. Creatinine and renal function. Nephrologie 1992;13(2):73–81 [in French].

4. Russell CD, Dubovsky EV. Quantitation of renal function using MAG3. J Nucl Med 1991;32(11):2061–3.

5. Russell CD, Thorstad BL, Yester MV, et al. Quantitation of renal function with technetium-99m MAG3. J Nucl Med 1988;29(12):1931–3.

6. Brenner DJ, Elliston CD. Estimated radiation risks potentially associated with full-body CT screening. Radiology 2004;232(3):735–8.

7. Mayo JR, Aldrich J, Muller NL. Radiation exposure at chest CT: a statement of the Fleischner Society. Radiology 2003;228(1):15–21.

8. Hackstein N, Buch T, Rau WS, et al. Split renal function measured by triphasic helical CT. Eur J Radiol 2007;61(2):303–9.

9. McCullough P. Outcomes of contrast-induced nephropathy: experience in patients undergoing cardiovascular intervention. Catheter Cardiovasc Interv 2006;67(3):335–43.

10. Martin DR, Sharma P, Salman K, et al. Individual kidney blood flow measured by contrast enhanced magnetic resonance first-pass perfusion imaging. Radiology 2008;246(1):241–8.

11. McDaniel BB, Jones RA, Scherz H, et al. Dynamic contrast-enhanced MR urography in the evaluation of pediatric hydronephrosis: part 2, anatomic and functional assessment of uteropelvic junction obstruction. AJR Am J Roentgenol 2005;185(6): 1608–14.

12. Jones RA, Perez-Brayfield MR, Kirsch AJ, et al. Dynamic contrast-enhanced MR urography in the evaluation of pediatric hydronephrosis: part 1, functional assessment. AJR Am J Roentgenol 2005; 185(6):1598–607.

13. Hackstein N, Kooijman H, Tomaselli S, et al. Glomerular filtration rate measured using the Patlak plot technique and contrast-enhanced dynamic MRI with different amounts of gadolinium-DTPA. J Magn Reson Imaging 2005;22(3): 406–14.

14. Huang AJ, Lee VS, Rusinek H. Functional renal MR imaging. Magn Reson Imaging Clin N Am 2004; 12(3):469–86, vi.

15. Lee VS, Rusinek H, Bokacheva L, et al. Renal function measurements from MR renography and a simplified multicompartmental model. Am J Physiol Renal Physiol 2007;292(5):F1548–59.

16. Peters AM. Graphical analysis of dynamic data: the Patlak-Rutland plot. Nucl Med Commun 1994;15(9): 669–72.

17. Hackstein N. Measurement of single kidney GFR using contrast enhanced GRE and Rutland-Patlak plot. J Magn Reson Imaging 2003;18:14–25.

18. Lee VS, Rusinek H, Noz ME, et al. Dynamic three-dimensional MR renography for the measurement of single kidney function: initial experience. Radiology 2003;227(1):289–94.

19. Votaw JR, Martin DR. Modeling systemic and renal gadolinium chelate transport with MRI. Pediatric Radiology 2008;38:28–34.

20. Cowper SE, Su LD, Bhawan J, et al. Nephrogenic fibrosing dermopathy. Am J Dermatopathol 2001; 23(5):383–93.

21. Hackstein N, Wiegand C, Rau WS, et al. Glomerular filtration rate measured by using triphasic helical CT with a two-point Patlak plot technique. Radiology 2004;230(1):221–6.

22. Peters AM, Henderson BL, Lui D. Indexed glomerular filtration rate as a function of age and body size. Clin Sci (Lond) 2000;98(4):439–44.

23. Hogg RJ, Furth S, Lemley KV, et al. National Kidney Foundation's Kidney Disease Outcomes Quality Initiative clinical practice guidelines for chronic kidney disease in children and adolescents: evaluation, classification, and stratification. Pediatrics 2003;111(6 Pt 1):1416–21.

24. Kucharczyk W, Henkelman RM. Visibility of calcium on MR and CT: can MR show calcium that CT cannot? AJNR Am J Neuroradiol 1994;15(6):1145–8.

25. Henkelman M, Kucharczyk W. Optimization of gradient-echo MR for calcium detection. AJNR Am J Neuroradiol 1994;15(3):465–72.

26. Martin G, Sundaram CP, Sharfuddin A, et al. Asymptomatic urolithiasis in living donor transplant kidneys: initial results. Urology 2007;70(1):2–5 [discussion: 5–6].

27. Grobner T. Gadolinium—a specific trigger for the development of nephrogenic fibrosing dermopathy and nephrogenic systemic fibrosis? Nephrol Dial Transplant 2006;21(4):1104–8.

28. Thomsen HS, Morcos SK, Dawson P. Is there a causal relation between the administration of gadolinium based contrast media and the development of nephrogenic systemic fibrosis (NSF)? Clin Radiol 2006;61(11):905–6.

29. Lauenstein TC, Salman K, Morreira R, et al. Nephrogenic systemic fibrosis: center case review. J Magn Reson Imaging 2007;26(5):1198–203.

30. Collidge TA, Thomson PC, Mark PB, et al. Gadolinium-enhanced MR imaging and nephrogenic systemic fibrosis: retrospective study of a renal replacement therapy cohort. Radiology 2007; 245(1):168–75.

31. Broome DR, Girguis MS, Baron PW, et al. Gadodiamide-associated nephrogenic systemic fibrosis: why radiologists should be concerned. AJR Am J Roentgenol 2007;188(2):586–92.

32. Sadowski EA, Bennett LK, Chan MR, et al. Nephrogenic systemic fibrosis: risk factors and incidence estimation. Radiology 2007;243(1): 148–57.

MR Imaging of the Aorta

Ichiro Sakamoto, MD*, Eijun Sueyoshi, MD,
Masataka Uetani, MD

KEYWORDS

• Aortic disease • Aortic aneurysm • Aortic dissection • MRI

Acquired disease of the aorta is widespread. In the past invasive angiography was required to depict structural abnormalities. Recent advances in noninvasive imaging methods, such as CT and MR imaging, have replaced most of invasive angiographic procedures, thus decreasing the cost and morbidity of diagnosis.[1–8] With its ability to delineate the intrinsic contrast between blood flow and vessel wall and to acquire images in multiple planes, MR imaging provides a high degree of reliability in the diagnosis of aortic diseases. Because of its noninvasive nature, MR imaging can be performed repeatedly, allowing the progression of the aortic disease to be evaluated over time. This article reviews and illustrates present MR imaging methods for evaluation of the aorta. Common diseases of the aorta also are discussed with a focus on their unique morphologic and functional features and characteristic MR imaging findings. Knowledge of pathologic conditions of common aortic diseases and proper MR imaging techniques enables accurate and time-efficient aortic evaluation.

COMPARISON WITH CT

Compared with MR angiography, CT angiography has the advantages of general availability and ease of performance, especially in urgent cases. Nevertheless, MR imaging has several distinct advantages over CT. First, MR imaging does not require the use of ionizing radiation. Because of the lack of radiation, MR imaging can be performed for repeatedly the follow-up of the patient without concern for radiation exposure. Second,

unlike CT angiography, MR angiography dose not require the use of nephrotoxic iodinated contrast material. Nephrotoxicity is a particularly relevant issue, because patients who have acquired aortic disease frequently suffer from renal insufficiency. In particular, MR angiography has advantages for patients undergoing endovascular treatment. Preprocedural planning using MR angiography excludes concerns related to iodine load and impaired renal function, thus enabling same-day or close performance of endovascular treatment.[7] Finally, cine MR imaging can be performed for dynamic evaluation of blood flow without using contrast material. Particularly, cine phase-contrast (cine PC) imaging can be used to determine flow velocity and direction. These cine MR techniques can be used to evaluate valvular and cardiac function.

BASIC TECHNICAL CONSIDERATIONS

Several different MR imaging techniques are used to depict the arteries. These techniques include black-blood imaging (conventional spin echo, fast spin echo), bright-blood imaging (time-of-flight imaging, PC imaging), and contrast-enhanced MR angiography. Recent advances in fast imaging, such as steady state free precession (SSFP) and subsecond contrast-enhanced MR angiography, enable quick examinations for initial screening evaluations of the aorta within several minutes. These improvements in MR technology and the aforementioned advantages of MR imaging over CT evaluation have increased the

This article originally appeared in *Radiologic Clinics of North America* 2007;45(3):485–97.
Department of Radiology and Radiation Biology, Nagasaki University Graduate School of Biomedical Sciences, 1-7-1 Sakamoto, Nagasaki 852-8501, Japan
* Corresponding author.
E-mail address: ichiro-s@net.nagasaki-u.ac.jp (I. Sakamoto).

role of MR angiography, even in the evaluation of some acute conditions.

Black-blood Vascular Imaging

The aorta can be well illustrated using black blood methods, namely, ECG-gated spin echo or fast spin echo, that exploit the inherent contrast between rapidly flowing blood and the aortic wall.[7,9–12] Unlike bright blood imaging, luminal signal void occurs because of the movement of spins and dephasing of turbulent flow. Spin echo imaging still constitutes the basis of any aortic study because this technique provides the best anatomic details of the aortic wall and pathologic conditions. Usually, a conventional study of the aorta in the axial plane is acquired first to display the orientation of the great arteries and to visualize mural lesions optimally perpendicular to their long axes. A main consideration in spin echo imaging is that each section corresponds to a different cardiac phase. Diastolic slow flow and entry or exit slice phenomena may produce high signal in the aortic lumen, which is difficult to differentiate from mural thrombus. Usually, T2-weighted imaging is of little usefulness in the study of the aorta because the low signal-to-noise ratio and the long acquisition time affect the image quality, mainly through motion artifact. With spin echo imaging the aortic caliber and also the vessel wall and perivascular tructures can be evaluated. Wall thickness can be demonstrated readily on T1-weighted imaging, and edema is seen as hyperintense intramural signal on T2-weighted imaging. Mural hyperenhancement of the vessel wall on T1-weighted images after injection of contrast material is considered to indicate active inflammation. ECG-gated double inversion recovery fast spin echo is a more recent black-blood method that allows breathhold acquisition.[13] By applying a nonselective inversion pulse followed by a section-selective inversion pulse, double inversion recovery fast spin echo provides better suppression of the signal from flowing blood (**Fig. 1**). This technique, however, is substantially less efficient in terms of scan time than fast spin echo technique because it is a sequential-slice imaging sequence.

Bright-blood Vascular Imaging

Several bright-blood techniques can be performed without the need for contrast agents.[7,14–17] One of the oldest techniques is the time-of-flight (TOF) effect, which is based on the phenomenon of flow-related enhancement of spins entering into a partially saturated imaging section. These unsaturated spins give more signal than surrounding

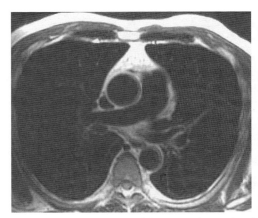

Fig. 1. Black-blood imaging of the aorta obtained at the level of the right pulmonary artery. Note the excellent suppression of the luminal blood signal and demonstration of the vessel wall. The image was obtained in 12 seconds with cardiac gating and breathholding.

stationary spins. With the two-dimensional (2D) technique, multiple thin, sequential sections are acquired by using a flow-compensated gradient echo (GRE) sequence. The acquired sections are viewed individually or are reformatted with the maximum intensity projection (MIP) technique to obtain a three-dimensional (3D) image. TOF imaging has several limitations:[18,19] (1) complex flow pattern producing loss of signal caused by intravoxel dephasing may mimic disease; (2) vessels not perpendicular to the acquired section plane may cause low signal intensity; (3) retrograde flow in collateral vessels may be saturated also, obscuring the true level of steno-occlusive lesions. Although arterial signal can be improved with cardiac gating, imaging times become long, and arterial signal on TOF MR angiography often remains inhomogeneous and unreliable for proper depiction of the aorta and its branches. Because of the long imaging times and aforementioned limitations, TOF imaging is being replaced rapidly with contrast-enhanced MR angiography.

The TOF effect can be useful when acquired in a 2D cine mode, for example, cine gradient echo (cine GRE).[7] Cine GRE images are acquired with ECG gating, thus resulting in high temporal resolution throughout the cardiac cycle, and can be displayed in cine format. The recently introduced SSFP (commercially known as "true fast imaging with steady precession (FISP)," "fast imaging employing steady state acquisition (FIESTA)," or "balanced fast field echo (FFE)" technique, with shorter TE and TR sequences, has become more widely available.[16,17] On SSFP, intraluminal signal generally is very high and homogenous even in cases of turbulent flow because this sequence depends mainly on a function of the T2/T1 ratio. Hence, in urgent situations, SSFP can be used to demonstrate quickly aortic abnormalities such as an intimal flap and a false lumen in aortic dissection.

One critical advantage of flow-based bright-blood techniques is the ability to perform a functional assessment of blood flow.[7,20,21] On cine GRE, turbulent flow produces rapid spin dephasing and results in flow jets extending distal to or downstream from the lesion, thus providing additional information in many pathologic conditions such as coarctation of the aorta, aortic valve insufficiency, and aortic dissection. Particularly in aortic dissection, the detection of entry and reentry sites is a special capability of this method that can be helpful in planning surgical and endovascular treatment. With the use of newer fast GRE pulse sequences with an ultrashort TR and TE, a flow jet may not be present despite the presence of a significant flow disturbance. The very short TE times may be insufficient for a sizable flow jet to form on this faster sequence. In cases of high suspicion, standard GRE sequences can be performed during free breathing (Fig. 2).[7] The longer TE will allow intravoxel dephasing to develop, and a flow jet should be seen if flow is turbulent.

Cine PC is another bright-blood technique that can be used for dynamic evaluation of blood flow.[7,22,23] Cine PC depends on the phase shifts that flowing protons experience as they travel along the gradient field. The data obtained with cine PC are processed into two sets of images: magnitude and phase-contrast. PC images display the direction of flow as bright or dark pixels, with their relative signal intensity representing their velocity. Hence, PC images can be used to assess flow direction, which may be important information for proper identification of a vascular structure or for quantifying blood flow.

Contrast-enhanced MR Angiography

Contrast-enhanced MR angiography, which first was described for imaging of aortoiliac disease in 1993, is the most widely accepted method for comprehensive evaluation of the aortic disease.[18,24–26] This technique can provide images that have high spatial resolution with a single breathhold and therefore is suitable for the depiction of aortic abnormalities such as aneurysm, dissection, penetrating atherosclerotic ulcer, and Takayasu arteritis.

Contrast-enhanced MR angiography uses the T1-shortening effect of a gadolinium-based contrast agent. By using a gadolinium chelate contrast agent, the T1 of blood is shortened so that the blood appears bright irrespective of flow patterns or velocities. Because signal enhancement and overall image quality of contrast-enhanced MR angiography depend on the intra-arterial concentration of the contrast agent, the correct timing of imaging after contrast material injection is crucial. Because image contrast depends mainly on central k-space data, collection of the central lines of k space during the plateau phase of arterial enhancement is essential for

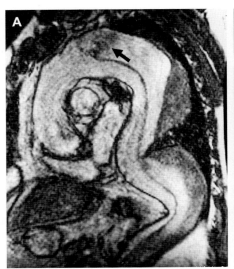 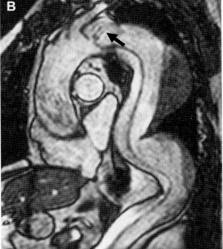

Fig. 2. Cine MR imaging in a patient who has aortic dissection. (A) Sagittal cine MR imaging obtained with standard GRE pulse sequence and during free breathing more clearly reveals a flow jet (arrows) through the entry than (B) that obtained with SSFP sequence and during breathholding.

optimal contrast-enhanced MR angiography.[27] The authors use 10 to 20 mL of contrast material delivered at a rate of 2 to 3 mL/s followed by 20 mL of saline solution delivered at the same rate. The dosage and delivery rate of the contrast material should be adjusted in individual patients, with special attention to the acquisition time. Several methods are used to determine the optimal delay between the start of intravenous contrast material injection and the start of image acquisition. Timing methods commonly used include injection of a test bolus using a small amount of contrast material, automatic triggering, and MR fluoroscopy.[28–30]

Imaging interpretation usually is done with the aid of a computer workstation on which individual source images are analyzed and postprocessing techniques, such as multiplanar volume reformation, MIP reformation, and volume rendering of the images, are performed. MIP images, in particular, can be obtained quickly, resemble catheter angiograms, and permit a 3D appreciation of anatomy (**Fig. 3**).

AORTIC DISEASE
Aortic Aneurysm

An aortic aneurysm is defined as a localized or diffuse dilatation involving all layers of the aortic wall and exceeding the expected aortic diameter by a factor of 1.5 or more.[11] Most thoracic and

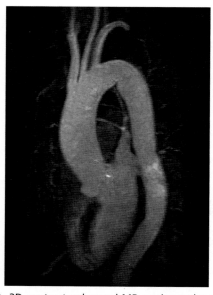

Fig. 3. 3D contrast-enhanced MR angiography of the thoracic aorta. Oblique sagittal MIP image clearly depicts the entire thoracic aorta and branch vessels from the aortic arch.

abdominal aneurysms are atherosclerotic in nature. Other causes of aortic aneurysms include infection, inflammation, syphilis, and cystic medial necrosis. Atherosclerotic aneurysms usually are fusiform, although saccular aneurysms are encountered occasionally.

The major goal in imaging an aortic aneurysm is the exact evaluation of the maximal diameter, the length, and involvement of major branch vessels.[31] All these features can be identified and characterized with MR imaging. Additionally, because the measurements are reproducible, MR imaging frequently can be used as a follow-up tool for monitoring the progression of disease. To obtain consistent results, vessel dimensions should be measured at the same anatomic locations on two subsequent examinations. Use of the sagittal or oblique sagittal plane allows accurate assessment of the location and extent of the aneurysm and avoids partial volume effects. 3D contrast-enhanced MR angiography is most suitable for depicting the location, extent, and exact diameter. This technique can provide precise topographic information concerning the extent of an aneurysm and its relationship to the aortic branches.[24,26,32,33] Although the resolution of contrast-enhanced MR angiography remains lower than that of multidetector CT, this technique is useful, especially in patients who have contraindications to iodinated contrast material. It is essential to recognize that measurement should be obtained from source images where the vessel wall is visible, because MIP images represent a cast of the lumen alone (**Fig. 4**). Standard spin echo images also are helpful in evaluating changes in the aortic wall and periaortic structures. Area of high signal intensity on spin echo images within the thrombus and aortic wall may indicate instability of the aneurysm (**Figs. 5** and **6**).[8] Aneurysms caused by a bacterial infection result in fragility of the vessel wall, thus causing saccular outpouching that most commonly involves the suprarenal portion of the aorta. In this condition, MR imaging can demonstrate the aneurysm itself and also wall thickening and periaortic abscess (**Fig. 7**).[34,35] Inflammatory abdominal aortic aneurysm is a variant of atherosclerotic aneurysm, characterized by inflammatory and/or fibrotic changes in the periaortic lesions. In this condition, MR imaging shows homogenous periaortic tissue with sparing of the posterior aspect of the aorta. This periaortic tissue shows variable enhancement after injection of contrast material, based on the degree of inflammation and fibrosis (**Fig. 8**).[36,37] Reduction in the thickness of periaortic tissue after surgical repair or endovascular stent grafting is seen occasionally.

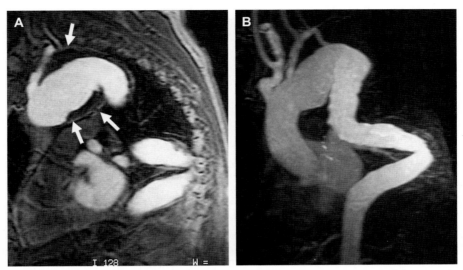

Fig. 4. 3D contrast-enhanced MR angiography in a patient with aortic arch aneurysm. (*A*) Source image of 3D contrast-enhanced MR angiography more clearly depicts involvement of the left subclavian artery by an aortic arch aneurysm than (*B*) the MIP image. Arrows in panel A indicates the aortic arch aneurysm with mural thrombus. As described in this article, in aneurysms with a large volume of mural thrombus, accurate evaluation of the branch vessel involvement by the aneurysm is difficult or impossible by MIP images alone.

If an aneurysm involves the ascending aorta or sinuses of Valsalva, concomitant aortic valve disease can be evaluated using cine MR technique. As described in the literature, the ability of contrast MR angiography to visualize the Adamkiewicz artery provides information that is important in planning the surgical repair of an aneurysm, thus avoiding postoperative neurologic deficit secondary to spinal cord ischemia.[38,39]

Aortic Dissection

Aortic dissection is a life-threatening condition requiring prompt diagnosis and treatment. This condition occurs when blood dissects into the

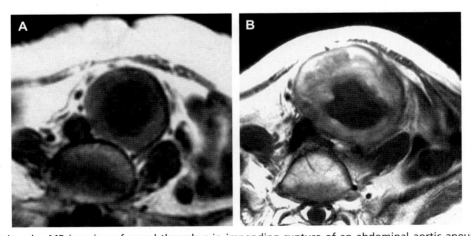

Fig. 5. Spin echo MR imaging of mural thrombus in impending rupture of an abdominal aortic aneurysm. (*A*) T1-weighted spin echo MR image obtained 24 months before impending rupture shows infrarenal abdominal aortic aneurysm with mural thrombus of homogenous low intensity. (*B*) T1-weighted spin echo MR image obtained at the time of impending rupture reveals an interval enlargement of the abdominal aortic aneurysm. A partial area of high signal intensity is also noted within the mural thrombus. In this case, a small amount of periaortic hemorrhage and hemorrhage into the mural thrombus were found at surgery.

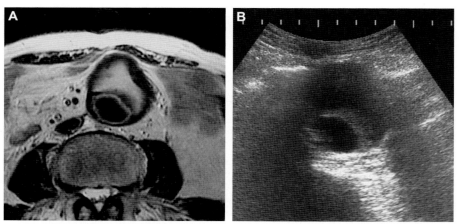

Fig. 6. Spin echo MR imaging of liquefactive thrombus in abdominal aortic aneurysm. (*A*) Most of mural thrombus is markedly high in signal intensity on T2-weighted spin echo images. (*B*) The area of high signal intensity in the mural thrombus is anechoic on ultrasound, indicating liquefaction of the thrombus.

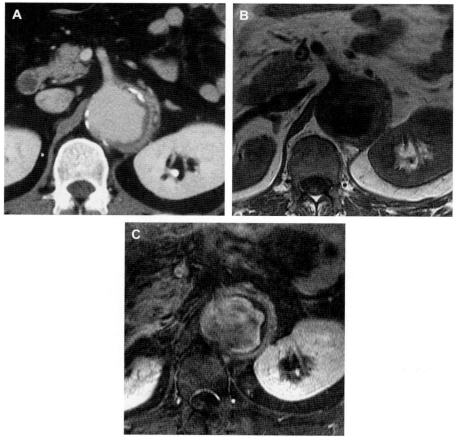

Fig. 7. MR imaging of infected aortic aneurysm. (*A*) Contrast-enhanced CT demonstrates an enlargement of the suprarenal abdominal aorta with a small amount of periaortic tissue adjacent to anterior to left lateral aspect of the aorta. Hyperenhancement of the periaortic tissue is also noted. T1-weighted spin echo MR images (*B*) before and (*C*) after injection of contrast material show the suprarenal abdominal aortic aneurysm with inhomogeneous hyperenhancement of the periaortic tissue.

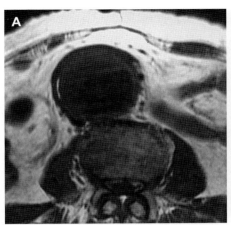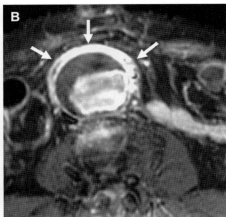

Fig. 8. MR imaging of inflammatory abdominal aortic aneurysm. (*A*) T1-weighted spin echo MR image shows infrarenal abdominal aortic aneurysm and periaortic tissue with sparing of posterolateral aspect of the aorta. (*B*) T1-weighted spin echo MR image after contrast material injection shows homogenous hyperenhancement of the periaortic tissue (*arrows*), indicating periaortic fibrosis and inflammation.

media of the aortic wall through an intimal tear. Classification of aortic dissections has been based traditionally on anatomic location (Stanford or DeBakey classification) and time from onset. The 14-day period after onset has been designated as the acute phase, because morbidity and mortality rates are highest (15%–25%), and surviving patients typically stabilize during this period. The Stanford classification simply distinguishes aortic dissection, irrespective of the site of the entry tear, into type A if the ascending aorta is involved or type B if the ascending aorta is spared. This classification is based fundamentally on prognostic factors: type A dissection necessitates urgent surgical repair, but most type B dissections can be managed conservatively. Hence, accurate recognition of anatomic details of the dissection with imaging is essential for successful management.[40]

In dissection, the diagnostic goals of imaging are a clear anatomic delineation of the intimal flap and its extension and the detection of the entry and reentry sites and branch vessel involvement. With current technology, MR imaging is the most accurate tool for detection of these features of the dissection. High spatial and contrast resolution and multiplanar acquisition provide excellent sensitivity and specificity of the disease and functional information with a totally noninvasive approach. In a patient suspected of having aortic dissection, the MR imaging examination usually begins with spin echo black-blood sequences that depict the intimal flap as a linear structure (**Fig. 9**). The true lumen can be differentiated from the false lumen because the true lumen shows a signal void, whereas the false lumen

shows higher signal intensity indicative of turbulent flow.[41] High signal intensity of pericardial effusion indicates a bloody component and is considered a sign of impending rupture of the ascending aorta into the pericardial space.

In stable patients, adjunctive GRE sequences or PC images can be performed to identify aortic insufficiency and intimal tear sites and to differentiate slow flow from thrombus in the false lumen (see **Fig. 9**). Further diagnostic refinement has been reported by gadolinium-enhanced 3D MR angiography in the diagnosis of aortic dissection and definition of its anatomic details.[42] Because 3D MR angiography is acquired rapidly without the need of ECG triggering, this technique can be performed even in severely ill patients. The lack of nephrotoxicity and other adverse effects enables the use of gadolinium in patients who have renal failure or low cardiac output. The analysis of gadolinium-enhanced 3D MR angiography should not be restricted to viewing MIP images, because MIP images occasionally fail to show the intimal flap (**Fig. 10**). Hence, it also should include a complete evaluation of reformatted images in all three planes to confirm or improve spin echo information and exclude artifacts. Combining the spin echo images with gadolinium-enhanced 3D MR angiography images completes the diagnosis and anatomic definition.[43]

Intramural Hematoma

Intramural hematoma is an atypical form of dissection without flow in the false lumen or a discrete intraluminal flap.[44,45] Intramural hematoma usually

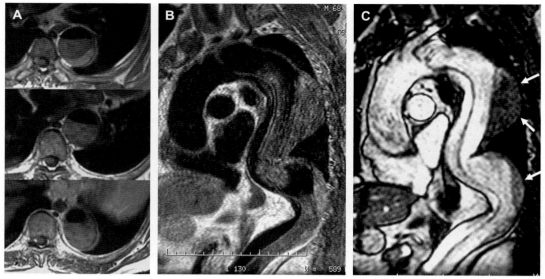

Fig. 9. MR imaging of aortic dissection. (*A*) Axial and (*B*) oblique sagittal spin echo images of type B dissection show a linear structure in the descending thoracic aorta, indicating the dissection flap. The true lumen is narrowed by compression of a dilated false lumen. Note the higher signal intensity in the false lumen, indicating turbulent flow and/or thrombus in the false lumen. Turbulent flow in the false lumen cannot be differentiated from thrombus using spin echo techniques alone. (*C*) On oblique sagittal cine MR imaging with SSFP technique, flowing blood in the false and true lumens is visualized as high intensity and partial thrombus in the false lumen as low intensity (*arrows*).

results from spontaneous rupture of the aortic wall vasa vasorum or from a penetrating atherosclerotic ulcer. Because the clinical signs and symptoms and the prognosis of this condition do not differ from classic aortic dissection, its standard treatment is considered to be similar to that of classic aortic dissection.[44] Complete resolution of the aortic hematoma is seen occasionally, but complications such as fluid extravasation with pericardial, pleural, and periaortic hematoma or aortic rupture may occur at the time of the onset or during the follow-up period.

Intramural hematoma can be identified as crescentic thickening of the aortic wall with abnormal signal intensity. Because of the short T1 relaxation time of fresh blood, differentiation from the

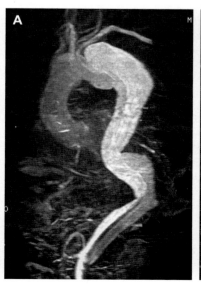

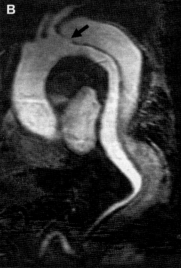

Fig. 10. 3D contrast-enhanced MR angiography of aortic dissection. (*A*) The anatomic details of the dissected aorta are difficult to recognize on the MIP image of 3D contrast-enhanced MR angiography alone. (*B*) Oblique sagittal re-formatted image clearly depicts the intimal flap and also the entry site (*arrow*).

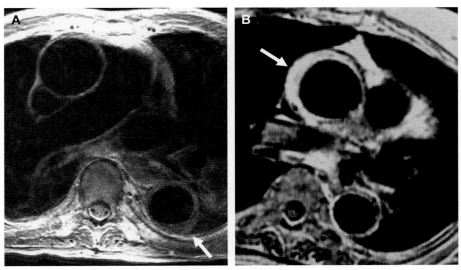

Fig. 11. Spin echo MR imaging of intramural hematoma. (*A*) On a T1-weighted spin echo MR image obtained 2 days after the onset, intramural hematoma of the descending thoracic aorta shows intermediate signal intensity (*arrow*) caused by the presence of oxyhemoglobin (acute stage). (*B*) In another patient, in a T1-weighted spin echo MR image obtained 40 days after the onset, an intramural hematoma of the ascending thoracic aorta shows high signal intensity (*arrow*) caused by the presence of methemoglobin (subacute stage).

adjacent mediastinal fat may be difficult. In such circumstances, precontrast fat saturation images can be helpful in differentiating intramural hematoma from surrounding mediastinal fat. Moreover, MR imaging may allow the assessment of the age of hematoma on the basis of the different degradation products of hemoglobin. T1-weighted spin echo MR imaging may show intermediate signal intensity caused by the presence of oxyhemoglobin in the acute stage and high signal intensity caused by the presence of methemoglobin in the subacute stage (**Fig. 11**).[8,46] The progression

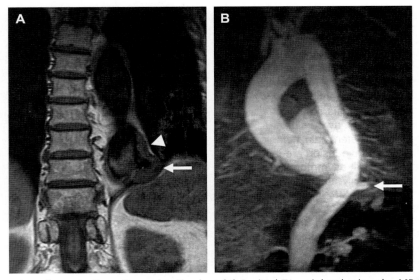

Fig. 12. MR imaging of penetrating atherosclerotic ulcer. (*A*) Sagittal T1-weighted spin echo MR image and (*B*) MIP image of 3D contrast-enhanced MR angiography clearly depict a penetrating atherosclerotic ulcer in the mid-portion of the descending thoracic aorta (*arrow*). Note mural thickening with intermediate signal intensity (*arrowhead* in A) indicating the formation of intramural hematoma.

A   **B**

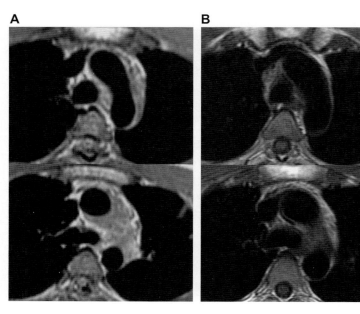

Fig. 13. Improvement of aortic wall thickening in early-phase Takayasu arteritis. T1-weighted spin echo MR images obtained (*A*) before and (*B*) after steroid therapy demonstrate marked reduction of the aortic wall thickening after the therapy.

of intramural hematoma to overt dissection and rupture has been reported in 32% of the cases, particularly when the ascending aorta is involved.

Penetrating Atherosclerotic Ulcer

Penetrating atherosclerotic ulcer is characterized by ulceration of an atherosclerotic plaque that disrupts the intima.[47,48] The ulcerated atheroma may extend into the media, resulting in an intramural hematoma, or it may penetrate through the media and form a saccular pseudoaneurysm with the risk of transmural aortic rupture. Penetrating atherosclerotic ulcer usually affects elderly individuals who have hypertension and extensive aortic atherosclerosis. It typically is located in the descending aorta, but locations in the aortic arch or in the abdominal aorta have been reported occasionally. Penetrating atherosclerotic ulcer should be considered a distinct entity with different management and prognosis, although clinical features of this condition may be similar to those of aortic dissection. Persistent pain, hemodynamic instability, and signs of expansion are indications for surgical treatment, but asymptomatic patients can be managed medically and followed up with imaging. The diagnostic MR imaging finding in penetrating atherosclerotic ulcer is a craterlike outpouching extending beyond the contour of the aortic lumen.[48–50] Mural thickening with high or intermediate signal intensity on spin echo sequences indicates the formation of intramural hematoma. On MR angiography, the penetrating atherosclerotic ulcer is recognized readily as a contrast-filled outpouching with a jagged edge (**Fig. 12**). The disadvantage of MR imaging,

compared with CT, is its inability to visualize dislodgment of intimal calcification, frequently seen in penetrating atherosclerotic ulcer.

Takayasu Arteritis

Takayasu arteritis is an idiopathic large vessel vasculitis affecting the aorta and its major branches as well as pulmonary arteries. The cause

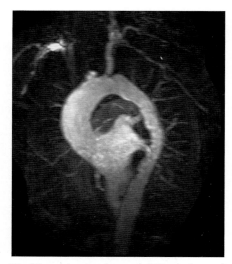

Fig. 14. 3D contrast-enhanced MR angiography of late-phase Takayasu arteritis. MIP image of 3D contrast-enhanced MR angiography shows occlusion of the right brachiocephalic and right common carotid arteries and mild stenosis of the orifice of the left subclavian artery. Note the irregular and diffuse narrowing of the proximal segment of the thoracic descending aorta.

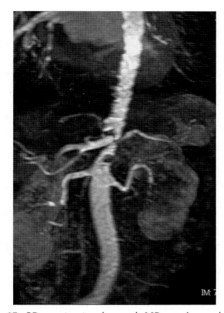

Fig. 15. 3D contrast-enhanced MR angiography of late-phase Takayasu arteritis. MIP image of 3D contrast-enhanced MR angiography shows marked and irregular narrowing of the abdominal aorta. This stenosing type of late-phase Takayasu arteritis is known as "atypical coarctation of the aorta."

of Takayasu arteritis is still unknown, although an autoimmune mechanism has been suspected. The arteritis is most common in Japan and other Asian countries, although it now is known worldwide. Women are affected about 10 times more often than men. Young women are particularly susceptible to the disease. Steno-occlusive lesions are characteristics of this disorder, but dilated forms are also common. Fever, malaise, easy fatigability, weakness of the upper extremity, dizziness, headache, and syncope are the symptoms frequently mentioned. There are many synonyms including "aortitis syndrome," "aortic arch syndrome," "pulseless disease," and "young female arteritis."

Angiography used to be the reference standard for delineating the vascular abnormalities, but CT and MR imaging now are considered to be alternative noninvasive techniques.[51–53] In fact, they provide more information about vascular changes in Takayasu arteritis. In particular, the thickness of the vessel wall is better demonstrated by these new modalities. MR imaging provides direct imaging in the axial, sagittal, and coronal planes, with good contrast resolution between the arterial lumen and its wall without use of contrast material.

The significant finding of acute-phase Takayasu arteritis is wall thickening of the aorta and its branches and the pulmonary arteries, which can be visualized better with multisectional scanning by MR imaging. Wall thickening of the vertically positioned aorta can be seen best on axial images; the horizontal portion of the right pulmonary artery can be evaluated best in the coronal and sagittal planes. Dramatic reduction of wall thickening in the aorta and pulmonary artery following steroid therapy may be documented by MR imaging (**Fig. 13**).[54]

In the late occlusive phase, 3D contrast-enhanced MR angiography can reveal short- or long-segment stenoses in the descending thoracic and abdominal aorta and major branch vessels (**Fig. 14**). The stenosing variety of late-phase Takayasu arteritis is known as "atypical coarctation of the aorta" (**Fig. 15**). Pulmonary arterial involvement (which as an incidence of approximately 70%) can also be depicted by 3D contrast-enhanced MR angiography or contrast-enhanced MR perfusion imaging (2D fast spoiled GRE sequence with single-slice technique) (**Fig. 16**).[55]

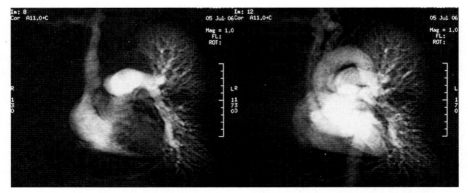

Fig. 16. Contrast-enhanced MR perfusion imaging of the lung in a patient who has late-phase Takayasu arteritis. Serial subtracted MR images of contrast-enhanced MR perfusion imaging of the lung show occlusion of the right main trunk of the pulmonary artery and a perfusion defect in the middle lung field of the left lung.

REFERENCES

1. Flamm SD, VanDyke CW, White RD. MR imaging of the thoracic aorta. Magn Reson Imaging Clin N Am 1996;4:217–35.
2. Leung DA, Debatin JF. Three-dimensional contrast-enhanced MRA of the thoracic vasculature. Eur Radiol 1997;7:981–9.
3. Krinsky G, Reuss PM. MR angiography of the thoracic aorta. Magn Reson Imaging Clin N Am 1998;6:293–320.
4. Reddy GP, Higgins CB. MR imaging of the thoracic aorta. Magn Reson Imaging Clin N Am 2000;8:1–15.
5. Ho VB, Corse WR, Hood MN, et al. MRA of the thoracic vessels. Semin Ultrasound CT MR 2003; 24:192–216.
6. Tatli S, Lipton MJ, Davison BD, et al. MR imaging of aortic and peripheral vascular disease. Radiographics 2003;23:S59–78.
7. Czum JM, Corse WR, Ho VB. MR angiography of the thoracic aorta. Magn Reson Imaging Clin N Am 2005;13:41–64.
8. Russo V, Renzulli M, Buttazzi K, et al. Acquired diseases of the thoracic aorta: role of MRI and MRA. Eur Radiol 2006;16:852–65.
9. Glazier HS, Gutierrez FR, Levitt G, et al. The thoracic aorta studied by MR imaging. Radiology 1985;157: 149–55.
10. Gomes AS. MR imaging of congenital anomalies of the thoracic aorta and pulmonary arteries. Radiol Clin North Am 1989;27:1171–81.
11. Fattori R, Nienaber CA. MRI of acute and chronic aortic pathology: pre-operative and postoperative evaluation. J Magn Reson Imaging 1999;10:741–50.
12. Russo V, Renzulli M, Palombara CL, et al. Congenital diseases of the thoracic aorta: role of MRI and MRA. Eur Radiol 2006;16:676–84.
13. Simonetti OP, Finn JP, White RD, et al. "Black blood" T2-weighted inversion recovery MR imaging of the heart. Radiology 1996;199:49–57.
14. Pelc LR, Pelc NJ, Rayhill SC, et al. Arterial and venous blood flow: noninvasive quantification with MR imaging. Radiology 1992;185:809–12.
15. Rebergen SA, van der Wall EE, Doornbos J, et al. Magnetic resonance measurement of velocity and flow: technique, validation, and cardiovascular application. Am Heart J 1993;126:1439–56.
16. Earls JP, Ho VB, Foo TK, et al. Cardiac MRI: recent progress and continued challenges. J Magn Reson Imaging 2002;16:111–27.
17. Pereles FS, McCarthy RM, Baskaran V, et al. Thoracic aortic dissection and aneurysm: evaluation with nonenhanced true FISP MR angiography in less than 4 minutes. Radiology 2002;223:270–4.
18. Prince MR, Yucel EK, Kaufman JA, et al. Dynamic gadolinium-enhanced three-dimensional abdominal MR arteriography. J Magn Reson Imaging 1993;3:877–81.
19. McCauley TR, Monib A, Dickey KW, et al. Peripheral vascular occlusive disease: accuracy and reliability of time-of-flight MR angiography. Radiology 1994; 192:351–7.
20. Didier D, Ratib O, Friedli B, et al. Cine gradient-echo MR imaging in the evaluation of cardiovascular disease. Radiographics 1993;13:561–73.
21. Ho VB, Kinney JB, Sahn DJ. Contributions of newer MR imaging strategies for congenital heart disease. Radiographics 1996;16:43–60.
22. Niezen RA, Doombos J, van der Wall EE, et al. Measurement of aortic and pulmonary flow with MRI at rest and during physical exercise. J Comput Assist Tomogr 1998;22:194–201.
23. Powell AJ, Maier SE, Chung T, et al. Phase-velocity cine magnetic resonance imaging measurement of pulsatile blood flow in children and young adults: in vitro and in vivo validation. Pediatr Cardiol 2000; 21:104–10.
24. Prince MR, Narasimham DL, Jacoby WT, et al. Three dimensional gadolinium-enhanced MR angiography of the thoracic aorta. Am J Roentgenol 1996;166: 1387–97.
25. Krinsky G, Rofsky N, Flyer M, et al. Gadolinium-enhanced three dimensional MR angiography of acquired arch vessels disease. Am J Roentgenol 1996;167:981–7.
26. Krinsky G, Rofsky N, De Corato DR, et al. Thoracic aorta: comparison of gadolinium-enhanced three dimensional MR angiography with conventional MR imaging. Radiology 1997;202:183–93.
27. Svensson J, Petersson JS, Stahlberg F, et al. Image artifacts due to a time-varying contrast medium concentration in 3D contrast-enhanced MRA. J Magn Reson Imaging 1999;10:919–28.
28. Hany TF, Mckinnon GC, Leung DA, et al. Optimization of contrast timing for breath-holding three-dimensional MR angiography. J Magn Reson Imaging 1997;7:551–6.
29. Foo TK, Saranathan M, Prince MR, et al. Automated detection of bolus arrival and initiation of data acquisition in fast, three-dimensional, gadolinium-enhanced MR angiography. Radiology 1997;203: 275–80.
30. Riederer SJ, Bernstein MA, Breen JF, et al. Three-dimensional contrast-enhanced MR angiography with real-time fluoroscopic triggering: design specifications and technical reliability in 330 patient studies. Radiology 2000;215:584–93.
31. Bonser RS, Pagano D, Lewis ME, et al. Clinical and patho-anatomical factors affecting expansion of thoracic aortic aneurysms. Heart 2000;84:277–83.
32. Debatin JF, Hany TF. MR-based assessment of vascular morphology and function. Eur Radiol 1998;8:528–39.
33. Neimatallah MA, Ho VB, Dong Q, et al. Gadolinium-based 3D magnetic resonance angiography of the

thoracic vessels. J Magn Reson Imaging 1999;10: 758–70.

34. Sueyoshi E, Sakamoto I, Kawahara Y, et al. Infected abdominal aortic aneurysm: early CT findings. Abdom Imaging 1998;23:645–8.

35. Macedo TA, Stanson AW, Oderich GS, et al. Infected aortic aneurysms: imaging findings. Radiology 2004;231:250–7.

36. Berletti R, D'Andrea P, Cavagna E, et al. Inflammatory and fibrotic changes in the periaortic regions: integrated US, CT and MR imaging in three cases. Radiol Med 2002;103:427–32.

37. Anbarasu A, Harris PL, McWilliams RG. The role of gadolinium-enhanced MR imaging in the preoperative evaluation of inflammatory abdominal aortic aneurysm. Eur Radiol 2002;12:S192–5.

38. Nijenhuis RJ, Jacobs MJ, van Engelshoven JM, et al. MR angiography of the Adamkiewicz artery and anterior radiculomedullary vein: postmortem validation. AJNR Am J Neuroradiol 2006;27:1573–5.

39. Yoshioka K, Niinuma H, Ehara S, et al. MR angiography and CT angiography of the artery of Adamkiewicz: state of the art. Radiographics 2006;26:S63–73.

40. Cigarroa JE, Isselbacher EM, DeSanctis RW, et al. Diagnostic standard and new direction. N Engl J Med 1993;328:35–43.

41. Chang JM, Friese K, Caputo GR, et al. MR measurement of blood flow in the true and false channel in chronic aortic dissection. J Comput Assist Tomogr 1991;15:418–23.

42. Fisher U, Vossherich R, Kopka L, et al. Dissection of the thoracic aorta: pre- and postoperative findings of turbo-FLASH MR images in the plane of the aortic arch. Am J Roentgenol 1994;163:1069–72.

43. Bogaert J, Meyns B, Rademakers FE, et al. Follow-up of aortic dissection: contribution of MR angiography for evaluation of the abdominal aorta and its branches. Eur Radiol 1997;7:695–702.

44. Nienaber CA, von Kodolitsch Y, Petersen B, et al. Intramural hemorrhage of the thoracic aorta: diagnosis and therapeutic implications. Circulation 1995;92:1465–72.

45. Ganaha F, Miller DC, Sugimoto K, et al. Prognosis of aortic intramural hematoma with and without penetrating atherosclerotic ulcer: a clinical and radiological analysis. Circulation 2002;106:342–8.

46. Murray JG, Manisali M, Flamm SD, et al. Intramural hematoma of the thoracic aorta: MR imaging findings and their prognostic implications. Radiology 1997;204:349–55.

47. Stanson AW, Kazmier FJ, Hollier LH, et al. Penetrating atherosclerotic ulcers of the thoracic aorta: natural history and clinicopathologic correlations. Ann Vasc Surg 1986;1:15–23.

48. Hayashi H, Matsuoka Y, Sakamoto I, et al. Penetrating atherosclerotic ulcer of the aorta: imaging features and disease concept. Radiographics 2000;20:995–1005.

49. Macura KJ, Szarf G, Fishman EK, et al. Role of computed tomography and magnetic resonance imaging in assessment of acute aortic syndromes. Semin Ultrasound CT MR 2003;24:232–54.

50. Yucel EK, Steinberg FL, Egglin TK, et al. Penetrating aortic ulcers: diagnosis with MR imaging. Radiology 1990;177:779–81.

51. Matsunaga N, Hayashi K, Sakamoto I, et al. Takayasu arteritis: protean radiologic manifestations and diagnosis. Radiographics 1997;17:579–94.

52. Matsunaga N, Hayashi K, Okada M, et al. Magnetic resonance imaging features of aortic diseases. Top Magn Reson Imaging 2003;14:253–66.

53. Nastri MV, Baptista LP, Baroni RH, et al. Gadolinium-enhanced three-dimensional MR angiography of Takayasu arteritis. Radiographics 2004;24:773–86.

54. Tanigawa K, Eguchi K, Kitamura Y, et al. Magnetic resonance imaging detection of aortic and pulmonary artery wall thickening in acute stage of Takayasu arteritis: improvement of clinical and radiologic findings after steroid therapy. Arthritis Rheum 1992;35: 476–80.

55. Sueyoshi E, Sakamoto I, Ogawa Y, et al. Diagnosis of perfusion abnormality of the pulmonary artery in Takayasu's arteritis using contrast-enhanced MR perfusion imaging. Eur Radiol 2006;16:1551–6.

Diagnostic Breast MR Imaging: Current Status and Future Directions

Elizabeth A. Morris, MD

KEYWORDS

• Breast MRI • Breast imaging • Breast intervention

Breast MRI has become an integral and necessary component of any breast imaging practice. The performance and clinical uses of breast MRI are now standardized and much more defined than they were several years ago. In the past few years, great strides have been made by societies in the realm of defining indications and findings on breast MRI.[1–3] The most important development, however, of the past few years was made in the area of breast intervention: new biopsy coils and a choice of MR-compatible biopsy needles are now available, making percutaneous biopsy of a suspicious MR lesion a possibility.[4] Additionally, more imaging sequences are now available from manufacturers with an increase in both image quality and speed of acquisition.[5] Breast MRI is now available in many practices and is one of the fastest growing areas in radiology. In fact, many of our current algorithms in the detection and treatment of breast cancer have been changed by the availability of breast MRI.

The basic strength of breast MRI lies in the detection of cancer that is occult on conventional imaging such as mammography and sonography. Many studies have shown that breast MRI is best used in situations where there is a known cancer, suspected cancer, or a high probability of finding cancer. For example, in the preoperative evaluation of the patient with a known cancer, the ability of MRI to detect multifocal (within the same quadrant of the breast) and multicentric (within different quadrants) disease that was previously unsuspected (**Fig. 1**) facilitates accurate staging.[6–9]

Incidental synchronous contralateral carcinomas have also been detected when screening the contralateral breast in patients with known cancer and may be the most compelling reason for performing breast MRI in the preoperative setting (**Fig. 2**).[10–12] In the patient with positive margins following an initial attempt at breast conservation (where MRI was not performed preoperatively), MRI can detect residual disease (**Fig. 3**);[13] and in the patient with inoperable locally advanced breast cancer, MRI may provide information to assess response to neoadjuvant chemotherapy (**Fig. 4**).[14–17] Suspected recurrence can be confirmed with MRI in the previously treated breast (**Fig. 5**)[18] and breast MRI is absolutely indicated in the patient with axillary node metastases with unknown primary (**Fig. 6**).[19,20] The final important indication is the use of MRI for screening in certain high-risk patients (**Fig. 7**),[17,21–27] which will be discussed elsewhere in this book.

RECENT GUIDELINES AND RECOMMENDATIONS

During the past few decades, as breast MRI has been incorporated into the clinical evaluation of the breast, it became apparent that standardization of image acquisition and terminology is extremely important. The American College of Radiology (ACR) Committee on Standards and Guidelines has published a document for the indications and performance of breast MRI in 2004. Recently, the Breast Imaging Reporting and Data

This article originally appeared in *Radiologic Clinics of North America* 2007; 45(5);863–80.
Memorial Sloan-Kettering Cancer Center, 1275 York Avenue, New York, NY 10021, USA
E-mail address: morrise@mskcc.org

Magn Reson Imaging Clin N Am 18 (2010) 57–74
doi:10.1016/j.mric.2009.09.005

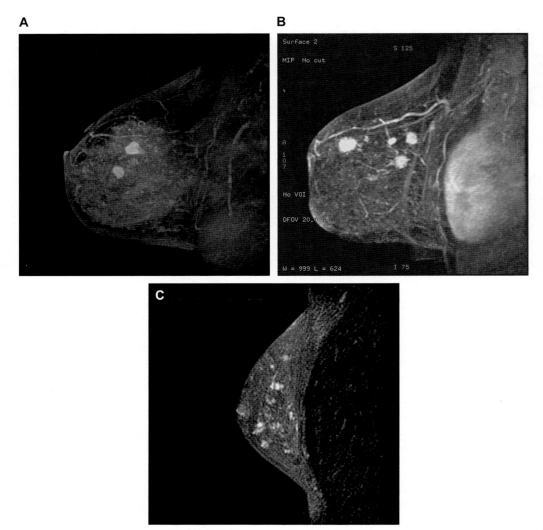

Fig. 1. Extent of disease evaluation. (*A*) Multifocal 43-year-old woman had routine mammography that was negative. Because of extreme breast density she underwent screening sonography, which demonstrated a suspicious lesion in the upper outer quadrant that subsequently was biopsied yielding invasive cancer. MRI demonstrates an additional invasive cancer inferiorly in the same quadrant compatible with multifocal disease. The patient underwent wide excision with negative margins. (*B*) Multicentric 45-year-old woman had negative mammography demonstrating dense breasts. Due to palpable fullness she underwent ultrasound that demonstrated two adjacent solid masses that were aspirated yielding suspicious cells. MRI demonstrates multiple masses extending over 8 cm suspicious for multicentricity. Biopsy of two lesions separated by a large distance was performed to confirm the need for mastectomy at initial surgery. (*C*) 46-year-old woman with prior contralateral mastectomy has routine screening MRI that demonstrated multiple suspicious masses in the remaining breast that proved to represent multicentric contralateral cancer. Mammography was dense and negative.

System (BI-RADS) lexicon[2] has added a section regarding breast MRI that has already been revised and further revisions are in progress. These efforts have been important in establishing the standards of reporting and the standards for patient selection. The existence of standardized guidelines in image acquisition and interpretation has helped disseminate this technology from academic centers into the community. Furthermore, the ACR is supporting efforts to establish a voluntary accreditation process for performing breast MRI. This will further standardize the acquisition of the MRI examination and provide high-quality imaging to women at those centers that are accredited. The revised recommendations for high-risk screening from the American Cancer

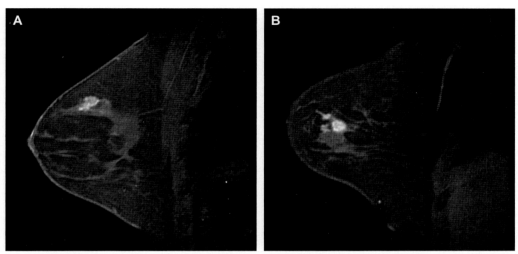

Fig. 2. Contralateral screening of a 35-year-old woman who presented with a palpable mass in the left breast at 12 o'clock. Mammogram was negative but a directed ultrasound demonstrated a mass that was biopsied yielding invasive carcinoma. (*A*) Left breast with known 1.5-cm poorly differentiated invasive ductal carcinoma. Sentinel node was positive. (*B*) Contralateral right breast with unsuspected lesion identified at targeted ultrasound proved to represent 1.6-cm poorly differentiated invasive ductal carcinoma with negative sentinel nodes. The patient elected to undergo bilateral mastectomy with immediate reconstruction.

Society (ACS) will no doubt accelerate this important accreditation process.

The ACS recently made a modification in the recommended screening guidelines to recommend annual screening MRI examination for certain high-risk women, which will be discussed briefly in this chapter.

SENSITIVITY AND SPECIFICITY ISSUES IN BREAST MR IMAGING

Breast MRI for cancer detection relies almost exclusively on the neovascularity associated with invasive carcinomas. The administration of an intravenous contrast agent such as gadolinium-diethylenetriamine pentaacetic acid (Gd-DTPA) allows these lesions to be well visualized, particularly if subtraction imaging or chemical fat suppression sequences are used. Leaky capillaries and arterio-venous shunts allow contrast agents to leave the lesion rapidly over time resulting in the characteristic washout time intensity curves that can be seen with most but not all malignancies.[28] Detection of invasive breast carcinoma is extremely reliable on MR imaging as the sensitivity approaches 100%. As the sensitivity for cancer detection is high, the negative predictive value of breast MRI is high. If no enhancement is present in the breast, and any possible technical mishap such as intravenous contrast extravasation has been excluded, there is an extremely high likelihood that no invasive carcinoma is

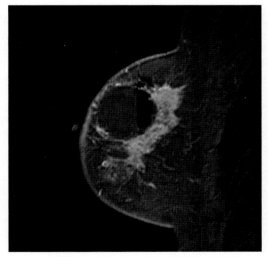

Fig. 3. Residual disease in a patient with positive margins. A 42-year-old patient desiring breast reduction surgery saw her plastic surgeon, who palpated a mass. Excisional biopsy confirmed invasive lobular carcinoma with positive margins. Mammography was unremarkable. MRI demonstrates a fresh postoperative seroma cavity with an air-fluid level and extensive residual masslike enhancement around the cavity compatible with residual disease. Targeted ultrasound was able to biopsy the adjacent hypoechoic area next to the seroma to confirm the presence of residual disease. At mastectomy, 7 cm of residual tumor was identified.

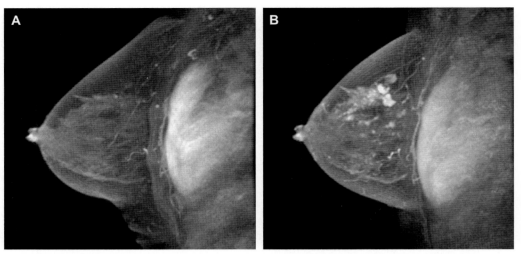

Fig. 4. Complete neoadjuvent chemotherapy response. (*A*) A 48-year-old woman with 4-cm invasive ductal carcinoma moderately to poorly differentiated underwent dose-dense adriamycin and cytoxan, paclitaxel to shrink the tumor for possible conservation. (*B*) Three months later following a full course there is no residual enhancement. Surgery however did demonstrate multiple foci of residual invasive disease; therefore, the MRI overestimated response. The patient was however able to achieve breast conservation therapy with negative margins.

present. Specificity is lower than sensitivity and therefore false positives can pose a problem in interpretation. False positives can be caused by high-risk lesions such as lobular carcinoma in situ (LCIS), atypical ductal hyperplasia (ADH), and atypical lobular hyperplasia (ALH), as well as benign masses such as fibroadenomas, papillomas, and lymph nodes. Additionally, fibrocystic changes, sclerosing adenosis, duct hyperplasia, and fibrosis can result in a benign biopsy. With experience, many of these lesions can be diagnosed as benign; however, false positives will always be an issue on MRI as they are on mammography and sonography.

Despite the reputation of high detection of cancer, false negative examinations with MRI do exist. It should be noted that false negatives have been reported with some well-differentiated invasive ductal carcinomas as well as invasive lobular carcinoma.[29] Moreover, not all DCIS is detected on MRI. Although the sensitivity is very high for invasive carcinoma, the sensitivity DCIS has been reported in prior literature to be somewhat lower, possibly secondary to more variable angiogenesis associated with DCIS lesions and the variable appearance. But, more recent evidence suggests that the sensitivity for DCIS detection may actually be higher than previously reported now that high-resolution scanning techniques are more available and widely used and the patterns of DCIS on MRI are more recognized.[30,31] Morphology may be more important than kinetics in the evaluation of DCIS; thus, a slightly modified

interpretation approach is taken when evaluating for DCIS. Although more work needs to be performed in the MR assessment of in-situ disease, MRI does not currently have as high a negative predictive value for DCIS as with invasive cancer. Therefore, MRI is not able to exclude DCIS with current technology and cannot be used to exclude

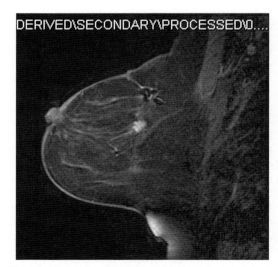

Fig. 5. Recurrence. A 68-year-old woman status post–breast conservation 2 years earlier for 0.6-cm invasive with an extensive intraductal component. Margins at initial surgery clear at 3 mm. First postsurgical MRI demonstrates suspicious mass compatible with recurrence. Completion mastectomy was performed.

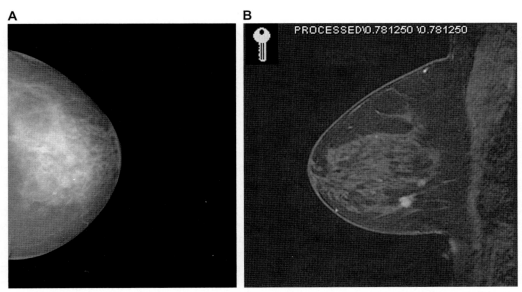

Fig. 6. Unknown primary. A 47-year-old woman presented with left axillary adenopathy with (A) negative mammogram and clinical examination. (B) MRI demonstrated an irregular mass in the lower breast that was not visible on ultrasound. MR needle localization was performed and pathology was 1-cm invasive ductal carcinoma.

the need for biopsy of suspicious calcifications. Nevertheless, MRI can detect mammographically occult DCIS and is able to play a valuable role possibly in the preoperative assessment of DCIS, where extent of disease may be underestimated by mammography.

Because of the potential issue of a false negative examination, a negative MRI examination should not deter biopsy of a suspicious lesion (BIRADS 4 or 5) on mammography or ultrasound. Mammographically suspicious findings, such as suspicious calcifications, spiculated masses, or

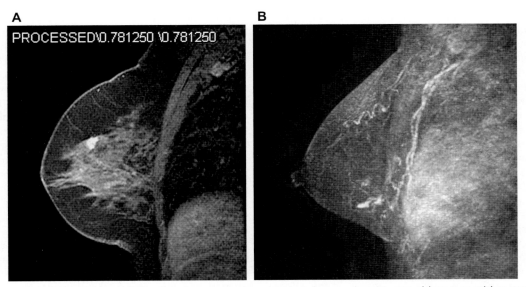

Fig. 7. High-risk screening. (A) Small node-negative invasive ductal cancer in a 34-year-old woman with a strong family history of breast cancer (two first-degree relatives). (B) Ductal carcinoma in situ in a 52-year-old patient with a personal history of contralateral invasive ductal carcinoma 8 years earlier. New linear enhancement on MRI was biopsied under MR guidance yielding DCIS.

areas of distortion warrant appropriate biopsy, regardless of a negative MR examination. The MRI should ideally be interpreted in conjunction with all other pertinent imaging studies such as mammograms and ultrasounds to arrive at the best treatment option for the patient. With these limitations, breast MRI is best used as an adjunct test to conventional imaging, complementing but never replacing basic mammography and sonography.

PREOPERATIVE STAGING
Background

Over the past 30 years, surgical treatment for breast cancer has evolved from total mastectomy in all cases to breast conservation therapy (BCT) in most cases. BCT has moved from being an experimental treatment to the mainstay of surgical therapy as observational studies and randomized controlled trials have demonstrated similar survival between the BCT and mastectomy groups. This has occurred with considerable refinement in patient selection, surgical technique with emphasis on clear margins, and postsurgical radiation and chemotherapy. To arrive at a point where BCT followed by radiation and chemotherapy has resulted in recurrence rates of approximately 10% or greater is remarkable given that is has been known all this while that residual disease is left in the breast. Elaborate treatment algorithms have evolved based on extent of disease evaluation based on clinical and mammographic examination. Surgeons and oncologists have accepted and become comfortable with the probability of recurrence in a significant but small number of patients. When these important studies were taking place, film screen mammography, which has significant limitations, was the standard of care. These days we now have better methods of evaluating tumor load in the breast with MRI, which is far superior to mammography. Controversy arises because the treatment of breast cancer is working well enough and clinicians who are vested in the treatment algorithm do not want to consider the extra information that MRI has to offer. Additionally, MRI has not undergone the rigorous evaluation and study design that these prior studies, many of them randomized controlled trials, have undergone. Certainly, the aim of incorporating breast MRI into the evaluation of cancer would not be to unnecessarily increase the mastectomy rate but rather triage those patients to the more appropriate therapy with full knowledge of the tumor load up front instead of having to guess.

If used carefully, breast MRI has the potential to decrease positive margin rates and recurrence rates in patients with newly diagnosed breast cancer who are candidates for BCT. Breast MRI may also help identify those patients in whom positive margins are likely to arise if surgery is undertaken and those patients who may best benefit from mastectomy as the first-line therapy.

Traditional preoperative planning for breast cancer involves clinical examination and mammogram. Assessment of lesion size, presence of multifocality or multicentricity, and involvement of adjacent structures such as pectoralis muscles and chest wall is therefore dependent on a modality that has limitations and is imperfect. It has been well documented that while mammography has benefits in overall screening of the average-risk population, it is less promising when certain individual groups of women are analyzed, such as women with dense breast tissue. Dense tissue is common, especially in younger women. It has been shown that 62% of women in their 30s, 56% of women in their 40s, 37% of women in their 50s, and 27% of women in their 60s had at least 50% density on mammography.[32] Aside from the inherent increased risk of breast cancer associated with increased density, mammographic detection of cancer is decreased[33,34] where up to 50% of cancer in some series can go undetected, particularly in young women who are at increased risk. This observation that breast density can hinder evaluation of additional disease is important in the realm of preoperative staging.

Breast MRI can give helpful information for staging on tumor size[35,36] and presence or absence of multifocal or multicentric disease, as well as whether the chest wall or pectoralis muscle is invaded.[37] It has been well documented that MR defines the anatomic extent of disease more accurately than mammography. Many studies have shown that MRI is able to detect additional foci of cancer in the breast that has been overlooked by our conventional techniques. Several investigators have shown that MRI is able to detect additional foci of disease (**Fig. 8**) in up to one third of patients, possibly resulting in a treatment change.[7,38–41] MRI can potentially provide valuable information for preoperative planning in the single-stage resection of breast cancer. By using breast MRI as a complementary test to the conventional imaging techniques, more precise information can be obtained about the extent of breast cancer, improving patient care. There is no evidence that the additional cancer found by MRI is any different or less significant that the cancer found by mammography, ultrasonography, or physical examination.[42]

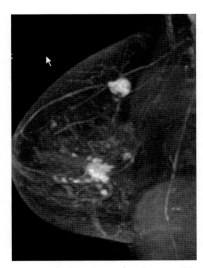

Fig. 8. Extent of disease evaluation. A 54-year-old woman with documented spiculated mass on mammography in the superior breast that was biopsied under ultrasound guidance yielding invasive ductal carcinoma. Additional disease not suspected on mammography or clinical examination in the inferior breast corresponded to a larger invasive ductal carcinoma with associated DCIS (note linear enhancement). Targeted ultrasound over this region with biopsy was able to document multicentric disease and the need for mastectomy as the first surgical procedure.

Contraindications to Breast Conservation Therapy

A joint committee of the American College of Surgeons, American College of Radiology, and College of American Pathologists published standards for breast conservation in1992, which have been routinely updated. Absolute contraindications include inability of the surgeon to obtain negative margins after a reasonable number of surgeries, first or second trimester pregnancy, inability to undergo radiation (prior chest radiation, lupus, scleroderma, and so forth), and clinical or mammographically detected multicentric cancer.

Multicentric cancer detected on mammography or clinical examination occurs in approximately 10% or less of cases of breast cancer. MRI is able to detect multicentricity in 13% to 37% of patients. As multicentricity on mammography is a contraindication to BCT, one could extrapolate that additional disease on MRI would obviate BCT. If one compares the type of tumor that is detected as multicentric disease on MRI, it is no different from that detected by mammography. By all measurable standards they appear to be the same. Therefore why would we put more emphasis on the additional cancer that was detected by one modality as opposed to the other? Because the treatment trials were performed with mammography.

Presumably some of this multicentric disease results in recurrence at a later date. Even if we could identify 5% to 10% of patients who harbor additional multicentric disease that could presumably cause a recurrence, this would justify the use of preoperative MRI.

Recurrence

It has been long known that all disease is not eradicated by surgery alone. The rationale for delivering whole breast radiation (or even partial breast radiation) is that the surgeon has removed the bulk of the disease but that radiation is needed to treat remaining subclinical disease. It has been shown from a study of 282 mastectomy specimens[43] (performed for unifocal breast cancer, assessed clinically and mammographically) that the majority of breasts (63%) have additional sites of cancer that were undetected by clinical examination or mammography. Additional foci of cancer were found pathologically in 20% within 2 cm of the index cancer (multifocal disease) and in 43% more than 2 cm away from the index cancer (disease that may or may not require mastectomy). There were 7% who had additional foci of carcinoma more than 4 cm away from the index cancer, likely representing cancer within a separate breast quadrant (multicentric disease likely requiring mastectomy).

Breast radiation therapy developed to fill a need to treat residual disease and has become a mainstay of the treatment of breast conservation of most patients whether or not residual disease exists. It has been well documented that radiation reduces local recurrence. However, until the use of MRI, it has not been possible to reliably identify those patients who harbor additional multifocal or multicentric cancer and who may be at increased risk of recurrence. While there has been a large body of work showing that MRI can document this additional disease there is a relative paucity of data to document that the recurrence rates are decreased with the addition of MRI. There is only one published paper that has addressed the impact of preoperative MRI on recurrence rates.[44] It demonstrates that if MRI is performed, recurrence rates are lower. Unfortunately the study is flawed in that both groups of women (those that had MRI and those that did not) are not identical. Additionally, the tumor stage and types were different in the two groups. More studies examining this important issue need to be performed.

Positive Surgical Margins

One of the most important factors associated with local recurrence after lumpectomy is the status of the surgical margin. Standard surgical practice is to obtain clear margins even if this requires a second or sometimes third surgical procedure. It is assumed that reexcision to achieve clear margins is as effective as complete tumor removal in a single procedure.

In a significant percentage of patients, the surgeon may not get all the cancer at surgery. The imaging lesion on mammography or ultrasonography or the palpable lesion may be removed but the pathologic margins come back as close or positive. In these cases the surgeon usually recommends reexcision unless there is advanced age/comorbidities. The purpose of the return trip to the operating room is to further excise (usually blindly unless the postoperative mammogram shows residual calcifications) more tissue to hopefully get negative margins at the second surgery.

Positive margins increase the health care costs, as a return trip to the operating room is required as well as increasing anxiety and concern in the patient. Unless residual calcifications are identified, reexcision is usually performed blindly. Too little or too much tissue may be removed when there is no information about how much residual disease exists. Positive margin rates have been reported as high as 70%, although more conservative estimates report 30% to 50% of women undergoing breast conservation therapy may require additional surgery for positive margins. There is a real potential for MRI to aid the surgeon in mapping the amount of residual disease.

Controversies in Using Breast MR Imaging in Cancer Staging

Controversy exists regarding the use of MRI to stage breast cancer.[45] Because breast cancer treatment has been successfully refined over the past decades there is appropriate concern about addition of MRI to the preoperative work-up of the known cancer.[46] The general argument is that with breast conservation surgery followed by radiation therapy, recurrence rates are low: reported recurrence rates at 10 years are conservatively 10%.[47] Early local recurrence is thought to be adversely related to patient outcome (likely reflecting residual disease not treated by surgery and radiation); however, recurrence that happens after 10 years is thought to probably not adversely affect patient outcome (likely a new primary).

In a study from Fox Chase Cancer Center[48] looking at Stage I and Stage II breast cancer treated with breast conserving therapy, axillary node dissection, and radiation therapy, the reexcision rate was 59%. Final margin status was negative in 77%, positive in 12%, and close (2 mm or less) in 11%. Recurrence rates at 5 years were not significantly different (negative 4%, positive 5%, close 7%); however, at 10 years there was a significant difference in recurrence rates (negative 7%, positive 13%, close 21%). First of all, these results underline the high proportion of patients undergoing a second surgery for margins that were not clear. Second, the importance of obtaining final negative margins is directly related to a low recurrence rate. Additionally, the results demonstrate that even from a specialty cancer center, recurrence rates can be significant.

Another controversial area in the performance of preoperative MRI has been the argument that MRI results in too many mastectomies and too many false positive biopsies. While it is true that before the advent of percutaneous MRI biopsy there were too many patients having mastectomies for MRI lesions that were not evaluated before surgery and later proved to be benign, the same cannot be said today. If one examines the literature of how preoperative MRI changed the surgical approach, MRI converts a patient to mastectomy approximately 15% of the time.[38] So it is the minority of patients undergoing preoperative evaluation who are converted to mastectomy. If you compare the number of MRI-prompted mastectomies with the number of women who have a recurrence at 10 years, they are surprisingly similar numbers. While there is no current evidence to directly suggest that MRI is detecting the disease that goes undetected, untreated, and ultimately results in a recurrence, it is an interesting question that warrants further examination. It is very likely in many cases that MRI is identifying disease that would likely cause a recurrence. Carefully designed studies are needed to evaluate this important question.

One recent study from Northwestern University in Chicago, Illinois,[39] evaluated the impact of breast MRI on the surgical management of 155 women with newly diagnosed breast cancer. MRI identified 124 additional lesions in 73 patients. Change in surgical management occurred in 36 (23%) of 155. Lumpectomy was converted to mastectomy in 10 (6%) of 155. In 8 (80%) of 10 this was beneficial to the patient. In 2 (20%) 10 borderline lesions for BCT were converted to mastectomy on the basis of MRI where MRI overestimated disease. Overall, MRI resulted in a beneficial change in surgical management in 10% of newly diagnosed breast cancers. In these authors' estimation, the detection of additional ipsilateral and contralateral cancers justifies the role of preoperative breast MRI. They also found the specificity improved during the course of the study with refinements in MR technique and increase in radiologist expertise. In their estimation, 10 women must undergo breast MRI to result in a benefit to 1 patient. They compare this to the prophylactic mastectomy data where six women must undergo bilateral mastectomy to benefit one woman. Therefore, as women with newly diagnosed breast cancer are high risk, this seems like a reasonable number. They also note that additional cancer identified on MRI regardless of size should be considered important. If surgeons believe it is important to clear lumpectomy margins of microscopic disease with further surgery to minimize the risk of local recurrence, it would follow that small foci detected on MRI should be considered important and also warrant excision.

Issues to Consider in Relation to Staging Controversy

Recurrence rates and positive margin rates vary throughout the country between practices and individual surgeons. Recurrence rates are cited as being low and decreasing, although no standardization or auditing occurs in most surgical practices. Positive margin rates necessitating return to the operating room for further reexcision are also not audited or standardized. Unlike breast imaging where benchmarks are published and auditing of a practice is routine, breast surgical practice is not as scrutinized or regulated. The impact of breast MRI on an individual surgical practice will depend on the positive margin rate as well as the recurrence rate of that individual practice.

From the radiology perspective, these issues raise many questions, such as what lesion size can we safely ignore on MRI. If we are committed to using radiation on all patients, perhaps MRI is too sensitive in detecting cancer in general. For our current treatment algorithms that involve the use of radiation, MRI is likely detecting subclinical disease that radiation therapy would adequately treat. In general, it is recognized that disease 1 cm or less will be treated with radiation. On the other hand, MRI may detect additional disease that would not be treated with adjuvant therapy, particularly invasive cancers that are 1 cm or greater. If we desire to continue in the treatment algorithms that have evolved and that use postoperative radiation therapy, the challenge is identifying what is and what is not significant disease. At this time, identification of significant disease that will not be treated with radiation therapy is not possible and all additional disease is treated

surgically. Performing breast MRI to possibly prevent recurrence may have benefit to a significant number of breast conservation patients, namely those who will recur (at least 10% by 10 years). Certainly it would be better to prevent recurrence with the attendant health care and personal costs if one could. Trials that involve radiologists as well as radiation oncologists and surgeons are needed to get information to potentially identify these patients so that optimum care is delivered to our patients.

Examining the Contralateral Breast in the Staging MR Imaging Examination

Probably the most compelling reason to perform breast MRI in the patient with known cancer is the assessment of the contralateral breast. It has been well documented that MRI is able to detect occult contralateral breast cancer in approximately 4% to 6% of patients. These cancers are sometimes the more significant lesion and may alter the staging of the patient. Furthermore, knowledge of the extent of disease in both breasts allows optimal treatment options to be discussed at the outset with the patient instead of many years later when the patient develops her contralateral primary. To ignore the opposite breast and assume that the adjuvant chemotherapy will treat unsuspected contralateral disease does not make clinical sense when we expend so much energy, time, and resources to treat the known cancer.

Who should Undergo Preoperative Breast MR Imaging?

All patients with a new diagnosis of breast cancer should arguably undergo bilateral MRI examination preoperatively. There are several reasons for this statement. First, the high rate of contralateral carcinoma justifies the use of routine bilateral MRI. Also, for those patients with true multicentric disease the appropriate therapy can be done up front. A conservative recurrence rate of 10% at 10 years certainly justifies the use of a single MRI examination at the time of treatment planning to identify those patients who may benefit from mastectomy. Last, the index lesion is better defined on MRI so that the surgeon may have a better chance at obtaining negative margins at the first attempt of conservation. One study from Stanford[49] demonstrates that bracketing of the lesion by MRI may facilitate complete removal of the lesion if a large DCIS component is not present. Therefore, performing preoperative MRI may increase the chance that the surgeon obtains a negative margin at the initial surgery. More data are needed to address this potential use of MRI to decrease the positive margin rate.

At the very least, perhaps the best patients for preoperative MRI are those who are known to have high rates of positive margins and recurrence. For example, young patients, all patients with dense or moderately dense breasts, and patients with difficult tumor histology such as infiltrating lobular carcinoma,[50,51] DCIS, and tumors with extensive intraductal component (EIC), where tumor size assessment is difficult on mammography or ultrasound (**Figs. 9** and **10**). EIC is when the invasive carcinoma has an associated greater than 25% component of DCIS. EIC is associated with positive margins and high recurrence rates. Interestingly, as MRI is more sensitive to DCIS detection than mammography, it may become the test of choice to evaluate patients preoperatively. Several trials are under way to assess this potential use of MRI.

NEOADJUVANT CHEMOTHERAPY RESPONSE

Neoadjuvant chemotherapy is given preoperatively to shrink the tumor before definitive surgery is performed. It is nearly always given in cases of locally advanced breast cancer, yet in recent years

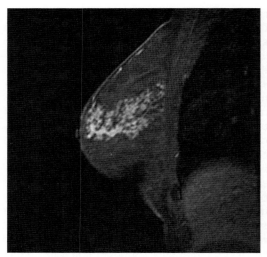

Fig. 10. Unsuspected DCIS in preoperative evaluation. A 57-year-old woman presents with spontaneous bloody nipple discharge. Mammogram was negative. Ductogram on the outside was performed with incomplete opacification of the ducts. MRI was recommended. In the upper outer quadrant of the right breast segmental clumped enhancement was identified. MR biopsy yielded invasive ductal carcinoma and DCIS. Mastectomy yielded extensive DCIS and multifocal invasive ductal carcinoma ranging in size from 0.2 to 0.4 cm with negative sentinel nodes.

it is being used to decrease tumor size in earlier stage cancer as well. The benefit of giving the chemotherapy up front is that one has the ability to determine whether the tumor is going to respond to that particular chosen chemotherapy regimen. A complete pathologic response (elimination of tumor) following neoadjuvant therapy is strongly predictive of excellent long-term survival. Minimal or no response suggests a poor long-term survival regardless of postoperative therapy.

Assessing response to neoadjuvant chemotherapy cancer can be complicated clinically and on mammography. MRI can be useful to overcome the limitations of breast density and fibrosis. MRI may find a role in being able to predict at an earlier time point, perhaps after several cycles of chemotherapy, which patients are responding to neoadjuvant chemotherapy. Early knowledge of suboptimal response may allow switching to alternative treatment regimens earlier rather than later. Unless the response is dramatic, it currently takes longer to predict response, as one must wait to see a volume change in the tumor that is measurable. Volume change may be difficult to assess on the mammogram and physical examination, as fibrosis, a response to chemotherapy, can mimic residual disease. Investigators[14–17] have

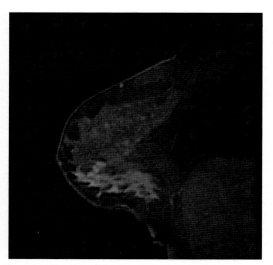

Fig. 9. Infiltrating lobular carcinoma (ILC) extent best shown on MRI. A 43-year-old woman felt a 3-cm area of palpable thickening in the 6 o'clock axis. Mammogram was unrevealing; however, ultrasound demonstrated a vague hypoechoic mass that was biopsied yielding invasive lobular carcinoma. MRI demonstrates a 7-cm area of regional enhancement suspicious for extensive disease. An attempt at conservation was made yielding 4 cm of tumor with positive margins. Further surgery (mastectomy) demonstrated extensive residual DCIS and residual ILC.

demonstrated that residual tumor measurements on MRI correlate with the pathologic residual disease following neoadjuvant chemotherapy. Patterns of response are being evaluated in the hope that these findings may predict recurrence and survival. Patterns of response may hold more information because the mere presence or absence of enhancement may be misleading, as fibrosis, a consequence of treatment, may enhance or residual tiny islands of tumor may exist after treatment that are below the detection level of MRI.

Besides volumetric measurements, MRI is able to exploit functional information about the tumor. Kinetic changes occur early in the tumors before volume alterations and another important application that MRI can provide to evaluate response is the use of MR spectroscopy (MRS). MRS evaluates the choline content in the cancer. Several preliminary studies have shown that choline can decrease before a change in the size or morphology of the cancer. It is proposed that choline may be able to predict very early on—perhaps in a day or two—following the first dose of chemotherapy whether or not the patient will have a response.[52] Information that is helpful to the oncologist in deciding the optimal chemotherapy regimen will hopefully give the patient the best chance for response.

ASSESSMENT OF RESIDUAL DISEASE

For patients who have not had a preoperative MRI examination and have undergone lumpectomy with positive margins, postoperative MRI can be helpful in the assessment of residual tumor load.[13] Postoperative mammography may be also indicated and is able to detect residual calcifications although it is very limited in the evaluation of residual uncalcified DCIS or residual mass. MRI is able to detect bulky residual disease at the lumpectomy site as well as residual disease in the same quadrant (multifocal) or different quadrant (multicentric). Determination of whether the patient would be best served with directed reexcision (residual disease at the lumpectomy site or multifocal disease) or whether the patient warrants mastectomy (multicentric disease) is where MRI can be helpful. Evaluation for microscopic residual disease directly at the lumpectomy site is not the role of MRI, as the surgeon will perform reexcision based on pathological margins and not based on MRI results.

The role of MRI is to define whether the patient should return to the operating room for a reexcision or would be better served with a mastectomy. Traditionally, a patient can have several trips to the operating room before the decision to perform mastectomy; therefore, MRI may save some patients from these repeated surgical procedures. If multicentric disease is identified on MRI before mastectomy, it is important to sample the lesion to document and verify this impression. A report[13] has shown that MRI identified multifocal or multicentric disease in approximately 35% of patients in whom it was not suspected.

The most appropriate time for scanning a patient to assess for residual disease is as soon as possible after surgery. Immediately after surgery there is a postoperative seroma cavity that is low in signal. Surrounding the cavity there is usually enhancement in the granulation tissue that is formed as a result of the surgical procedure. The enhancement is generally thin and uniform when there is no residual disease or if there is minimal/microscopic residual disease. Bulky residual disease will be easily seen as bulky asymmetrical enhancement around the cavity. More importantly, however, is the assessment of the remainder of the breast for additional disease that would preclude the patient from receiving conservation therapy. The longer one waits following surgery, the more chance there is for the seroma cavity to collapse and cause diagnostic difficulties.[53] Once the seroma cavity collapses the enhancing seroma wall is all that is left and the appearance can mimic a spiculated mass or area of distortion with suspicious morphology and enhancement. When the breast is imaged early following surgery, then these diagnostic dilemmas usually do not arise.

TUMOR RECURRENCE AT THE LUMPECTOMY SITE

Tumor recurrence after breast conservation occurs at an estimated rate of 1% per year, although with recent improvements in chemotherapy and use of tamoxifen, recurrence at 10 years is under 10%. Recurrence directly at the lumpectomy site occurs earlier than elsewhere in the breast and usually peaks several years following conservation therapy. Early recurrence is generally thought to represent untreated disease that was present at the time of lumpectomy.

Evaluation of the lumpectomy site by mammography may be limited because of postoperative scarring. Physical examination has been reported to have greater sensitivity than mammography in the detection of recurrence. Mammography, however, is still an important tool and should be performed and is able to detect 25% to 45% of recurrences. Mammography is more likely to detect recurrent tumors associated with calcifications than recurrences without calcifications, as the postsurgical distortion limits evaluation for residual masses.

MRI is able to supplement mammography and sonography to detect recurrent disease that may be suspected but not detected by conventional means. All recurrences on MRI in one study enhanced with nodular enhancement in all cases of invasive carcinoma and linear enhancement was observed in the cases of DCIS recurrence. The majority of scars showed no enhancement in this study. Practically, however, active scar can enhance for many years following surgery. Therefore, purely the presence or absence of enhancement alone should not constitute the entire evaluation of whether recurrence is present or not. Morphological analysis and relationship of findings to operative site should factor significantly into the analysis.

OCCULT PRIMARY BREAST CANCER

Patients presenting with axillary metastases suspicious for breast primary and a negative physical examination and negative mammogram must undergo breast MRI. In patients with this rare clinical presentation, MRI has been able to detect cancer in 90% to 100% of cases, if a tumor is indeed present. The tumors are generally small in size, under 2 cm, thus they may evade detection by conventional imaging and physical examination.

The identification of the site of malignancy is important therapeutically. Patients traditionally undergo mastectomy, as the site of malignancy is unknown. Thus, if a site of malignancy can be identified, the patient can be spared mastectomy and offered breast conservation therapy, thereby having a significant impact on patient management. In one study, the results of the MR examination changed therapy in approximately one half of cases, usually allowing conservation in lieu of mastectomy. In our practice, if a site of malignancy is not identified on MRI, the patient receives full breast radiation with careful follow-up with MRI examination.

HIGH-RISK SCREENING

An important recent recommendation of breast MRI is in the screening of high-risk patients who have at least a 20% to 25% or greater lifetime risk of developing breast cancer. As mammography has an overall false negative rate of up to 15% in a general population, it is evident that all cancers are not detected by conventional means. The rate of false negative examinations may be even higher in premenopausal women with dense breasts (reaching 50%) and therefore exploration into

alternative screening methods such as full breast ultrasound and MRI has occurred. Of the available methods, MRI has proven to have the most promise, mostly due to the high-resolution capabilities, full documentation of the examination, and the potential to detect preinvasive DCIS and small invasive cancers that are usually node negative. Studies that include patients with an overall cumulative lifetime risk of developing breast cancer of approximately 30% show that MRI is able to detect cancer in approximately 1% to 3% of patients.

The use of breast MRI in the high-risk population is limited to those women with documented BRCA 1 or 2 gene or those women with a family member who is a documented carrier but they themselves are untested; any woman with a greater than 20% to 25% lifetime risk (as defined by the BRCAPRO or other models dependent on family history); women with a history of mantle radiation; women with a breast cancer syndrome such as Li-Fraumeni, Cowden, and Bannayan-Riley-Ruvalcaba. There is very little information that exists for screening patients who are at increased risk based on a prior benign biopsy yielding lobular carcinoma in situ (LCIS), atypical ductal hyperplasia (ADH), or atypical lobular hyperplasia (ALH). Furthermore, no information exists for screening "dense, difficult to examine" breasts in patients who are not high risk. There is evidence that women with dense breasts are at increased risk of developing breast cancer and therefore these recommendations may change in the future as more data accumulate. Screening by MRI in this population where the incidence of breast cancer is low would very likely result in too many false positive biopsies to justify its use, although no data exist to support this view.

BRCA 1 and 2 carriers are a group of high-risk patients who have an up to 70% risk of developing breast cancer over their lifetime. The onset of inherited breast cancer is earlier than sporadic cases and the prevalence of bilaterality is higher. Other studies that have included patients at a lower risk than the heterozygote patients[54] have demonstrated that MRI still finds occult breast cancer although at lower rates. It appears that the lower the patient's risk, the lower the prevalence of MRI-detected cancer; however, no screening studies have been performed on the average risk population to determine if this is indeed true. The recommendation to not screen average-risk women with MRI is based solely on expert opinion.

WHEN OTHER REPORTS ARE INCONCLUSIVE

When mammography and ultrasound are inconclusive, MRI can sometimes be helpful in the assessment of the breast.[55] By no means should this indication comprise the majority of a breast MRI practice. In fact, the mammographic and sonographic workup should be exhausted before resorting to MRI. MRI should not be used in place of inadequate conventional workup. That said, there are certainly cases where MRI can greatly help. Usually MRI is used in these situations to exclude the presence of disease. Caution should be exercised, however, as a negative MRI in this setting can be over-reassuring and misleading particularly if the conventional workup has been assigned a BI-RADS 0. Use of BI-RADS 0 varies across practices. In our practice we try not to use BI-RADS 0 after a diagnostic workup where MRI is recommended for further evaluation. This is so the entire evaluation does not rest with the MRI results. In the event that the MRI shows nothing, a decision still needs to be rendered regarding the mammographic and sonographic findings. This way the radiologist reading the MRI does not have to reinterpret the entire workup before MRI.

POTENTIAL PITFALLS IN OVERUSE/ OVER-RELIANCE ON MR IMAGING

As with any examination, breast MRI interpretation is dependent on the experience of the reader. A real concern is when inexperienced interpreters generate large numbers of false positive biopsies. Examination of the literature however demonstrates that the positive biopsy rate of MR recommended biopsies is quite high, approaching 45%[4]; however, these numbers come from centers with a lot of experience in MRI interpretation. However, the reputation of MRI as generating too many false positive biopsies is unjustified if one looks at the positive predictive values for biopsy. Indeed, even in a community practice just staring out in their biopsy practice, a positive biopsy rate indicating cancer detection was found in 25% of women recommended for biopsy on the basis of MRI.[56] The biopsy rate is similar to that generated by routine mammography and is certainly better than that generated by ultrasonography.[57,58] What is interesting about the analysis of these biopsy studies is that many of the lesions recommended for biopsy under MRI guidance turn out to be high-risk lesions such as atypical lobular hyperplasia (ALH), atypical ductal hyperplasia (ADH), and lobular carcinoma in situ (LCIS) in 10% to 15% of reported biopsies. Often the presence of a high-risk lesion is an important data point for the patient and referring clinician.

Concern has also been raised about the possibility of inexperienced readers recommending close interval follow-up or biopsies in too many patients. Short-term follow-up recommendation of breast MRI examinations varies in the literature from 5% to 30%. It is clearly apparent that the more experience a radiologist has, the fewer follow-ups are recommended. Additionally, the more comparison MRI examinations a patient has, the lower the recommendation for short-term follow-up. As with mammography, being able to document the stability of a particular finding allows the reader to assign a benign interpretation to the examination in lieu of short-tem follow-up or even biopsy. As patients undergoing breast MRI examination are likely high risk, there may be more of a tendency by the reader to recommend biopsy over short-term follow-up. A minimal number of MRI examinations should be performed by an individual radiologist to gain experience to recognize normal enhancement versus suspicious enhancement. That number has not yet been defined but it is evident that the more examinations a radiologist is responsible for the more comfortable they become with benign enhancement. What these data indicate is that it is important to audit your practice to document the positive biopsy rate as well as the follow-up rate.

HORMONAL-RELATED ENHANCEMENT

As MRI is performed with intravenous contrast, normal fibroglandular parenchyma can demonstrate contrast enhancement.[59] Background enhancement refers to the normal enhancement of the patient's fibroglandular parenchyma. In general, background enhancement is bilateral, symmetrical, and diffuse; however, sometimes it may be focal, regional, and/or asymmetric. Background enhancement may not be directly related to the amount of fibroglandular parenchyma present. Patients with extremely dense breasts may demonstrate little or no background enhancement whereas patients with mildly dense breasts may demonstrate marked background enhancement. In general, younger patients with dense breasts are more likely to demonstrate background enhancement.

In general, background enhancement is progressive over time; however, significant and rapid enhancement can occur on the first post–contrast image even when obtained in the first few minutes following contrast injection. Background enhancement on MRI is analogous to density on mammography in so far as it can "obscure" suspicious possibly malignant enhancing lesions by decreasing conspicuity of enhancing cancers. A description of background enhancement should be included in the breast

MRI report because it indicates the likelihood that the interpreting radiologist will be able to discern small or subtle enhancement.

Background enhancement is a combination of both volume of tissue that is enhancing as well as intensity of enhancement. The background enhancement assessed volumetrically is described as MINIMAL (less than 25% of glandular tissue demonstrating enhancement) (**Fig. 11**), MILD (25% to 50% of glandular tissue demonstrating enhancement) (**Fig. 12**), MODERATE (50% to 75% of glandular tissue demonstrating enhancement) (**Fig. 13**), and MARKED (more than 75% of glandular tissue demonstrating enhancement) (**Fig. 14**). It should be noted that small areas of very intense enhancement may be described as moderate or marked where the volume requirement is not met.

In general, background enhancement is more prominent in the luteal phase of the cycle if the patient is premenopausal. Therefore, for elective examinations (ie, high-risk screening), every effort should be made to schedule the patient in the second week of her cycle (days 7 to 14) to minimize the issue of background enhancement. Despite scheduling the patient at the optimal time of her cycle, enhancement may still occur. Women in whom cancer has been diagnosed and MRI is performed for staging (ie, diagnostic) should be imaged with MRI regardless of the timing of the menstrual cycle or menstrual status.

Enhancing focus is a tiny, round, pin-point "dot" of enhancement that demonstrates increased signal on postcontrast images (**Fig. 15**). A corresponding finding is not usually identified on the precontrast image. A focus is distinguished from

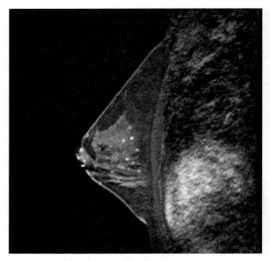

Fig. 12. Mild background enhancement.

a mass by a lack of distinguishing features—lack of internal enhancement, lack of assessment by margin analysis, or shape. An enhancing focus may be benign or malignant. Multiple enhancing foci, which are thought to be due in many cases to fibrocystic disease, are more prevalent in premenopausal women and are almost always benign. Foci can be found, however, in women regardless of age and menopausal status.

In general, foci are less than 5 mm in size; however, applying a strict size criteria is not favored. Size of enhancing lesions can be a helpful in assessing the need for biopsy. A recent study has shown that there is a very low likelihood that lesions under 5 mm represent malignancy.[60] As the size of an MR lesion increases so does the

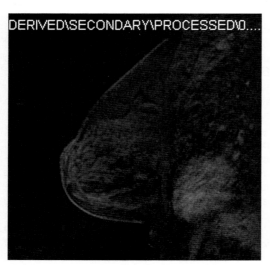

Fig. 11. Minimal background enhancement.

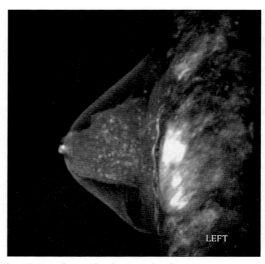

Fig. 13. Moderate background enhancement.

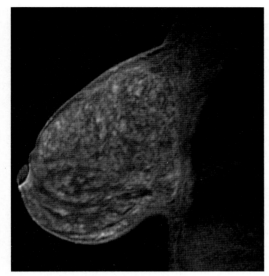

Fig. 14. Marked background enhancement.

chance of malignancy. Therefore, a helpful guideline that is useful for interpretation of lesions less than 5 mm is as follows: if the lesion is smaller than 5 mm, there should be other suspicious features to warrant biopsy (ie, have rim enhancement, spiculated or irregular margins, clumped appearance). If a lesion is larger than 5 mm, size alone may direct the need for biopsy as a significant proportion of lesions larger than 5 mm prove to be cancer at biopsy. In this situation, the lesion may need to demonstrate benign features to avert biopsy.

IMAGE ACQUISITION

There is no gold standard technique for performing breast MR imaging. Many techniques are available

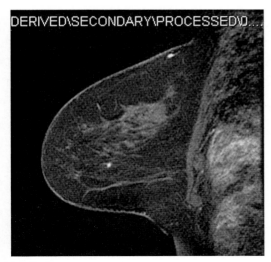

DERIVED\SECONDARY\PROCESSED\J....

Fig. 15. Focus.

and widely used depending on hardware and software capabilities and personal preferences. There are however a few minimal technical requirements that should be adhered to when considering your designated protocol. The basic sequence for breast MRI involves a T1-weighted sequence that is obtained within 2 minutes with high resolution (~1 mm in plane resolution) before and at least 3 times after gadolinium-DTPA administration. High-resolution techniques favor morphologic analysis of lesions and rapid acquisition is used for assessing enhancement profiles. A high-signal fluid sequence (T2-weighted or STIR) is useful for lesion analysis. For example, breast cysts that can be simple or hemorrhagic in addition to myxoid fibroadenomas and lymph nodes that can be very high in signal intensity on this sequence.

Certain minimal technical requirements have been proposed by the International Working Group[3] with the aim of detecting small cancers by assessing lesion morphology and enhancement kinetics. A dedicated breast coil must be used with localization or biopsy capability for MRI-only detected lesions. So far in the literature, only high-field systems have been validated, as these provide adequate high signal to noise and allow fat suppression to be performed.

Parallel imaging applied to breast MRI allows both high spatial and temporal resolution so that neither one needs to be sacrificed. Additionally, these sequences allow simultaneous high-resolution sagittal imaging of both breasts without increasing imaging time. The increased efficiency that parallel imaging affords can be invested in decreasing exam time, improving image quality, and improving spatial and temporal resolution. Parallel imaging is advantageous in that resolution is increased with a concomitant decrease in scan time, artifacts, and acoustic noise. Parallel imaging is a major advantage to those who prefer sagittal small field of view imaging of the breast to axial large field of view imaging. Even for those who prefer axial bilateral imaging, parallel imaging techniques offer advantages and these techniques will likely become the standard techniques in the future.

The suppression of signal from fat is important for increasing conspicuity of breast lesions relative to the breast background tissue that can contain variable amounts of fat. One can suppress signal from fat by performing a fat suppression technique or subtracting the postcontrast image from the precontrast image. For diagnostic purposes, if subtraction is the only method used, misregistration from patient movement between the pre- and the postcontrast images may result, possibly rendering the examination not interpretable.

NEW DEVELOPMENTS IN MR IMAGING TECHNOLOGY

MRI can provide more information other than vascularity of breast lesions. On MRI, inherent information about the chemical composition of a lesion can be assessed with MRS.

Proton MR Spectroscopy (1H MRS) provides biochemical information about the tissue under investigation.[61] The value of 1H MRS is typically based on the detection of elevated levels of choline compounds, which is a marker of tumor. Proton MRS (1H MRS) is FDA approved and is widely used in the brain and prostate. In vivo 1H MRS studies aimed at improving the discrimination between benign and malignant breast lesions have been done at several centers and have shown to be highly sensitive for all breast cancers, regardless of histology.[61–63] In addition to being used for breast cancer diagnosis, in vivo proton MRS has also been assessed in monitoring breast cancer response to chemotherapies.

A major criticism of breast MRI is that the specificity is relatively low, resulting in benign biopsies. Methods to improve the positive predictive value of MRI biopsy recommendations would improve the acceptability and cost-effectiveness of this imaging technique. MRS has been suggested as an adjunct to breast MRI. Studies performed on 1.5-T MR scanners have reported sensitivities of 70% to 100% and specificities of 67% to 100% for breast MRS. One of these studies suggests that MRS may be a useful supplement to breast MRI, reducing the number of benign biopsies without compromising the diagnosis of breast cancer.[63]

Currently breast MRS is available on several vendor MR machines. On 1.5 T, a 1-cm lesion can be analyzed by manually placing an ROI around the lesion and the small area can be interrogated for chemical content. Usually, as lesions on MRI are visualized as enhancement this is done after enhancement. The radiologist, physicist, or technologist must manually perform this task. The acquisition of spectral data takes approximately 10 minutes and the spectral data (in graph form) is later analyzed for chemical content (usually for choline compounds).

FUTURE ALGORITHMS FOR BREAST CONSERVATION THERAPY

The trend on breast cancer treatment these days to less-invasive therapy needs a reliable modality to map disease. Particularly when partial breast radiation is being tested and used in the clinical setting, exclusion of multicentric disease is imperative as these areas will not be treated with targeted radiation. Additionally, percutaneous treatment options are gaining in interest particularly high-intensity focused ultrasound (HIFUS) where an altrasound bean can thermally ablate tumor without surgical incision.[64] This technology is extremely interesting and may allow more people to have BCT; however, it will rely on meticulous pretreatment planning. The days where all tumor must be surgically removed may be a distant memory in the future.

SUMMARY

Breast MRI has become an integral component in breast imaging. Indications have become clearer and better defined. Guidelines and recommendations are evolving and many are recognized and published. Future applications are exciting and may possibly improve our ability to diagnose breast cancer, improving the patient's treatment options and ultimately patient outcome.

REFERENCES

1. Saslow D, Boetes C, Burke W, et al. American Cancer Society guidelines for breast screening with MRI as an adjunct to mammography. CA Cancer J Clin 2007;57:75–89.
2. American College of Radiology. Breast Imaging Reporting and Data System (BI-RADS). Reston (VA): American College of Radiology; 2003.
3. Harms SE. Technical report of the international working group on breast MRI. J Magn Reson Imaging 1999;10(6):979.
4. Lehman CD, Deperi ER, Peacock S, et al. Clinical experience with MRI-guided vacuum-assisted breast biopsy. AJR Am J Roentgenol 2005;184: 1782–7.
5. Sodickson DK, Griswold MA, Jakob PM. SMASH imaging. Magn Reson Imaging Clin N Am 1999;7: 237–54.
6. Esserman L, Hylton N, Yassa L, et al. Utility of magnetic resonance imaging in the management of breast cancer: evidence for improved preoperative staging. J Clin Oncol 1999;17:110–9.
7. Berg WA, Gutierrez L, NessAiver MS, et al. Diagnostic accuracy of mammography, clinical examination, US, and MR imaging in preoperative assessment of breast cancer. Radiology 2004;233: 830–49.
8. Van Goethem, Shelfout K, Dijckmans, et al. MR mammography in the pre-operative staging of breast cancer in patients with dense breast tissue: comparison with mammography and ultrasound. Eur Radiol 2004;14(5):809–16.

9. Liberman L. Breast MR imaging in assessing extent of disease. Magn Reson Imaging N Am 2006;14: 339–49.

10. Liberman L, Morris EA, Kim CM, et al. MR imaging findings in the contralateral breast of women with recently diagnosed breast cancer. AJR Am J Roentgenol 2003;180:333–41.

11. Lee SG, Orel SG, Woo IJ, et al. MR imaging screening of the contralateral breast in patients with newly diagnosed breast cancer: preliminary results. Radiology 2003;226:773–8.

12. Lehman CD, Gastonis C, Kuhl CK, et al. ACRIN Trial 6667 Investigators Group. MRI evaluation of the contralateral breast in women with recently diagnosed breast cancer. N Engl J Med 2007;356: 1295–303.

13. Orel SG, Reynolds C, Schnall MD, et al. Breast carcinoma: MR imaging before re-excisional biopsy. Radiology 1997;205(2):429–36.

14. Hylton N. MR imaging for assessment of breast cancer response to neoadjuvant chemotherapy. Magn Reson Imaging N Am 2006;14:383–9.

15. Partridge SC, Gibbs JE, Lu Y, et al. MRI measurements of breast tumor volume predict response to neoadjuvant chemotherapy and recurrence-free survival. AJR Am J Roentgenol 2005;184:1774–81.

16. Schott AF, Roubidoux MA, Helvie MA, et al. Clinical and radiologic assessment to predict breast cancer pathologic complete response to neoadjuvant chemotherapy. Breast Cancer Res Treat 2005;92: 231–8.

17. Yeh E, Slanetz P, Kopans DB, et al. Prospective comparison of mammography, sonography, and MRI in patients undergoing neoadjuvant chemotherapy for palpable breast cancer. AJR Am J Roentgenol 2005;184:868–77.

18. Preda L, Villa G, Rizzo S, et al. Magnetic resonance mammography in the evaluation of recurrence at the prior lumpectomy site after conservative surgery and radiotherapy. Breast Cancer Res 2006;8:R53.

19. Morris EA, Schwartz LH, Dershaw DD, et al. MR imaging of the breast in patients with occult primary breast cancer. Radiology 1997;205:437–40.

20. Orel SG, Weinstein SP, Schnall MD, et al. Breast imaging in patients with axillary node metastases and unknown primary malignancy. Radiology 1999; 212:543–9.

21. Kuhl CK, Schmutzler RK, Leutner CC, et al. Breast MR imaging screening in 192 women proved or suspected to be carriers of a breast cancer susceptibility gene: preliminary results. Radiology 2000; 215:267–79.

22. Warner E, Plewes DB, Shumak RS, et al. Comparison of breast magnetic resonance imaging, mammography, and ultrasound for surveillance of women at high risk for hereditary breast cancer. J Clin Oncol 2001;19:3524–31.

23. Morris EA, Liberman L, Ballon DJ, et al. MRI of occult breast carcinoma in a high-risk population. AJR Am J Roentgenol 2003;181:619–26.

24. Podo F, Sardanelli F, Canese R, et al. The Italian multi-centre project on evaluation of MRI and other imaging modalities in early detection of breast cancer in subjects at high genetic risk. J Exp Clin Cancer Res 2002;21:115–24.

25. Kuhl CK, Schrading S, Leutner CC, et al. Mammography, breast ultrasound, and magnetic resonance imaging for surveillance of women at high familial risk for breast cancer. J Clin Oncol 2005;23: 8469–76.

26. Leach MO, Boggis CR, Dixon AK, et al. MARIBS study group. Screening with magnetic resonance imaging and mammography of a UK population at high familial risk of breast cancer: a prospective multicentre cohort study (MARIBS). Lancet 2005; 365:1769–78.

27. Kriege M, Brekelmans CT, Boetes C, et al. Magnetic Resonance Imaging Screening Study Group. Efficacy of MRI and mammography for breast-cancer screening in women with a familial or genetic predisposition. N Engl J Med 2004;351:427–37.

28. Knopp MV, Weiss E, Sinn HP, et al. Pathophysiologic basis of contrast enhancement in breast tumors. J Magn Reson Imaging 1999;10:260–6.

29. Boetes C, Strijk SP, Holland R, et al. False-negative MR imaging of malignant breast tumors. Eur Radiol 1997;7:1231–4.

30. Hwang ES, Kinkel K, Esserman LJ, et al. Magnetic resonance imaging in patients diagnosed with ductal carcinoma-in-situ: value in the diagnosis of residual disease, occult invasion and multicentricity. Ann Surg Oncol 2003;10:381–8.

31. Menell JH, Morris EA, Dershaw DD, et al. Determination of the presence and extent of pure ductal carcinoma in situ by mammography and magnetic resonance imaging. Breast J 2005;11:382–90.

32. Stomper PC, D'Souza DJ, DiNitto PA, et al. Analysis of parenchymal density on mammograms in 1353 women 25-79 years old. AJR Am J Roentgenol 1996;167:1261–5.

33. Kerlikowski K, Grady D, Barclay J, et al. Effect of age, breast density, and family history on the sensitivity of first screening mammography. JAMA 1996; 276:33–8.

34. Kolb TM, Lichy J, Newhouse JH. Occult cancer in women with dense breasts: detection with screening US-diagnostic yield and tumor characteristics. Radiology 1998;207:191–9.

35. Bluemke DA, Gatsonis CA, Chen MH, et al. Magnetic resonance imaging of the breast prior to biopsy. JAMA 2004;292:2735–42.

36. Achouten van der Velden AP, Boetes C, Bult P, et al. The value of magnetic resonance imaging in diagnosis and size assessment of in situ and

small invasive breast carcinoma. Am J Surg 2006; 192:172–8.

37. Morris EA, Schwartz LH, Drotman MB, et al. Evaluation of pectoralis major muscle in patients with posterior breast tumors on breast MR imaging: preliminary experience. Radiology 2000;214:67–72.

38. Bedrosian I, Mick R, Orel SG, et al. Changes in the surgical management of patients with breast carcinoma based on preoperative magnetic resonance imaging. Cancer 2003;98:468–73.

39. Bilimoria KY, Cambic A, Hansen NM, et al. Evaluating the impact of preoperative breast magnetic resonance imaging on the surgical management of newly diagnosed breast cancers. Arch Surg 2007;142:441–5.

40. Deurloo EE, Klein Zeggelink WF, Teertstra HJ, et al. Contrast-enhanced MRI in breast cancer patients eligible for breast-conserving therapy: complimentary value for subgroups of patients. Eur Radiol 2006;16:692–701.

41. Schelfout K, Van Goethem M, Kersschot E, et al. Contrast-enhanced MR imaging of breast lesion and effect on treatment. Eur J Surg 2004;30:501–7.

42. Schnall M. MR imaging evaluation of cancer extent: is there clinical relevance? Magn Reson Imaging N Am 2006;14:379–81.

43. Holland R, Veling SH, Mravunac M, et al. Histologic multifocality of Tis, T1-2 breast carcinomas. Implications for clinical trials of breast-conserving surgery. Cancer 1985;56:979–90.

44. Fischer U, Baum F, Luftner-Nagel S. Preopertive MR imaging in patients with breast cancer: preoperative staging, effects on recurrence rates, and outcome analysis. Magn Reson Imaging N Am 2006;14:351–62.

45. Morrow M. Magnetic resonance imaging in breast cancer: one step forward, two steps back? JAMA 2004;292:2779–80.

46. Morrow M. Limiting breast surgery to the proper minimum. Breast 2005;14:523–6.

47. Morrow M, Freedman G. A clinical oncology perspective on the use of breast MR. Magn Reson Imaging N Am 2006;14:363–78.

48. Freedman G, Fowble B, Hanlon A, et al. Patients with early stage invasive cancer with close or positive margins treated with conservative surgery and radiation have an increased risk of breast recurrence that is delayed by adjuvant systemic therapy. Int J Radiat Oncol Biol Phys 1999;44(5):1005–15.

49. Wallace AM, Daniel BL, Jeffrey SS, et al. Rates of re-excision for breast cancer after magnetic resonance imaging-guided bracket wire localization. J Am Surg Coll 2005;200:527–37.

50. Quan ML, Sclafani L, Heerdt AS, et al. Magnetic resonance imaging detects unsuspected disease in patients with invasive lobular cancer. Ann Surg Oncol 2003;10:1048–53.

51. Kepple J, Layeeque R, Klimberg VS, et al. Correlation of magnetic resonance imaging and pathological size of infiltrating lobular carcinoma of the breast. Am J Surg 2005;190:623–7.

52. Meisamy S, Bolan PJ, Baker EH, et al. Neoadjuvant chemotherapy of locally advanced breast cancer: predicting response with in vivo (1) H MR spectroscopy—a pilot study at 4T. Radiology 2004;233:424–31.

53. Frei K, Kinkel K, Bonel HM, et al. MR imaging of the breast in patients with positive margins after lumpectomy: influence of the time interval between lumpectomy and MR imaging. AJR Am J Roentgenol 2000;175:1577–84.

54. Lehman CD, Blume JD, Weatherall P, et al. International Breast MRI Consortium Working Group. Screening women at high risk for breast cancer with mammography and magnetic resonance imaging. Cancer 2005;203:1898–905.

55. Lee CH, Smith RC, Levine JA, et al. Clinical usefulness of MR imaging of the breast in the evaluation of the problematic mammogram. AJR Am J Roentgenol 1999;173:1323–9.

56. Friedman P, Sanders L, Russo J, et al. Detection and localization of occult lesions using breast magnetic resonance imaging: initial experience in a community hospital. Acad Radiol 2005;12:728–38.

57. Berg WA. Supplemental screening sonography in dense breasts. Radiol Clin North Am 2004;42(5):845–51.

58. LaTrenta LR, Menell JH, Morris EA, et al. Breast lesions detected with MR imaging: utility and histopathologic importance of identification with US. Radiology 2003;227:856–61.

59. Kuhl CK, Bieling HB, Gieseke J, et al. Healthy premenopausal breast parenchyma in dynamic contrast-enhanced MR imaging of the breast: normal contrast medium enhancement and cyclical phase dependency. Radiology 1997;203:137–44.

60. Liberman L, Mason G, Morris EA, et al. Does size matter? Positive predictive value of MRI-detected breast lesions as a function of lesion size. AJR Am J Roentgenol 2006;186:426–30.

61. Mountford C, Lean C, Malycha P, et al. Proton spectroscopy provides accurate pathology on biopsy and in vivo. J Magn Reson Imaging 2006;24:459–77.

62. Bolan PJ, Nelson MT, Yee D, et al. Imaging in breast cancer: magnetic resonance spectroscopy. Breast Cancer Res 2005;7:149–52.

63. Bartella L, Morris EA, Dershaw DD, et al. Proton MR spectroscopy with choline peak as malignancy marker improves positive predictive value for breast cancer diagnosis: preliminary study. Radiology 2006;239:686–92.

64. Jolesz FA, Hynynen K, McDannold N, et al. MR imaging-controlled focused ultrasound ablation: a noninvasive image-guided surgery. Magn Reson Imaging Clin N Am 2005;13:545–60.

Imaging of Lymphoma of the Musculoskeletal System

Sinchun Hwang, MD

KEYWORDS

- Lymphoma • Bone muscle • Cutaneous • Radiography
- CT • MR imaging • PET

Musculoskeletal involvement by lymphoma may occur as a part of disseminated disease or an isolated manifestation (ie, primary lymphoma of bone or muscle). Clinical features, prognosis, and treatment of lymphoma differ for isolated, primary lymphoma and disseminated disease, but their imaging features are similar. This article reviews imaging features of lymphoma of bone, muscles, and subcutaneous tissue. Evaluation of bone marrow changes with MR imaging and positron emission tomography (PET) will be discussed as well as post-treatment changes.

The evaluation of musculoskeletal lymphoma often requires more than one imaging modality and may include radiography, bone scintigraphy, CT, MR imaging, and/or PET. Lymphoma is a heterogenous disease, and thus its imaging features vary among the different modalities. Radiography, bone scintigraphy, CT, PET, and MR imaging each provide different information about the disease process. Radiography and CT depict bone destruction. Bone scintigraphy depicts the osteoblastic reaction and bone formation. PET depicts 2-(18F) fluoro-2-deoxy-D-glucose (FDG)-avid lesions in the bone marrow, and MR imaging detects changes by tumor and treatment in the bone marrow composition. For example, marrow involvement of lymphomas is detected better with PET and MR imaging, whereas cortical bone destruction and pathologic fractures are visualized easily with radiography and CT. Plasma cell myeloma and plasmocytoma are included in the 2001 World Health Organization (WHO) Classification Scheme for Lymphoma but will not be discussed explicitly in this article.

LYMPHOMA OF THE BONE

Primary lymphoma of bone (PLB) is rare, comprising less than 1% of all lymphomas,[1] 5% of extranodal non-Hodgkin lymphoma (NHL) and 3% to 5% of all primary bone tumors.[2,3] PLB initially was described as reticulum cell sarcoma by Oberling in 1928,[4] to distinguish it from other primary malignant bone tumors. Parker and Jackson[5] reported the first case series of NHL in adults in 1939. The term PLB was introduced by Ivins and Dahlin in 1963.[6] The diagnostic criteria for PLB include lymphoma within a single bone with or without regional nodal metastases and the absence of distal lesions within 6 months following the diagnosis.[7] When PLB involves more than one bone without distal metastases, it is recognized as a subgroup of PLB and termed primary multifocal osseous lymphoma or multifocal primary lymphoma of bone.[2,8,9] PLB has a predilection for the pelvis and appendicular skeleton, with the femur and tibia being the most common sites. Multifocal PLB also tends to involve vertebrae more often than PLB.[2,3] Within long bones, diaphyses and metaphyses commonly are involved. The location of the involved bone does not appear to have a statistically significant effect on the overall survival rate of PLB.[10]

Multiorgan involvement with involvement of the bone or relapsed lymphoma with involvement of

---

This article originally appeared in *Radiologic Clinics of North America* 2008;46(2):379–96.

Department of Radiology, Memorial Sloan-Kettering Cancer Center, 1275 York Avenue, New York, NY 10065, USA

E-mail address: hwangs1@mskcc.org

Magn Reson Imaging Clin N Am 18 (2010) 75–93
doi:10.1016/j.mric.2009.09.006

the bone has imaging and immunocytologic features similar to those of PLB and will not be discussed separately.

Clinical Features

The most common symptom is bone pain (61%), but B symptoms (fever, night sweat, and weight loss) are rare (13%) in PLB.[11] Palpable masses and an elevated level of lactate dehydrogenase (LDH) (31%)[11] may be present. Most cases of PLB and multifocal osseous lymphoma involvement result from NHL. PLB is more common in males (male-to-female ratio 1.5-2.3:1).[2,3,12] The median age is 42 to 54 years.[2,3,11–13] PBL is rare in children younger than 10 years of age.[14] The overall survival rate for PLB is better than the survival rates for other primary bone tumors. For example, in a study of 82 patients who had PLB, Beal and colleagues[11] reported that the 5-year survival rate (with combined radiation and chemotherapy, radiation alone or chemotherapy alone) was 88%, and in a study of 77 patients who had PLB, Barbieri and colleagues[13] reported that the 15-year survival rate (with radiation, with or without chemotherapy) was 88.3%. In contrast, a study of 1702 patients who had osteosarcoma by Bielack and colleagues[15] found 5-year and 15-year survival rates of 65% and 57%, respectively. In adults, favorable prognostic factors for overall survival include age younger than 40 years, lack of B symptoms, normal LDH level, and female gender.[11]

Imaging

Lymphoma can occur in bone marrow, cortical bone, or both, and also may extend outside of bone. When tumor is confined only to bone marrow, infiltration of the bone marrow with lymphoma cells may have no imaging correlate on MR imaging or PET and often is diagnosed by bone marrow biopsy. When a cortical lesion is associated with an extraosseous soft tissue mass, it may be difficult to distinguish lymphoma of bone with extraosseous extension from soft tissue lymphoma invading the bone. This distinction, however, does not influence staging or treatment significantly.

Radiography

Radiographic manifestation of osseous lymphoma is variable and nonspecific and tends to underrepresent the extent of osseous lesions, especially when lesions are confined to the marrow cavity. Therefore, additional imaging such as MR imaging or PET usually is obtained for further evaluation. The radiographic pattern can be normal, predominantly lytic, sclerotic, or mixed lytic–sclerotic. In particular, osseous lymphoma is known for having a deceivingly normal appearance on

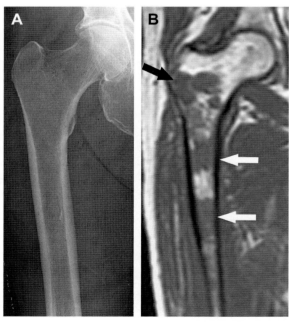

Fig. 1. Normal radiographic appearance and multiple marrow involvement of non-Hodgkin lymphoma at MR imaging. (*A*) Frontal radiograph of the right proximal femur is normal. (*B*) Coronal T1 weighted image reveals multiple low-signal-intensity lesions (*arrows*) in the medullary canal of the proximal femur.

radiography while displaying extensive abnormality on cross-sectional modalities and bone scintigraphy (**Figs. 1–3**).[12] When it is visible on radiography, it most often displays a lytic pattern.[12,14] Lytic osseous lymphoma may be well circumscribed, or it may be characterized by a wide zone of transition (permeative or moth-eaten). Cortical destruction, extraosseous soft-tissue masses, and periosteal reaction indicate advanced local disease (**Fig. 4**).[2] Periosteal reactions are usually aggressive patterns, including linear, lamellated, or disrupted, and disrupted periosteal bone formation is considered to be an indicator of poor prognosis.[2] Pathologic fractures are not rare at the time of diagnosis (17% to 22%).[12,14] Differential diagnostic considerations of lytic osseous lymphoma include both malignant and benign categories. In adults, they may include metastases, chondroblastic osteosarcoma, multiple myeloma, plasmacytoma, osteomyelitis, and giant cell tumor (especially in the end of long bones). In children, differential diagnostic considerations may include Ewing sarcoma, primitive neuroectodermal tumor (PNET), infection, and eosinophilic granuloma.

A sclerotic pattern of osseous lymphoma was reported in 2% of PLB in a study of 237 patients[12]; it is seen more frequently in Hodgkin lymphoma (HL) (**Fig. 5**) and reported in 24% of 15 patients whose radiography was performed in one study.[16] Diffuse sclerosis may be related to fibrosis, with dense ivory vertebrae being a classic presentation,[17] and sclerosis can develop following chemotherapy or radiation.[2] Diffuse sclerotic osseous lesions also have been associated with other neoplastic and non-neoplastic processes such as primary bone tumor (osteosarcoma), metastases (from prostate or breast cancer), Paget's disease, and sarcoidosis.

Bone Scan

Bone scintigraphy is superior to radiography in the detection of multifocal osseous involvement (**Fig. 6**), but it is less effective than MR imaging and PET in the detection of marrow involvement and lesions without bone remodeling. At bone scintigraphy, increased radiotracer uptake is the most common finding.[12] Bone scintigraphy, however, is not specific for tumor, because radiotracer uptake also is seen in benign processes such as fractures. The results of bone scintigraphy do not correlate with clinical outcomes.[8]

CT

CT is an excellent imaging modality for assessing osseous involvement of lymphoma, including cortical and trabecular destruction, periosteal

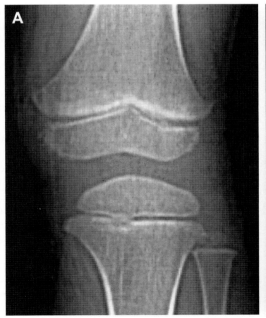
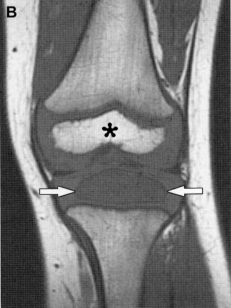

Fig. 2. Normal radiographic appearance and epiphyseal involvement of non-Hodgkin lymphoma at MR imaging. (*A*) Frontal radiograph of a 7-year-old patient with knee pain is normal. (*B*) Coronal T1 weighted image shows diffuse marrow involvement of the proximal epiphysis of the tibia (*arrows*). Note that the normal marrow of the distal femoral epiphysis is fatty (*) after physiologic conversion from red to yellow marrow.

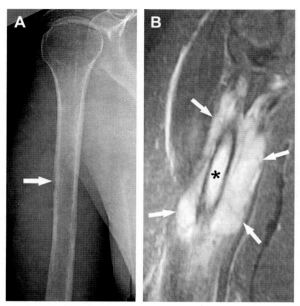

Fig. 3. A large mass on MR imaging without osseous destruction on radiograph. (*A*) Frontal radiograph of the humerus shows a subtle lucent focus (*arrow*) at the deltoid attachment. Otherwise, no osseous destruction is evident. (*B*) Coronal STIR image demonstrates a humeral lesion (*) and a large extraosseous mass (*arrows*) encasing the humerus.

reaction, sequestra, and extraosseous extension. (**Figs. 7, 8**) Contrast-enhanced CT is also occasionally useful in studying marrow involvement and planning targeted biopsy

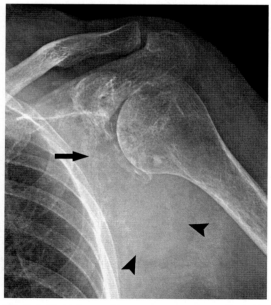

Fig. 4. Lytic radiographic appearance of non-Hodgkin lymphoma. Frontal view of the shoulder shows a permeative lytic lesion in the glenoid (*arrow*) and an extraosseous mass in the axilla (*arrowheads*).

(**Fig. 9**). Osseous destruction is variable on CT, and the relative absence of cortical destruction is an imaging feature favoring lymphoma over other malignant and benign tumors that destroy the cortex, such as osteosarcoma and eosinophilic granuloma. Intramedullary lesions and extraosseous masses with a lack of cortical destruction suggest tumor spread by means of vascular channels of the cortex.[18] Extraosseous tumor growth of lymphoma with relative preservation of the cortex is known in lymphoma and best seen on CT and MR imaging (**Fig. 10**). This feature, however, also is observed in other malignancies such as Ewing sarcoma and PNET.

Sequestra, fragments of dead bone, are also features noted in osseous lymphoma at CT.[18] Although sequestra most are often associated with osteomyelitis, they also are seen in nonmatrix forming bone tumors such as fibrosarcoma, malignant fibrous histiocytoma, and eosinophilic granuloma.[12] CT is also superior to radiography and MR imaging in detecting and characterizing periosteal reactions.

MR Imaging

Normal bone marrow consists largely of lipids and water. Because MR imaging is remarkably effective in detecting lipids and free mobile protons (ie, water), it offers major advantages in the evaluation of changes in bone marrow affected by lymphoma. The signal intensity of tumor within

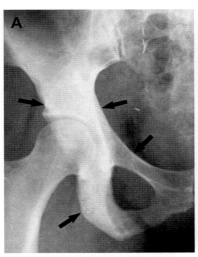

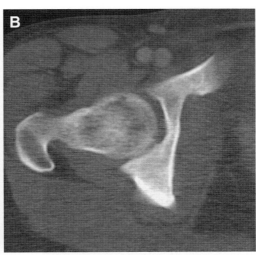

Fig. 5. Sclerotic radiographic appearance of Hodgkin lymphoma. (A) Frontal radiograph and (B) CT axial image of the right hip demonstrate diffuse sclerosis in the acetabulum, pubis, and ischium (arrows in A).

bone marrow is low to slightly high (relative to that of muscle) on T1 weighted images and high on T2 weighted images (Fig. 11). Although this imaging feature is helpful in detecting tumor, it is not specific for lymphoma. A T1 weighted sequence is best for evaluating the extent of tumor in terms of size and multifocal marrow involvement. Short tau inversion recovery or T2 weighted fat

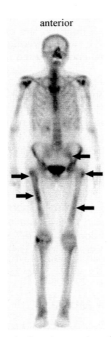

anterior

Fig. 6. Multifocal involvement of non-Hodgkin lymphoma on bone scan. Anterior whole-body bone scan demonstrates multiple areas of increased radio-tracer uptake in the femora and left ilium (arrows). A pathologic compression fracture of T6 vertebra was also present in the posterior view (not shown). Subsequent MR imaging and positron emission tomography (not shown) confirmed multifocal osseous involvement. Foci of increased uptake in the shoulders, sternomanubrial region, and right knee are degenerative in origin.

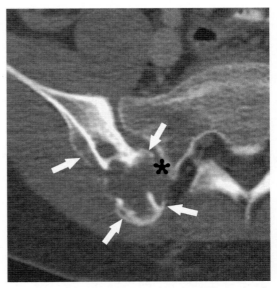

Fig. 7. Cortical destruction and periosteal reaction in Hodgkin lymphoma. Axial CT image of the right pelvis reveals a destructive lesion in the right posterior ilium, extending into the sacroiliac joint (*). Periosteal reaction (arrows) is evident at the edge of the cortical destruction.

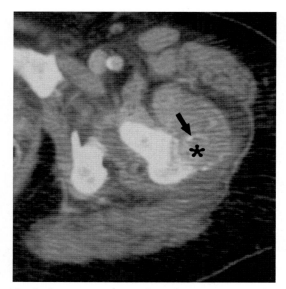

Fig. 8. Extraosseous extension of osseous non-Hodgkin lymphoma. Axial CT image of left proximal femur demonstrates a destructive lesion arising from the greater trochanter. Extraosseous soft tissue mass (*) contains bony fragments (*arrow*).

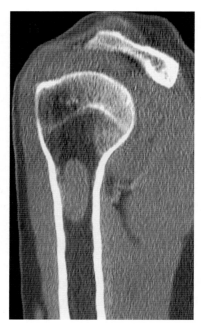

Fig. 9. Marrow involvement of non-Hodgkin lymphoma on contrast-enhanced CT. A coronal reformatted contrast-enhanced CT image shows an enhancing marrow lesion in the proximal humerus. It may be difficult to differentiate lymphoma in bone marrow from enhancing red marrow on CT.

suppression images are also sensitive in detecting marrow lesions, but peri-lesional edema may not be distinguishable from tumor and may result in overestimation of osseous lesions. The signal intensity of osseous lymphoma on STIR and T2 weighted images is more variable (intermediate to high) (**Fig. 12**). Low signal intensity of lymphoma on T2 weighted images also has been reported in a few studies.[3,19] Extraosseous soft tissue masses are of low signal intensity on T1 weighted images and of high signal intensity on T2 weighted images, and contrast enhancement of extraosseous masses is predominantly diffuse and homogenous (see **Fig. 11**).[19] Extraosseous extension of tumor without cortical destruction is visualized well on MR imaging (**Fig. 13**). Involvement of lymphoma in bone marrow often can be multifocal or diffuse. Although bone marrow biopsy is a well-established method for diagnosing bone marrow involvement in lymphoma, MR imaging, as a noninvasive imaging tool, allows evaluation of larger areas of marrow and can guide biopsies to focal regions of involvement (**Fig. 14**).

MR imaging is less specific than histologic analysis in distinguishing viable tumor from post-treatment changes. In attempts to increase the accuracy of MR imaging in identifying treatment response and post-treatment changes, various complementary techniques have been evaluated, including the use of a quantitative T1 relaxation time, quantitative chemical-shift imaging, diffusion-weighted echo–planar imaging, and dynamic contrast-enhanced imaging.[20–23] Studies, however, have been limited by numbers of patients and technical complexities. With recent technical advances in MR imaging allowing faster scanning, whole-body MR imaging is becoming a promising tool for the diagnosis and staging of osseous involvement of lymphoma. The potential role of whole-body MR imaging is pending the results of larger studies.[24] Few detailed studies have been performed comparing PET and MR imaging for the evaluation of bone marrow disease in lymphoma.

LYMPHOMA OF MUSCLES

Skeletal muscle involvement of lymphoma usually occurs as a part of disseminated disease. Although it is rare, lymphoma can occur in skeletal muscle as primary lymphoma of muscle (PLM). Samuel and colleagues[25] found eight cases of PLM in a database of over 6000 patients who had NHL, and Komatsuda and colleagues[26] reported 31 cases (both HL and NHL) among 2147 patients who had lymphoma. PLM usually occurs in patients over 60 years of age and is predominantly NHL (large B-cell type); thighs, chests, and arms are the

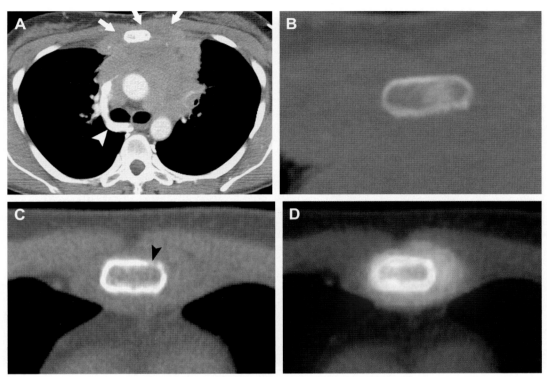

Fig. 10. Osseous and extraosseous involvement of lymphoma without cortical destruction. (*A*) Axial CT image of a patient with Hodgkin lymphoma shows a large mediastinal mass. The mass obstructs the superior vena cava, causing reflux of intravenous contrast into the azygous vein (*arrowhead*). The mass also infiltrates the anterior chest wall (*arrows*) and encases the sternum. (*B*) Magnified axial CT image of the sternum reveals a sclerotic lesion within the sternum without cortical destruction. (*C*) Axial CT image of a different patient with non-Hodgkin lymphoma shows a parasternal mass. Except for a subtle lucency in the anterior sternum (*arrowhead*), the cortex is intact. (*D*) Axial fused positron emission tomography–CT image of the sternum shows diffuse FDG uptake within the sternum and parasternal mass.

most commonly reported sites.[25,27,28] B symptoms and elevation of LDH can be seen. Samuel and colleagues[25] reported that three of eight patients had B symptoms and that LDH was elevated in all six patients who were tested.

Imaging

On imaging, the appearance of lymphoma in muscle is variable. It can appear as muscle enlargement (diffuse or focal), infiltration, or a focal mass, and it may involve more than one muscle. When it is multifocal, lymphomatous involvement may or may not be contiguous.[27] The tumor may extend beyond the muscular compartment and fascial planes.

MR Imaging

MR imaging is superior to other imaging modalities in delineating anatomic borders and the internal architecture of soft tissue. In particular, MR imaging has advantages for evaluating concurrent cortical marrow involvement. The signal intensity of lymphoma in muscle is intermediate (relative to muscle) on T1 weighted images and high on T2 weighted images (**Fig. 15**). Muscle enlargement, however, may not be apparent despite signal abnormality (**Fig. 16**).[29] Infiltration of adjacent subcutaneous tissue and fascial planes is not uncommon (see **Fig. 16**).[27,30] Contrast enhancement can be homogeneous or heterogeneous.

CT

CT is used for evaluating soft-tissue masses as an alternative modality when MR imaging is not available or MR imaging is limited because of patient compliance issues such as claustrophobia and motion. CT also serves as a tool to guide biopsy of soft-tissue masses. Lymphoma in muscle can be homogeneously iso-dense to muscle on non-contrast CT (**Fig. 17**), and it may be difficult to detect lesions even with intravenous contrast

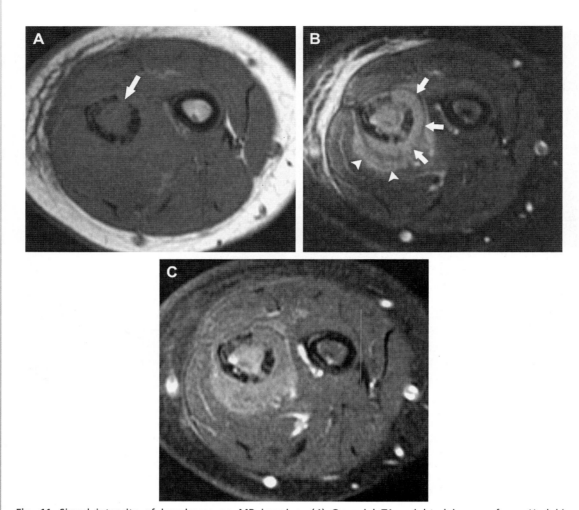

Fig. 11. Signal intensity of lymphoma on MR imaging. (*A*) On axial T1 weighted image of non-Hodgkin lymphoma in the forearm, the signal intensity of tumor within the ulna is intermediate to slightly high relative to the signal intensity of muscle. Cortical destruction (*arrow*) may be present as it is in this patient. (*B*) On axial T2 weighted image with fat suppression, the signal intensity of tumor is high. The extraosseous mass (*arrowheads*) also extends beyond the periosteum (*arrows*). (*C*) On axial T1 weighted MR image, diffuse contrast enhancement is seen within the tumor.

administration (see **Fig. 17**).[29] The calcifications are usually absent.[30]

Ultrasound

Ultrasound (US) has a minor role in the staging of malignant soft tissue masses. Because it is readily available and non-invasive, however, without requiring intravenous contrast and ionizing radiation, US often is used as the initial imaging modality for a symptomatic mass. In addition, US provides real-time guidance during biopsies, allowing safe and accurate tissue sampling with avoidance of neurovascular structures and necrotic areas. The sonographic appearance of soft tissue lymphoma is solid, heterogeneous,

and hypoechoic, and the borders of lesions may be defined well or poorly (**Fig. 18**).[27] Hypervascularity on color and power Doppler US is variable and not specific for malignancy.[31]

Differential Diagnosis

Imaging features of lymphoma in skeletal muscle are nonspecific, and it can be difficult to differentiate lymphoma from various neoplastic and non-neoplastic conditions such as primary soft tissue sarcoma, metastases, trauma, and myositis. When muscle involvement is diffuse, it can mimic muscle edema from deep vein thrombosis, infectious myositis, and inflammatory myositis. In contrast, when tumor is focal, primary soft tissue

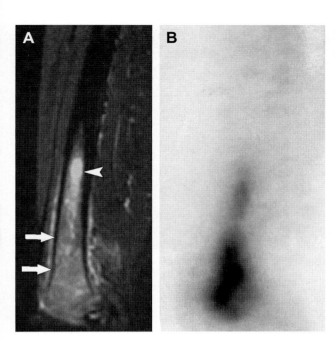

Fig. 12. Signal heterogeneity of osseous non-Hodgkin lymphoma on MR imaging. (*A*) Sagittal STIR image of the thigh demonstrates heterogeneous signal intensity within marrow of the distal femur. Signal intensity in the distal metadiaphysis (*arrows*) is lower than signal intensity in the distal diaphysis (*arrowhead*). (*B*) Sagittal positron emission tomography image also shows heterogenous uptake in the distal femur.

sarcoma, hematoma, and metastases are important differential considerations. Primary soft tissue sarcoma tends to be more heterogeneous in density than lymphoma on CT.

LYMPHOMA OF CUTANEOUS AND SUBCUTANEOUS TISSUE

Primary cutaneous lymphoma refers to lymphoma in the skin without extracutaneous involvement of lymphoma at the time of diagnosis.[32,33] The skin is the second most common site of extranodal involvement of NHL after the gastrointestinal tract.[32] Depending on cellular origin, primary cutaneous lymphoma is classified as either cutaneous T cell lymphoma (CTCL) or cutaneous B cell lymphoma (CBCL). Mycosis fungoides is the most common type of CTCL.[32] CTCL generally appears as eczema-like skin rashes or plaque-like lesions affecting any part of the body, with or without localized or diffuse lymphadenopathy. CBCL often produces nodule-like lesions. Imaging features of cutaneous lymphoma are nonspecific and include soft tissue thickening, infiltration, or

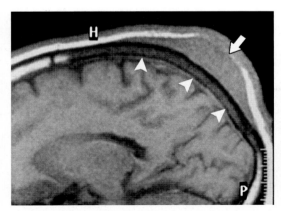

Fig. 13. Non-Hodgkin lymphoma involving the parietal bone and adjacent scalp without cortical destruction. Sagittal T1 weighted image of the head demonstrates low signal intensity in the parietal bone (*arrowheads*) and adjacent scalp mass (*arrow*) compatible with tumor involvement. There is no cortical destruction.

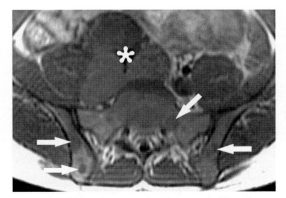

Fig. 14. Multifocal osseous involvement of lymphoma on MR imaging. Axial T weighted image of the pelvis demonstrates multiple marrow lesions in the iliac bones and sacrum (*arrows*). Right common iliac adenopathy (*) is also evident.

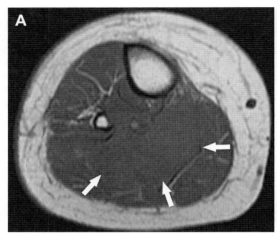
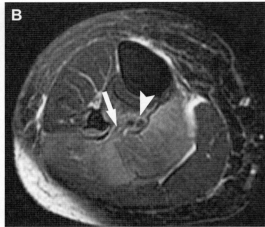

Fig. 15. Muscle lymphoma of the calf on MR imaging. (*A*) Axial T1 weighted image shows a mass (*arrows*) in the posterior compartment. The signal intensity of the mass is intermediate relative to that of muscle. (*B*) Axial STIR image demonstrates high signal intensity within the mass, which increases the lesion conspicuity. The mass extends through deep fascia (*arrow*) of the posterior compartment and encases the posterior tibial vessels (*arrowhead*). (*Courtesy of* Robert A. Lefkowitz, MD, New York, NY.)

a mass (**Figs. 19, 20**).[33,34] The Ann Arbor staging classification for lymphoma is of limited value for most primary cutaneous lymphomas, and specialized staging criteria, including the TMN classification, were introduced for these entities.[35] Imaging is important for identifying extracutaneous manifestations of lymphoma, and it usually includes CT of the chest, abdomen, and pelvis with contrast, alone, or with whole-body PET, or, alternatively, integrated whole-body PET CT.[35]

MUSCULOSKELETAL LYMPHOMA AND AIDS

In patients who have HIV and AIDS, lymphoma is a common neoplastic complication. For example, NHL is the second most common type of tumor in patients who have AIDS after Kaposi's sarcoma.[36] The risk of NHL is reported to be 60 times greater in patients who have AIDS than in the general population,[37] and lymphoma is considered one of the diagnostic criteria for AIDS. NHL in AIDS tends to be highly aggressive and widely disseminated in bones and muscles, and bone marrow involvement is seen in almost one third of affected patients.[38] The imaging appearance of NHL in AIDS is similar to that of lymphoma in the general population.

Staging of Musculoskeletal Lymphoma

Lymphoma of bone or muscle without regional nodal involvement and without disseminated

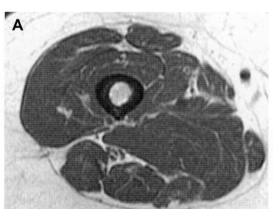
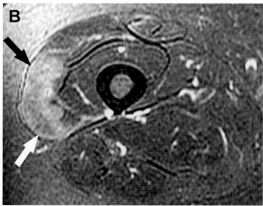

Fig. 16. Subtle muscle lymphoma of the thigh on MR imaging. (*A*) Axial T1 weighted image of the right thigh shows no obvious muscle enlargement or mass. (*B*) Axial STIR image at the same level shows a high signal intensity mass (*arrows*) involving the vastus lateralis muscle. (*Courtesy of* Robert A. Lefkowitz, MD, New York, NY.)

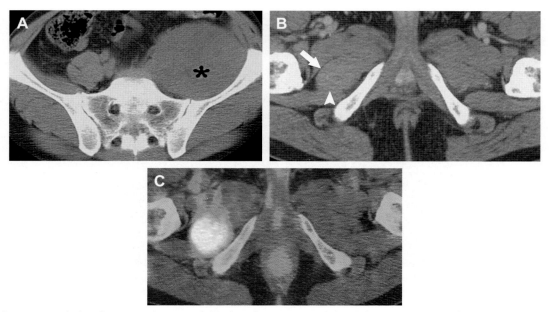

Fig. 17. Muscle involvement of non-Hodgkin lymphoma on CT. (*A*) Axial noncontrast CT shows a large mass involving the left iliopsoas muscle (*). The mass is iso-dense to the normal muscles. (*B*) Axial contrast-enhanced CT of a different patient shows a subtle bulging of the right adductor muscle (*arrow*) and loss of the fat plane (*arrowhead*) with the adjacent quadratus femoris muscle. Note that the enhanced bulged muscle is iso-dense to enhanced normal muscles. (*C*) Axial-fused CT–positron emission tomography image shows intense FDG uptake within the muscles, confirming tumor involvement.

disease is classified as stage 1E, whereas lymphoma of bone or muscle with regional nodal involvement and without disseminated disease is classified as stage 2E, according to the Cotswolds modification of the Ann Arbor staging classification.[39]

RESPONSE TO TREATMENT AND TREATMENT-RELATED CHANGES

Although CT remains the most commonly used imaging modality for the initial evaluation of

lymphoma, it has obvious limitations in differentiating viable tumor from post-treatment changes or in assessing bone marrow. PET and MR imaging offer advantages for monitoring treatment response in patients who have musculoskeletal lymphoma.

Monitoring Treatment Response with FDG–Positron Emission Tomography and MR Imaging

In patients who have FDG PET-avid disease at initial staging, FDG PET allows the assessment

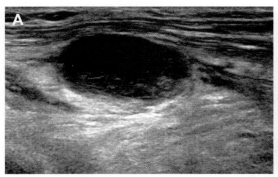
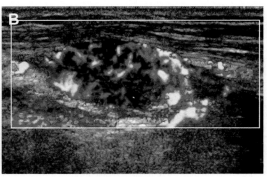

Fig. 18. Muscle lymphoma on ultrasound. (*A*) Longitudinal gray scale image demonstrates a well-circumscribed heterogeneously hypoechoic mass within the flexor compartment of the forearm. (*B*) On power Doppler image, the mass is hypervascular. (*Courtesy of* Ronald S. Adler, PhD, MD, New York, NY.)

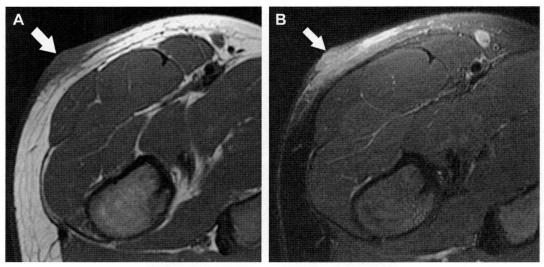

Fig. 19. Cutaneous non-Hodgkin lymphoma on MR imaging. (*A*) Axial T1 weighted image and (*B*) axial T2 weighted image with fat suppression demonstrate nodular thickening of the cutaneous and subcutaneous tissue (*arrows*) in the anterior right groin.

of treatment response,[40,41] and it has been incorporated into the revised International Working Group Response Criteria.[42] Response to treatment is defined by a decrease in uptake as identified both on a semiquantitative standardized uptake value scale and by visual inspection. FDG PET shows tumor response earlier than do other imaging modalities, as a decrease in tracer uptake may be detected even before a decrease in tumor volume can be seen. Studies have shown that early response in the course of chemotherapy (as early as the second cycle of chemotherapy) on FDG PET is predictive of event-free and overall survival,[40,41] and FDG PET has potential for identifying patients who may benefit from more aggressive therapies early in the course of treatment.

On MR imaging, a decrease in tumor size, a decrease in signal intensity on T2 weighted images, and a decrease in tumor contrast enhancement may be encountered after treatment

(**Fig. 21**). Only the change in size of a mass like lesion is incorporated in the response criteria.[42,43] Residual lesions from necrosis, inflammation, and/ or fibrosis of treated tumor are difficult to distinguish from viable tumor.[44,45] On CT, a decrease in size and a decrease in contrast enhancement of tumors indicates clinical response. They are not necessarily specific for residual tumor viability, however. In the author's experience, post-treatment changes may persist for anywhere from a few months to years on MR imaging or CT.

Evaluation of Bone Marrow with MR Imaging After Treatment

Post-treatment changes in marrow may be encountered on MR imaging examinations obtained for reasons other than response assessment, such as evaluation of newly developed back pain. Post-treatment changes reflect

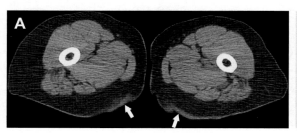
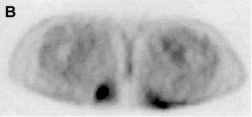

Fig. 20. Mycosis fungoides on CT and positron emission tomography (PET). (*A*) Axial CT image demonstrates mild skin thickening and subcutaneous infiltration of the posterior thighs (*arrows*). (*B*) Axial PET image reveals intense FDG uptake within the thickened skin and subcutaneous infiltration.

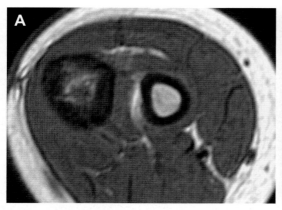
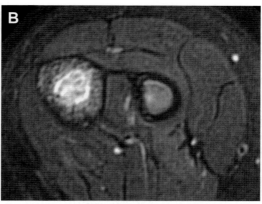

Fig. 21. Post-treatment changes of osseous lymphoma (the same patient in **Fig. 11**) on MR imaging. (*A*) Axial T1 weighted image and (*B*) axial fat-suppressed T2 weighted image show resolution of the extraosseous mass and cortical destruction (see **Fig. 11**). There is new diffuse cortical thickening. Given residual signal abnormality in the ulna, viable tumor is difficult to exclude. There was no FDG-avid disease in the positron emission tomography study (not shown).

changes in marrow composition during and after the course of treatments such as chemotherapy, administration of granulocyte-colony stimulating factor (G-CSF), stem cell transplantation, and radiation therapy. Occasionally, they may be related to post-treatment complications such as infarct and fractures. Knowledge of the marrow signal changes of red marrow hyperplasia and post-treatment effects on MR imaging are crucial for avoiding misdiagnosis of tumor at staging and follow-up.

After initiation of chemotherapy, the signal intensity of marrow becomes low on T1 weighted images and high on T2 weighted images, reflecting edema.[46] After chemotherapy, conversion from yellow to red marrow occurs in the reverse sequence of physiologic conversion from red to yellow marrow. Throughout the body, red marrow regenerates from the central skeleton to the peripheral, usually in a bilateral and symmetric fashion. In long bones, regeneration of red marrow occurs from metaphysis to diaphysis. The signal intensity of red marrow tends to be higher than that of muscle on T1 weighted images and intermediate to slightly high on fat-suppressed T2 weighted images and STIR sequences (**Fig. 22**). Contrast enhancement of red marrow is mild. Reconversion of yellow to red marrow also can be stimulated by injection of G-CSF or profound chemotherapy-induced anemia. When it is diffuse, red marrow may be difficult to differentiate from tumor.

During and after chemotherapy, G-CSF often is administered to increase the number of neutrophil

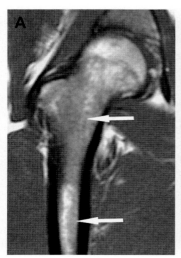
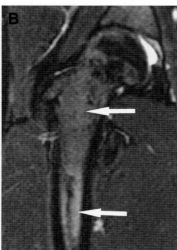

Fig. 22. Signal intensity of red marrow on MR imaging. (*A*) On coronal T1 weighted image of the proximal femur, the signal intensity of red marrow (*arrows*) in the proximal femur is high to intermediate relative to that of muscle. (*B*) On coronal fat-suppressed T2 weighted image, the signal intensity of red marrow (*arrows*) is intermediate to slightly high.

counts in the setting of chemotherapy-induced neutropenia, and the drug stimulates the bone marrow to produce granulocytes and stem cells. On MR imaging, multiple areas of red marrow develop in a discrete or diffuse pattern (**Fig. 23**), and the marrow signal intensity is identical to the signal of physiologic red marrow. The dose of G-CSF does not appear related to the extent of red marrow reconversion.[47] Awareness of marrow-stimulating therapy in the course of chemotherapy and the clinical status of individual patients (such as decreased tumor burden in other parts of body) can help to diagnose red marrow reconversion.

Radiation therapy (RT) often is used to treat localized disease such as PLB and to offer pallia-tive relief and local control of multifocal disease such as an impending or pathologic fracture. Radi-ation-induced changes can be acute or chronic.

Immediately following RT, vascular congestion, hemorrhage, and edema ensue within irradiated marrow. An increase in signal intensity on T2 weighted and STIR sequences within a few days after RT is considered to represent marrow edema and hemorrhage, and yellow marrow is seen as early as 8 days after the start of RT.[48] Chronic changes include fatty replacement of marrow, which is evidenced by high-signal intensity within irradiated marrow on T1 weighted images (**Fig. 24**). In a study of 31 patients, complete conversion to yellow marrow within the radiation field was seen 6 to 8 weeks after the start of pelvic RT in 90% of patients.[48] The ability of marrow to regenerate depends greatly on many factors, however, including patient age and radiation dose.[49]

Evaluation of Bone Marrow with FDG-Positron Emission Tomography

The introduction of FDG PET imaging contributed significantly to the evaluation and staging of lymphoma, and at the author's hospital PET re-placed gallium scans entirely. Focal or diffuse marrow uptake may be encountered in patients who have lymphoma (**Fig. 25**). In untreated patients, FDG uptake in marrow greater than FDG uptake in the liver is suggestive of bone marrow involvement.

In the post-treatment setting, diffuse FDG uptake in marrow after chemotherapy usually

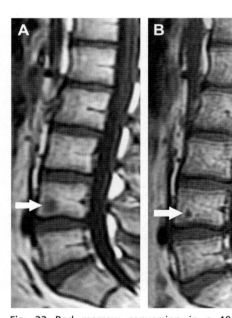

Fig. 23. Red marrow conversion in a 19-year-old patient with lymphoma after granulocyte-colony stimulating factor (G-CSF) treatment. (*A*) Sagittal T1 weighted image of the lumbar spine before G-CSF treatment demonstrates mildly fatty marrow and a focal lesion in the L4 vertebra (*arrow*). The focal lesion was also FDG-avid on positron emission tomog-raphy (not shown), compatible with tumor. (*B*) Sagittal T1 weighted image after G-CSF treatment shows diffuse decrease in signal intensity throughout bone marrow. The focal lesion in the L4 vertebra (*arrow*) is smaller, and pelvic adenopathy (not shown) also has resolved. Given improved disease at different sites, this decrease in signal intensity likely represents red marrow hyperplasia resulting from G-CSF treatment.

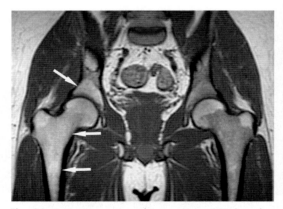

Fig. 24. Fatty marrow replacement on MR imaging after radiation therapy for a right pelvic tumor (patient does not have lymphoma). Coronal T1 weighted image of the pelvis demonstrates diffuse high signal intensity within the irradiated field of the right ilium, right acetabulum, and right proximal femur, compatible with fatty marrow replacement (*arrows*). Note the high-to-intermediate signal inten-sity of normal red marrow in the contralateral pelvis and left proximal femur.

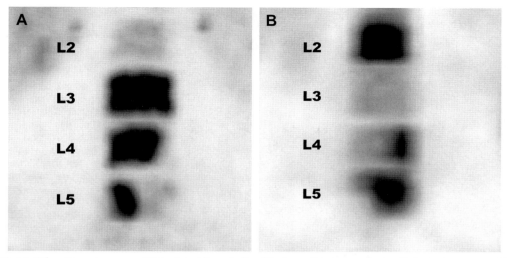

Fig. 25. Multifocal lymphoma on PET before (*A*) and after (*B*) chemotherapy and growth factor treatment. The L2 vertebra was not involved by lymphoma in the pretreatment PET scan (*A*), and after chemotherapy and growth factor treatment (*B*), there is new diffuse FDG uptake reflecting red marrow proliferation. The L3 vertebra showed diffuse FDG uptake in the pretreatment scan (*A*), and the uptake is resolved after treatment (*B*). The L4 and L5 vertebrae showed partial uptake in the right side of the vertebral bodies in the pretreatment scan (*A*). After treatment (*B*), the FDG uptake is decreased in the right side of L4 and L5 vertebrae, while it is increased in the left side, reflecting treatment response to the growth factor.

indicates rebound of normal marrow, and in patients treated with G-CSF, intense FDG uptake in marrow is accompanied by increased FDG uptake in the spleen. Clinical response of tumor at other sites is also helpful to support a diagnosis of rebound marrow. For example, after treatment, it would be very unusual to see a worsening of marrow disease (and hence an increase in SUV relative to the baseline scan SUV) when tumor in other organs had decreased.

Bone marrow evaluation with FDG PET raises two concerns, however. First, it is difficult to

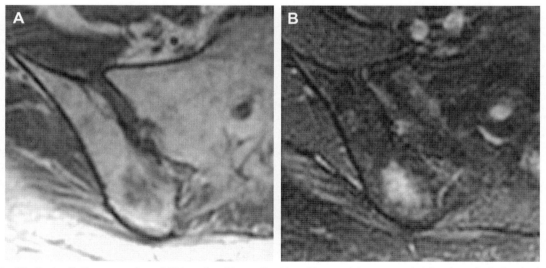

Fig. 26. Postradiation necrosis on MR imaging. The patient is a 47-year-old woman who developed a lesion in the right posterior ilium a few years after radiation therapy for sarcoma. (*A*) Axial T1 weighted image demonstrates a lesion of slightly high-to-intermediate signal intensity in the right posterior ilium, and the border of the lesion is irregular and feathery. (*B*) Axial T2 weighted image demonstrates high T2 signal in the lesion. Open biopsy showed fat necrosis and osteoporosis.

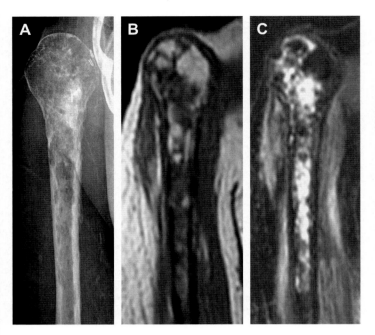

Fig. 27. Radiation osteitis in a 28-year-old woman treated with radiation therapy (RT) for soft tissue sarcoma of the right shoulder. (A) Frontal radiograph of the right humerus demonstrates diffuse mixed radiolucent and sclerotic appearance of the irradiated bone caused by areas of osteopenia and trabecular thickening (ie, radiation osteitis). The scapula also was resected in this patient because of RT-induced osteosarcoma (not shown). (B) Coronal T1 weighted image and (C) coronal fat-suppressed T2 weighted image demonstrate mixed areas of varied T1 and T2 signal intensity within the irradiated bone. The radiographic appearance had been stable for years, and no mass was identified on MR imaging.

identify low-level disease in marrow at the time of staging on FDG PET. It is recognized that the sensitivity of FDG PET is insufficient and that PET cannot replace bone marrow biopsy.[50] The

second concern is more theoretic and relates to the question of whether residual disease may be present in bone marrow that rebounds after chemotherapy. The author's current approach in

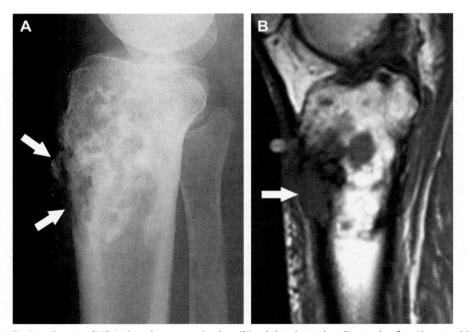

Fig. 28. Radiation therapy (RT)-induced sarcoma in the tibia. (A) A lateral radiograph of a 48-year-old woman shows a lytic lesion with cortical destruction (arrows) arising from the tibia. The patient received RT to the same area 26 years ago for treatment of osseous lymphoma. A patchy area of mixed lucency and sclerosis in the proximal tibia reflects RT-related treatment changes within the previous lymphoma. (B) Sagittal T1 weighted image confirms a tumor (arrow) arising from the tibia. Biopsy showed undifferentiated high-grade sarcoma.

complicated cases is to wait until rebound activity normalizes and perform a repeat PET scan to see if there is persistent focal uptake. In cases of strong clinical suspicion, a repeat bone marrow biopsy should be considered.

COMPLICATIONS OF CHEMOTHERAPY AND RADIATION

Chemotherapy and radiation impair the ability of marrow and bone to regenerate and to heal, causing various complications. Chemotherapy can induce anemia, leukopenia, and osteoporosis (by means of premature gonadal failure or directly interfering with bone formation and repair). In adults and children, avascular necrosis, osteoporosis, and fractures may occur during and after prolonged administration of steroids. RT is known for its risks of growth impairment in children, insufficiency fractures, osteonecrosis, and radiation osteitis (**Figs. 26, 27**).[51,52] RT-induced tumors are a rare but well-known complication,[53] and they can be benign osteochondroma or sarcoma (**Fig. 28**). The most common histologic types of RT-induced sarcoma of bone include high-grade osteosarcoma, fibrosarcoma, and malignant fibrous histiocytoma, and they are known to be radioresistant.

SUMMARY

Imaging plays a crucial role in staging and in the assessment of treatment response in patients who have lymphoma of the musculoskeletal system. On radiography, lymphoma of the bone is most commonly lytic, but the affected bone also can appear deceivingly normal, even when a large tumor is present. On CT and MR imaging, osseous destruction is variable. Relative preservation of the cortex in the presence of a large extraosseous tumor is not specific for lymphoma, but it is a helpful finding for differential diagnostic consideration of lymphoma at initial presentation. On CT, lymphoma of muscle can be homogeneous in attenuation, and it may not show contrast enhancement, making tumor detection more difficult. MR imaging and PET are the most effective imaging modalities in detecting multifocal lesions, including marrow lesions. Post-treatment changes often are encountered on MR imaging and PET, and when considered in light of the patient's therapy regimen (eg, radiation therapy and G-CSF) they usually can be differentiated from tumor. Post-treatment changes include diffuse FDG uptake in marrow after chemotherapy, indicating rebound of normal marrow, and MR imaging signal abnormalities that may persist for anywhere from a few months to years after treatment.

REFERENCES

1. Fairbanks RK, Bonner JA, Inwards CY, et al. Treatment of stage IE primary lymphoma of bone. Int J Radiat Oncol Biol Phys 1994;28:363–72.
2. Krishnan A, Shirkhoda A, Tehranzadeh J, et al. Primary bone lymphoma: radiographic MR imaging correlation. Radiographics 2003;23(6):1371–83.
3. Hermann G, Klein MJ, Abdelwahab IF, et al. MRI appearance of primary non-Hodgkin's lymphoma of bone. Skeletal Radiol 1997;26(11):629–32.
4. Oberling C. Les reticulosarcomes et les reticuloendotheliosarcomes de la moelle osseuse (sarcomas d'Ewing). Bulletin de l'Association francaise pour l'etude du cancer 1928;17:259–96.
5. Parker F Jr, Jackson JH Jr. Primary reticulum cell sarcoma of bone. Surg Gynecol Obstet 1939;68:45–53.
6. Ivins JC, Dahlin DC. Malignant lymphoma (reticulum cell sarcoma) of bone. Proc Staff Meet Mayo Clin 1963;28(38):375–85.
7. Coley BL, Higinbotham NL, Groesbeck HP. Primary reticulum cell sarcoma of bone; summary of 37 cases. Radiology 1950;55(5):641–58.
8. Melamed JW, Martinez S, Hoffman CJ. Imaging of primary multifocal osseous lymphoma. Skeletal Radiol 1997;26(1):35–41.
9. Ostrowski ML, Unni KK, Banks PM, et al. Malignant lymphoma of bone. Cancer 1986;58(12):2646–55.
10. Mankin HJ, Hornicek FJ, Harmon DC, et al. Lymphoma of bone: a review of 140 patients. Therapy 2006;3(4):499–507.
11. Beal K, Allen L, Yahalom J. Primary bone lymphoma: treatment results and prognostic factors with long-term follow-up of 82 patients. Cancer 2006;106(12):2652–6.
12. Mulligan ME, McRae GA, Murphey MD. Imaging features of primary lymphoma of bone. AJR Am J Roentgenol 1999;173(6):1691–7.
13. Barbieri E, Cammelli S, Mauro F, et al. Primary non-Hodgkin's lymphoma of the bone: treatment and analysis of prognostic factors for stage I and stage II. Int J Radiat Oncol Biol Phys 2004;59(3):760–4.
14. Glotzbecker MP, Kersun LS, Choi JK, et al. Primary non-Hodgkin's lymphoma of bone in children. J Bone Joint Surg Am 2006;88(3):583–94.
15. Bielack SS, Kempf-Bielack B, Delling G, et al. Prognostic factors in high-grade osteosarcoma of the extremities or trunk: an analysis of 1702 patients treated on neoadjuvant cooperative osteosarcoma study group protocols. J Clin Oncol 2002;20(3):776–90.

16. Ostrowski ML, Inwards CY, Strickler JG, et al. Osseous Hodgkin disease. Cancer 1999;85(5): 1166–78.

17. Bullough P. Hodgkin's lymphoma. In: Orthopedic pathology. New York: Mosby; 2004. p. 477.

18. Mulligan ME, Kransdorf MJ. Sequestra in primary lymphoma of bone: prevalence and radiologic features. AJR Am J Roentgenol 1993;160(6): 1245–8.

19. Heyning FH, Kroon HM, Hogendoorn PC, et al. MR imaging characteristics in primary lymphoma of bone with emphasis on nonaggressive appearance. Skeletal Radiol 2007;36(10):937–44.

20. Vande Berg BC, Michaux L, Scheiff JM, et al. Sequential quantitative MR analysis of bone marrow: differences during treatment of lymphoid versus myeloid leukemia. Radiology 1996;201:519–23.

21. Gerard EL, Ferry JA, Amrein PC, et al. Compositional changes in vertebral bone marrow during treatment for acute leukemia: assessment with quantitative chemical shift imaging. Radiology 1992;183:39–46.

22. Yasumoto M, Nonomura Y, Yoshimura R, et al. MR detection of iliac bone marrow involvement by malignant lymphoma with various MR sequences including diffusion-weighted echo–planar imaging. Skeletal Radiol 2002;31:263–9.

23. Dyke JP, Panicek DM, Healey JH, et al. Osteogenic and Ewing sarcomas: estimation of necrotic fraction during induction chemotherapy with dynamic contrast-enhanced MR imaging. Radiology 2003; 228:271–8.

24. Johnston C, Brennan S, Ford S, et al. Whole-body MR imaging: applications in oncology. Eur J Surg Oncol 2006;32:239–46.

25. Samuel LM, White J, Lessells AM, et al. Primary non-Hodgkin's lymphoma of muscle. Clin Oncol 1999; 11(1):49–51.

26. Komatsuda M, Nagao T, Arimori S. An autopsy case of malignant lymphoma associated with remarkable infiltration in skeletal muscles. Rinsho Ketsueki 1981; 22(6):891–5.

27. Beggs I. Primary muscle lymphoma. Clin Radiol 1997;52(3):203–12.

28. Lanham GR, Weiss SW, Enzinger FM. Malignant lymphoma. A study of 75 cases presenting in soft tissue. Am J Surg Pathol 1989;13(1):1–10.

29. Panicek DM, Lautin JL, Schwartz LH, et al. Non-Hodgkin lymphoma in skeletal muscle manifesting as homogeneous masses with CT attenuation similar to muscle. Skeletal Radiol 1997;26(11):633–5.

30. Lee VS, Martinez S, Coleman RE. Primary muscle lymphoma: clinical and imaging findings. Radiology 1997;203(1):237–44.

31. Kaushik S, Miller TT, Nazarian LN, et al. Spectral Doppler sonography of musculoskeletal soft tissue masses. J Ultrasound Med 2003;22(12):1333–6.

32. Willemze R, Jaffe ES, Burg G, et al. WHO-EORTC classification for cutaneous lymphomas. Blood 2005;105(10):3768–85.

33. Lee HJ, Im JG, Goo JM, et al. Peripheral T-cell lymphoma: spectrum of imaging findings with clinical and pathologic features. Radiographics 2003; 23(1):7–26.

34. Malloy PC, Fishman EK, Magid D. Lymphoma of bone, muscle, and skin: CT findings. AJR Am J Roentgenol 1992;159(4):805–9.

35. Kim YH, Willemze R, Pimpinelli N, et al. TNM classification system for primary cutaneous lymphomas other than mycosis fungoides and Sezary syndrome: a proposal of the International Society for Cutaneous Lymphomas (ISCL) and the Cutaneous Lymphoma Task Force of the European Organization of Research and Treatment of Cancer (EORTC). Blood 2007;110(2):479–84.

36. Restrepo CS, Lemos DF, Gordillo H, et al. Imaging findings in musculoskeletal complications of AIDS. Radiographics 2004;24(4):1029–49.

37. Beral V, Peterman T, Berkelman R, et al. AIDS-associated non-Hodgkin lymphoma. Lancet 1991;337: 805–9.

38. Haskal ZJ, Lindan CE, Goodman PC. Lymphoma in the immunocompromised patient. Radiol Clin North Am 1990;28:885–99.

39. Lister TA, Crowther DM, Sutcliffe SB, et al. Report of a committee convened to discuss the evaluation and staging of patients with Hodgkin's disease; Cotswolds meeting. J Clin Oncol 1989;7:1630–6.

40. Lin C, Itti E, Haioun C, et al. Early 18F-FDG PET for prediction of prognosis in patients with diffuse large B cell lymphoma: SUV-based assessment versus visual analysis. J Nucl Med 2007;48(10): 1626–32.

41. Hutchings M, Loft A, Hansen M, et al. FDG PET after two cycles of chemotherapy predicts treatment failure and progression-free survival in Hodgkin lymphoma. Blood 2006;107(1):52–9.

42. Cheson BD, Pfistner B, Juweid ME, et al. Revised response criteria for malignant lymphoma. J Clin Oncol 2007;25:579–86.

43. Rahmouni A, Luciani A, Itti E. MRI and PET in monitoring response in lymphoma. Cancer Imaging 2005;5 Spec No A:S106–12.

44. Lin C, Luciani A, Itti E, et al. Whole-body MRI and PET/CT in haematological malignancies. Cancer Imaging 2007;7 Spec No A:S88–93.

45. Yuki M, Narabayashi I, Yamamoto K, et al. Multifocal primary lymphoma of bone: scintigraphy and MR findings before and after treatment. Radiat Med 2000;18(5):305–10.

46. Altehoefer C, Laubenberger J, Lange W, et al. Prospective evaluation of bone marrow signal changes on magnetic resonance tomography during high-dose chemotherapy and peripheral

blood stem cell transplantation in patients with breast cancer. Invest Radiol 1997;32(10):613–20.

47. Fletcher BD, Wall JE, Hanna SL. Effect of hematopoietic growth factors on MR images of bone marrow in children undergoing chemotherapy. Radiology 1993;189(3):745–51.

48. Blomlie V, Rofstad EK, Skjonsberg A, et al. Female pelvic bone marrow: serial MR imaging before, during, and after radiation therapy. Radiology 1995;194(2):537–43.

49. Sacks EL, Goris ML, Glatstein E, et al. Bone marrow regeneration following large-field radiation: influence of volume, age, dose, and time. Cancer 1978;42: 1057–65.

50. Pakos EE, Fotopoulos AD, Ioannidis JP. 18F-FDG PET for evaluation of bone marrow infiltration in staging of lymphoma: a meta-analysis. J Nucl Med 2005;46:958–63.

51. Mammone JF, Schweitzer ME. MRI of occult sacral insufficiency fractures following radiotherapy. Skeletal Radiol 1995;24:101–4.

52. Mitchell DG, Rao VM, Dalinka MK, et al. Femoral head avascular necrosis: correlation of MR imaging, radiographic staging, radionuclide imaging, and clinical findings. Radiology 1987;162:709–15.

53. Weatherby RP, Dahlin DC, Ivins JC. Postradiation sarcoma of bone: review of 78 Mayo Clinic cases. Mayo Clin Proc 1981;56:294–306.

MR Imaging in Osteoarthritis: Hardware, Coils, and Sequences

Thomas M. Link, MD

KEYWORDS

- Osteoarthritis • MR imaging • Sequences
- Hardware • Field strength

MR imaging must be tailored for imaging of osteoarthritis (OA) by using scanners with adequate field strength, coils that allow imaging with high spatial resolution, and optimized imaging sequences that best visualize tissues involved by OA. These tissues encompass cartilage, menisci, ligaments, and bone marrow. Among these tissues, cartilage has an outstanding role, and imaging cartilage is particularly challenging in terms of the required signal-to-noise-ratio (SNR), spatial resolution, and contrast. The requirements for cartilage imaging dictate the overall requirements in hardware and in sequence profiles.

This article (1) outlines requirements concerning field strength, analyzing scanners with different field strengths from 0.2 T to 7 T, (2) investigates the potential of open and extremity MR imaging, (3) examines the role of weight-bearing MR imaging, (4) reviews coil technology, and (5) analyzes sequence protocols and their role in imaging the different tissues involved in OA.

FIELD STRENGTH

Considerations concerning field strength required for OA imaging always should take into account that cartilage imaging is critical for adequate whole-organ OA analysis. Previous studies have shown that imaging with low field strength clearly has limitations in assessing cartilage morphology and therefore is not recommended for OA imaging.[1–3] Woertler and colleagues[3] compared the diagnostic performance of a dedicated orthopedic MR imaging system (0.18 T) and a conventional MR imaging system (1.0 T) in the detection of articular cartilage lesions created in an animal model. Using receiver operating characteristics (ROC) analysis with three different radiologists, these investigators found that the high-field-strength system demonstrated a significantly better diagnostic performance than the low-field-stength system in the detection of less-than-full-thickness articular cartilage lesions ($P < .001$). Ahn and colleagues[4] studied cadaver patellae using a 0.2-T extremity-only magnet and found that high-grade cartilaginous lesions could be evaluated reliably with low-field-strength MR imaging by using a combination of imaging sequences. Limitations were encountered analyzing less-than-full-thickness cartilage lesions, however. Based on the results of these previous studies, the use of MR imaging scanners with a field strength of at least 1.0 T is recommended for imaging cartilage.

The current standard is 1.5-T imaging, and most of the studies establishing MR imaging for assessment of OA were conducted at this field strength.[5–8] Semiquantitative scores to grade OA and techniques to quantify cartilage volume were developed at 1.5 T.[6,9,10] The early studies analyzing quantitative parameters to characterize the biochemical composition of cartilage, such as T2 relaxation time and T1rho mapping, as well as delayed gadolinium-enhanced MR imaging

This article originally appeared in *Radiologic Clinics of North America* 2009;47(4):617–32.

Department of Radiology and Biomedical Imaging, University of California at San Francisco, 400 Parnassus Avenue, A-367, San Francisco, CA 94131, USA

E-mail address: tmlink@radiology.ucsf.edu

of cartilage (dGEMRIC), also were performed at 1.5 T.[11–13]

Although 1.5-T imaging is standard, a number of studies have demonstrated that 3.0-T MR imaging allows better visualization of cartilage lesions[14–19] and therefore may be better suited for the overall assessment of OA. Using optimized high-resolution MR imaging sequences in an animal model, Link and colleagues showed that cartilage lesions were visualized better and diagnostic performance was improved at 3.0 T compared with 1.5 T. Interestingly, however, standard lower-spatial-resolution intermediate (IM)-weighted fast spin echo (FSE) sequences did not improve diagnostic performance at 3.0 T. **Fig. 1** shows two corresponding IM-weighted fat-saturated MR images obtained at 1.5 and 3.0 T demonstrating a superficial cartilage defect at the patella in a pig knee, which is visualized better at 3.0 T.[18] Although this study was performed at the knee, additional studies performed at human cadaver ankles[14,15] also showed better diagnostic performance in assessing cartilage lesions and a higher sensitivity for assessing ligamentous and tendon pathology at 3.0 T than at 1.5 T.

Recently Kijowski and colleagues[17,20] performed a retrospective study comparing the diagnostic performance of 1.5-T and 3.0-T MR imaging protocols for evaluating the articular cartilage of the knee joint in symptomatic patients. Analyzing 241 knee MR images at 1.5 T and 226 MR images at 3.0 T, these investigators found that the sensitivity, specificity, and accuracy of MR imaging for detecting cartilage lesions were 69.3%, 78.0%, and 74.5%, respectively, at 1.5 T and were 70.5%, 85.9%, and 80.1%, respectively, at 3.0 T. The MR imaging protocol had significantly higher specificity and accuracy ($P < .05$) but not higher sensitivity ($P = .73$) for detecting cartilage lesions at 3.0 T than at 1.5 T. The investigators concluded that 3.0-T MR imaging protocols were superior to the 1.5-T protocol for evaluating the articular cartilage of the knee joint in symptomatic patients (**Figs. 2** and **3**).

Bauer and colleagues[16] compared the precision and accuracy of 3.0-T and 1.5-T MR imaging in the quantification of cartilage volume by using direct volumetric measurements as a reference standard in a cadaver model. These investigators calculated accuracy errors for MR imaging–based volume calculations of 3.0% at the femur for standard fat-suppressed spoiled gradient-echo (SPGR) sequences at 3.0 T, versus 16% for the standard fat-suppressed SPGR sequence at 1.5 T. Effective signal-to-noise ratio and effective contrast-to-noise ratio also were substantially improved at 3.0 T. This study provides evidence that cartilage volumetric measurements obtained at 3.0 T are more accurate than those obtained at 1.5 T. Eckstein and colleagues[21] performed an in vivo study in patients who had OA and normal volunteers to evaluate the precision of quantitative MR imaging assessments of human cartilage morphology at 3.0 T and to correlate the measurements at 3.0 T with validated measurements at 1.5 T. They found that with a slice thickness of 1.5 mm,

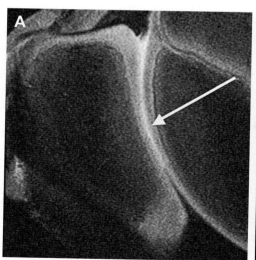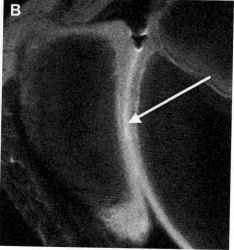

Fig. 1. Sagittal MR images of a pig knee with artificially created patellar cartilage defect obtained at (*A*) 1.5 T and (*B*) 3.0 T using fat-suppressed IM-weighted FSE sequences (4000/35 milliseconds; TR/TE for both 1.5; 3.0 T). Superficial cartilage defect at the patella (*arrows*) is well shown on the 3.0-T image (*B*) but is not well visualized on the 1.5-T image (*A*).

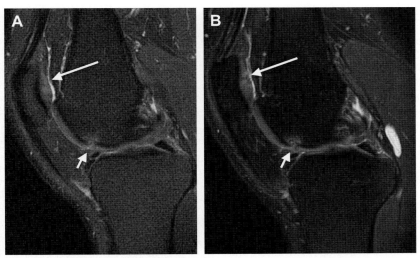

Fig. 2. Sagittal MR image of the knee obtained in a middle-aged runner with knee pain at (*A*) 1.5 T and (*B*) 3.0 T using fat-suppressed IM-weighted FSE sequences (3200/46 and 4300/51 milliseconds). Cartilage defects at the patella (*long arrow*) and osteochondral lesion at the trochlea (*short arrow*) are better visualized at 3.0 T than at 1.5 T.

measurements tended to be more reproducible at 3.0 T than at 1.5 T, and they concluded that imaging at 3.0 T may provide superior ability to detect changes in cartilage status over time and to determine responses to treatment with structure-modifying drugs.

To achieve the best possible imaging technique for assessing OA, the National Institute of Health–sponsored Osteoarthritis Initiative (OAI) therefore adopted imaging at 3.0 T. The OAI is a nationwide, multicenter research study that provides a large dataset of clinical information, questionnaires, radiographs, and MR imaging studies obtained from nearly 5000 participants (4796 participants at baseline) who are followed up every 12 months for a period of 48 months. The overall aim of the OAI is to develop a public domain research resource to facilitate the scientific evaluation of biomarkers for OA as potential surrogate end points for disease onset and progression. The OAI recruits participants who have knee OA (the progression cohort) and participants who have

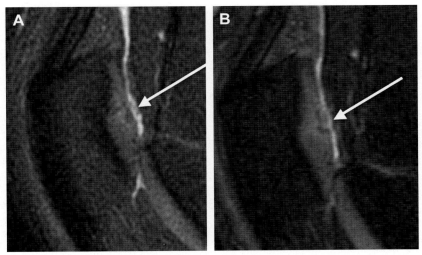

Fig. 3. (*A*) 1.5-T and (*B*) 3.0-T sagittal fat-suppressed IM-weighted FSE MRI of the patella (3200/46 and 4300/51 milliseconds). Fissures at the patella (*arrow*) are shown in greater detail, and the surface of the cartilage is evaluated substantially better at 3.0 T than at 1.5 T.

risk factors but no symptoms of OA (the incidence cohort). The imaging protocol includes morphologic and quantitative MR imaging sequences performed at 3.0 T with five identical scanners from the same manufacturer.[22]

To date, MR imaging at 7.0 T is a research application, and only limited studies have been performed in human participants.[23,24] Currently available sequence protocols have not been shown to be superior to 3.0 T in the assessment of OA. Future research work clearly will need to focus on developing adequate surface coils and optimized sequences for imaging at 7.0 T.

EXTREMITY AND OPEN MR IMAGING

Peripheral extremity magnets have lower installation, maintenance, and management costs than whole-body systems, and these systems are beneficial for patients who have claustrophobia. Moreover, they do not require the amount of shielding necessary for a whole-body system and potentially can be used in private offices, thus making MR imaging widely available. Dedicated extremity scanners operating at higher field strength have been developed to overcome the limitations of 0.2-T MR imaging scanners in visualizing cartilage and other anatomic structures such as ligaments (**Fig. 4**). Using a dedicated peripheral extremity-only MR imaging system operating at 1.0 T, Roemer and colleagues[25] examined 34 knees using fat-suppressed FSE proton density (PD)-weighted sequences. They found good to excellent interobserver performance in assessing OA-associated abnormalities, including cartilage lesions (**Fig. 5**). These high-field peripheral scanners may offer a low-cost alternative providing

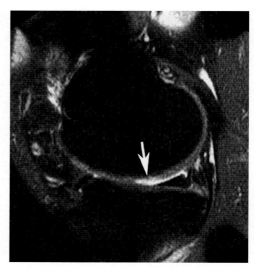

Fig. 5. Sagittal fat-suppressed PD-weighted MR image at 1.0 T depicts a focal cartilage defect (*arrow*) at the central weight-bearing medial femoral condyle. (*Courtesy of* Ali Guermazi, MD, Boston University.)

adequate image quality for assessing cartilage pathology. Currently, peripheral extremity scanners operating at 1.5-T field strength are available also.

Depending on the open MR imaging configuration, patients can be placed in the scanner in either a supine or weight-bearing position. Open MR imaging scanners allow the functional aspects of joint function to be assessed and may therefore be useful in investigating conditions associated with abnormal articulation in certain joint positions that may lead to accelerated OA. For example, femoroacetabular impingement is a condition in which labral and cartilage damage results from an abnormal morphology of the head–neck junction (cam-type impingement) or an abnormally deep acetabulum (pincer-type impingement). This impingement typically occurs with flexion, abduction, and external rotation. Open MR imaging can be used to assess these functional aspects of the hip joint. Yamamura and colleagues[26] demonstrated that, although impingement occurred frequently during daily activities, it was not associated with accelerated OA of the hip in male and female Japanese participants.

Open MR imaging scanners also can be used to assess patella kinematics and patellofemoral contact areas, which may play a role in development of femoropatellar OA. Hinterwimmer and colleagues[27] studied a sample of 15 patients who had genu varum and mild OA and 15 healthy volunteers in an open MR imaging scanner.

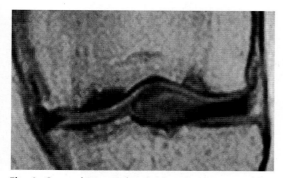

Fig. 4. Coronal T1-weighted spin echo sequence (520/24 milliseconds) of the right knee obtained at 0.2 T with a dedicated extremity scanner in a patient who has subchondral bone infarcts. The limitations of image SNR and spatial resolution that limit visualization of cartilage abnormalities are demonstrated clearly.

Three-dimensional (3D) gradient echo sequences of the knee were obtained in 0°, 30°, and 90° with and without activity of the extensor muscles. Contact areas between patella and femur cartilage were defined by intersection of opposing cartilage volumes. These investigators, however, were not able to demonstrate significant differences in patella kinematics and patellofemoral contact areas ($P > .05$) between varus knees with mild OA and healthy knees either at the different flexion angles or under extending muscle activity.

WEIGHT-BEARING MR IMAGING

Weight-bearing MR imaging can be performed using open MR imaging systems that have vertically orientated magnets or with whole-body MR imaging systems that use special loading devices for the knee, such as the one described by Nishii and colleagues.[28] Although the vertical alignment of the magnets in a double-doughnut system allows true weight-bearing MR imaging studies, the field strength and image quality of these scanners are limited, affecting cartilage imaging in particular. Image quality in whole-body systems generally is superior, and loading devices also have been applied successfully in 3.0-T scanners.[28] Static loading conditions usually are obtained by applying an axial compression force of approximately 50% of body weight during imaging.

Anterior cruciate ligament (ACL) tears have been identified as an important factor in the pathogenesis of OA, and it also has been found that patients who have ACL repair experience accelerated OA.[29] Logan and colleagues[30] used a vertical open MR imaging system to study the tibiofemoral kinematics of ACL-deficient weight-bearing in 10 patients. The tibiofemoral motion was assessed through the arc of flexion from 0° to 90° in the ACL-deficient and normal contralateral knees. These investigators found that ACL tears change tibiofemoral kinematics, producing anterior subluxation of the lateral tibial plateau. They hypothesized that altered kinematics may explain, at least in part, the increased incidence of secondary OA in patients who have had an ACL tear. In another study, the same investigators[31] used the same weight-bearing technique in an open MR imaging system to study 10 patients who had isolated reconstruction of the ACL (hamstring autograft) in one knee and a normal contralateral knee. They found that ACL reconstruction reduces sagittal laxity to within normal limits but does not restore normal tibiofemoral kinematics; the abnormal kinematics, again, may explain the relatively high rate of accelerated OA in this patient population.

Currently there has been substantial interest in studying changes in cartilage volume and biochemical matrix in response to load-bearing. It has been suggested that failure to respond to normal load-bearing may be caused by the disorder or degeneration of articular cartilage with collagen disorganization or abnormal water content.[28] Nishii and colleagues[28] used T2 relaxation time measurements to study the biochemical composition of the normal hyaline knee cartilage under loading. Using 3.0-T MR imaging and applying an axial compression force of 50% of body weight during imaging, they obtained sagittal T2 maps of the medial and lateral femorotibial joints of 22 healthy volunteers. They compared the T2 values of the femoral and tibial cartilage at the weight-bearing area in the unloading and loading conditions. These investigators found that under loading conditions, mean cartilage T2 values generally decreased. At the medial joint compartment, a significant decrease in T2 values with loading was observed at the femoral region in direct contact with the opposing tibial cartilage. A significant decrease in T2 values with loading also was observed at the medial and lateral tibia, at regions both covered and not covered by the meniscus.

In addition, the role of the meniscus during weight-bearing is critical in preventing OA. While axial compression forces are applied, MR imaging directly visualizes changes of the meniscus in morphology, deformity, extrusion, and, potentially, biochemistry (**Fig. 6**). These findings may help elucidate the evolution and pathophysiology of OA, but at present the experience in direct visualization of meniscal abnormalities with weight-bearing MR imaging is limited.

SURFACE COILS

In addition to adequate field strength, dedicated surface coils are important prerequisites to achieve good image quality and visualization of the joint tissues involved in OA. Currently, surface coils for the wrist, shoulder, knee, and ankle are standard; most of these coils are multichannel phased-array coils. For visualization of smaller structures such as the fingers and toes, smaller (so-called "microscopy") coils have been developed. These coils allow imaging with small fields of view and high spatial resolution.

Fig. 7 shows the effect of the coil on the image quality. In panel *A*, a non-dedicated two-element paddle coil was used; in panel *B*, a dedicated three-element shoulder coil was applied. The

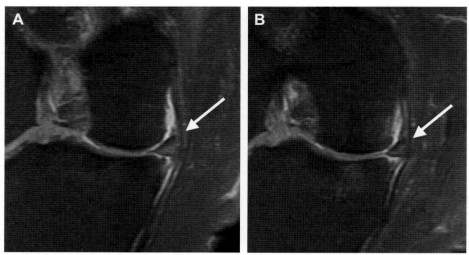

Fig. 6. Coronal MR image of the knee in a patient who has mild knee OA obtained using fat-suppressed PD-weighted FSE sequences (3000/10.3 milliseconds) (*A*) without and (*B*) with loading (50% body weight) in a whole-body 3.0-T MR scanner. Note that the medial meniscal extrusion (*arrow*) is increased under loading conditions and also that the shape of the meniscus is changed slightly.

effect on visualization of the cartilage is evident. Even if a high-quality, high-field scanner is used, inadequate coils limit image quality substantially, as shown by Lutterbey and colleagues.[32] These investigators found that using the standard body coil at 3.0 T for imaging of the knee gave a lower image performance than achieved using a 1.5-T scanner with a dedicated knee coil.

Multichannel phased-array coils give high SNR and allow parallel imaging, which can provide better image quality with the same acquisition time or can shorten acquisition time by maintaining image quality. With parallel imaging, each of the coil elements/channels provides image information separately; the information then is fused to obtain one image (**Fig. 8**).

In an in vitro study performed in human cadaver ankles, Bauer and colleagues[33] compared an autocalibrating parallel imaging technique at 3.0 T with standard acquisitions at 3.0 T for small

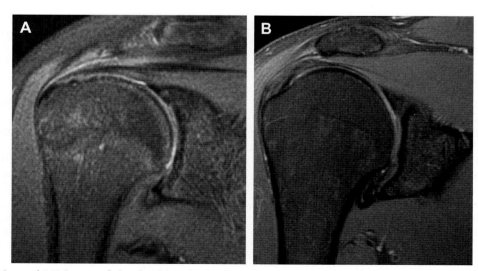

Fig. 7. Coronal MR image of the shoulder obtained at 3.0 T using fat-suppressed IM-weighted FSE sequences (3300/51 milliseconds) with (*A*) a non-dedicated paddle coil and (*B*) a three-element shoulder phased-array coil. Differences in image quality, especially in the visualization of the cartilage and bone marrow, are evident.

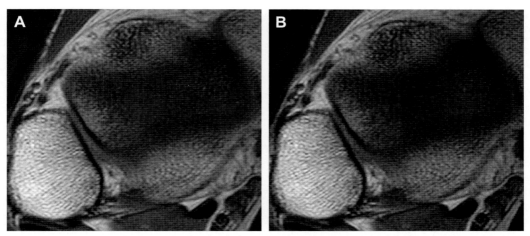

Fig. 8. MR image of a human cadaver ankle joint obtained at 3.0 T using a T1-weighted (675/15.7 milliseconds) FSE sequence (*A*) without and (*B*) with parallel imaging. Images in *B* were obtained with a 44% shorter acquisition time. There is no difference in image quality, particularly in visualizing the ligaments.

field-of-view imaging of the ankle. Using parallel imaging techniques, these investigators obtained a reduction in scan time of approximately 44%. All images were analyzed for image quality by two radiologists. Macroscopic findings after dissection served as a reference for the pathologic evaluation. This study did not find a significant difference in ligament and cartilage visualization or in image quality between standard and generalized, autocalibrating, partially parallel acquisitions reconstructions at 3.0 T. The authors concluded that parallel imaging can provide more flexibility in protocol design by either shortening image acquisition time or improving image quality with the same acquisition time.

Zuo and colleagues[34] evaluated the feasibility and reproducibility of quantitative cartilage imaging with parallel imaging at 3.0 T and determined the impact of the acceleration factor on morphologic and relaxation measurements. They found that morphologic parameters and relaxation time maps from parallel imaging showed results comparable with those obtained by the conventional technique. Intraclass correlation coefficients of the two methods for measuring cartilage volume and mean cartilage thickness were very high both for T1rho, and T2 measurements, and the reproducibility was excellent. In summary, for both quantitative and morphologic OA imaging, multichannel phased-array coils with parallel imaging techniques are recommended.

SEQUENCE PROTOCOLS

Because different tissues are involved in OA and both morphologic and quantitative analyses are

required, a number of different sequences have been tailored and developed for "whole-organ" assessment of OA. The workhorse sequences for morphologic imaging of the joints are FSE sequences. In particular fluid-sensitive fat-suppressed sequences have been found useful to assess cartilage, bone marrow, ligaments, menisci, and tendons. Most experience and good results in morphologic imaging of cartilage and subchondral pathology were gathered with (1) two-dimensional (2D) PD-, IM-, and T2-weighted FSE and (2) 3D SPGR or fast low-angle shot (FLASH) gradient echo sequences. Additional fat suppression in these sequences was found useful to visualize cartilage pathology better and to reduce chemical shift artifacts.

There is some controversy about how exactly to define T2-, IM-, and PD-weighted sequences. In general established terminology, IM-weighted sequences have echo times (TE) in the range of 30 to 60 milliseconds, T2-weighted sequences have TEs of 70 to 80 milliseconds, and PD-weighted sequences have TEs of 10 to 30 milliseconds.[19,35] In the author's experience, fat-suppressed IM-weighted FSE sequences are most useful for imaging joints with OA, because they are fluid sensitive, provide good visualization of cartilage, menisci, and ligaments, and also allow assessment of the bone marrow. These sequences also provide better visualization of anatomic structures than T2-weighted FSE sequences. PD-weighted sequences with lower TE values may be more helpful in assessing the menisci and give additional information concerning tendons and ligaments, but they are less fluid sensitive.

Intermediate- and T2-Weighted Fast Spin-Echo Sequences

The sequence most frequently used for OA assessment in clinical practice is an IM-weighted fat-suppressed FSE sequence, which allows good visualization of cartilage defects, bone marrow edema pattern, menisci, and tendons (**Fig. 9**). The standard parameters used for this sequence are a repetition time (TR) of 3000 to 4000 milliseconds; a TE of 30 to 60 milliseconds; and an echo train length of 8. This TE range is chosen because it provides higher intrinsic contrast of the cartilage and is less prone to magic angle effects than "true" PD-weighted pulse sequences obtained at shorter TEs. Slice thickness varies between 2 and 4 mm; 3 mm usually is used in a clinical setting. To maintain an acceptable acquisition time and to achieve a good SNR, the matrix size is in the order of 256 × 256 pixels but may be increased if imaging is performed at 3.0 T. Sequence parameters must be adjusted to the joint; the parameter most affected is the field of view. A clinically acceptable acquisition time is in the order of 3 to 6 minutes.

With IM- and T2-weighted FSE sequences, normal hyaline cartilage has intermediate signal intensity, and fluid is bright, allowing good contrast to identify surface abnormalities as well as pathologies of the cartilage matrix. Using 3.0-T MR

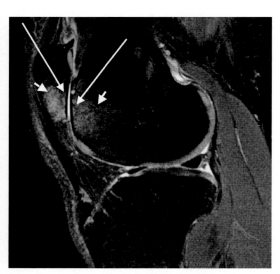

Fig. 9. Sagittal fat-suppressed IM-weighted FSE (3200/30 milliseconds) MR image of the knee obtained in a 48-year-old man who had advanced degenerative disease of the femoropatellar joint. Cartilage lesions (*long arrows*), bone marrow edema pattern (*short arrows*) at the trochlea and patella, osteophytes, tendons, menisci, and ligaments are well visualized with this fluid-sensitive sequence.

imaging, Saadat and colleagues[36] analyzed the performance of IM-weighted sequences in relation to histology in patients who had advanced OA before undergoing total knee arthroplasty (**Fig. 10**). Intraoperatively obtained specimens underwent histologic analysis, and sections were matched with preoperative MR images. Findings on preoperative MR imaging were compared with the corresponding region in histologic sections. Parameters assessed included thinning of cartilage (differentiating <50%, >50%, and full-thickness lesions), surface integrity (including fissuring and fraying), and abnormalities in cartilage signal pattern. Histologic findings related to the pattern of bone marrow edema and cartilage swelling were documented also. The overall sensitivity, specificity, and accuracy of their imaging findings were 72%, 69%, and 70%, respectively, for cartilage thinning, 69%, 74%, and 73%, respectively, for surface irregularities, and 36%, 62%, and 45%, respectively, for intracartilaginous signal abnormalities. The authors concluded that MR imaging using fat-suppressed IM-weighted FSE sequences was useful in assessing cartilage thickness and surface lesions, but changes in cartilage signal were not useful for characterizing the severity of cartilage degeneration. Thus signal abnormalities visualized on IM-weighted FSE sequences of the cartilage matrix may have limited value in characterizing cartilage degeneration and softening. In this study, the areas of bone marrow edema pattern corresponded to fibrovascular tissue ingrowths.

Multiple clinical studies have found that IM- and T2-weighted FSE sequences have high sensitivity and specificity in assessing tissue abnormalities that may be related to OA.[14,37–40] The diagnostic performance for cartilage lesions improves when different imaging planes are used. Bredella and colleagues[41] studied how the use of a combination of different imaging planes affects the detection and grading of articular cartilage defects in the knee. They found that the sensitivity of a sagittal T2-weighted FSE sequence was only 40%, and the specificity was 100%. The sensitivity of a combination of axial and coronal fat-suppressed T2-weighted FSE sequences and sagittal T2-weighted FSE sequences was 94%, specificity was 99%, and accuracy was 98%, using arthroscopy as a standard of reference.

Three-Dimensional Spoiled Gradient-Echo and Fast Low-Angle Shot Sequences

3D SPGR and FLASH sequences are well suited for depicting the cartilage volume and, to some extent, the cartilage surface. Sequence

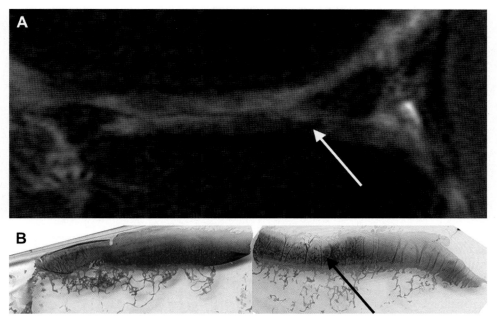

Fig. 10. (*A*) Sagittal MR image of the knee obtained in a patient undergoing total knee replacement at 3.0 T using a fat-suppressed IM-weighted FSE sequence (4300/51 milliseconds) shows focal cartilage thinning and fraying (*arrow*). The MR image also shows additional abnormal signal of the cartilage. (*B*) Corresponding histologic slide (hematoxylin and eosin staining) obtained after surgery demonstrates the same focal cartilage thinning and fraying (*arrow*).

parameters used to visualize cartilage are in the range of TR: 20 to 35 milliseconds, TE: 7 to 12 milliseconds, and flip angle: 12° to 30°; parameters need to be optimized according to the field strength. The bright signal of cartilage in the SPGR and FLASH images limits the visualization of internal cartilage pathology to some extent; fissures, for example, may not be as well visualized. These gradient-echo sequences are not suited for visualizing bone marrow pathology and are very limited in assessing menisci, ligaments, and tendons. They have been found useful, however, in segmenting cartilage for quantitative measurement of volume and thickness.[9,21,42]

A number of studies have compared SPGR versus IM- or T2-weighted FSE sequences[18,19,43] and have found that the two sequence types have similar overall diagnostic performance in detecting focal cartilage lesions. 3D SPGR and FLASH sequences provide high spatial resolution but usually require fairly long imaging time, and motion artifacts can degrade image quality. These gradient-echo sequences also are very sensitive to susceptibility artifacts, a consideration after previous surgery and in particular after cartilage repair procedures. In their clinical practice, the author and colleagues have found IM-weighted FSE sequences easier to use and more practically applicable than SPGR or FLASH sequences. More recent studies also suggest that SPGR sequences may be less suited than IM-weighted FSE sequences for visualizing subtle cartilage abnormalities (**Fig. 11**).[14,15]

Other Sequences

In addition to these sequences, 3D double-echo steady-state sequences (DESS) also have shown good results in detecting cartilage lesions (**Fig. 12**). This mixed T1/T2*-weighted sequence provides high spatial resolution with the cartilage appearing more intermediate in signal. In an experimental study, Woertler and colleagues[3] found that fat-suppressed 3D FLASH and water-excited 3D DESS sequences performed similarly in detecting cartilage surface lesions. Ruehm and colleagues[44] analyzed patellar cartilage abnormalities in 58 consecutive patients using a 3D DESS and a T2-weighted FSE sequence. These authors concluded that the DESS sequence was less accurate in detecting cartilage surface abnormalities but was more accurate in diagnosing cartilage softening. 3D DESS sequences usually are obtained with thin sections, allowing relatively high-quality reconstructions in additional imaging planes.

A number of sequences have been developed to improve morphologic depiction of cartilage. These sequences include driven equilibrium Fourier

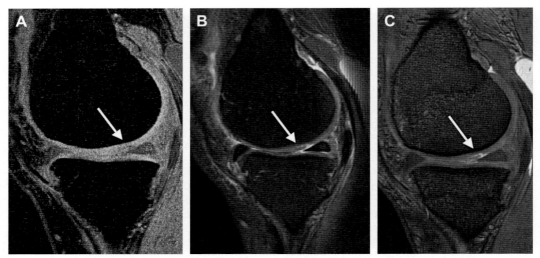

Fig. 11. Sagittal MR images of the knee obtained in a middle-aged runner using (*A*) fat-suppressed SPGR (21/12.5 milliseconds, flip angle: 15°), (*B*) IM-weighted FSE (4300/51 milliseconds), and (*C*) a non–fat-suppressed fluid-sensitive fast imaging employing steady-state acquisition (FIESTA; 5.9/1.9 milliseconds, flip angle: 15°) sequence. Cartilage delamination (*arrow*) is well visualized on the fluid-sensitive sequences (*B* and *C*) but not on the SPGR sequence (*A*) in which the cartilage appears uniformly bright.

transform (DEFT) and steady-state free precision (SSFP) imaging. DEFT imaging makes use of a much higher cartilage-to-fluid contrast; the signal of synovial fluid is higher than in SPGR sequences, and the signal of cartilage is higher than in T2-weighted FSE sequences.[45] Yoshioka and colleagues[43] used this sequence in 35 OA knees and correlated imaging findings with arthroscopy. In their study the fat-suppressed 3D

DEFT images showed results similar to SPGR and IM-weighted FSE sequences with high sensitivity but relatively low specificity. Gold and colleagues[46] compared 3D DEFT and T2-weighted FSE sequences in 104 consecutive patients who had knee pain and used arthroscopy in 24 patients as a standard of reference. These investigators found that the 3D DEFT sequences provided excellent synovial fluid-to-cartilage contrast while

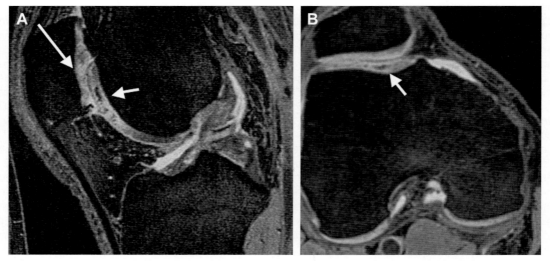

Fig. 12. (*A*) Sagittal 3D DESS MR image (16.3/4.7 milliseconds, flip angle: 25°) of the knee obtained in a 50-year-old man. (*B*) Axial reconstruction from the image dataset. Note femoropatellar cartilage degeneration with surface irregularity (*long arrow*) and signal changes (*short arrow*). Low-intensity signal changes at the trochlea are consistent with chondrocalcinosis.

preserving signal from cartilage, giving this method a high cartilage SNR. In addition 3D DEFT showed the full cartilage thickness better than T2-weighted FSE sequences, but T2-weighted FSE sequences had better fat suppression and fewer artifacts than 3D DEFT sequences.

SSFP imaging has been described as an efficient, high-signal method for obtaining 3D images and may be useful for depicting cartilage, because cartilage signal is higher than in conventional sequences.[47] Kornaat and colleagues[48] used this sequence in volunteers at 1.5 and 3 T and found that SSFP-based techniques showed higher SNR and increased contrast-to-noise efficiency at 3.0 T than SPGR sequences. **Fig. 11** shows images of cartilage delamination at the medial femoral condyle of the knee obtained with an SSFP sequence (fast imaging employing steady state acquisition, FIESTA) and SPGR and IM-weighted FSE sequences. Bauer and colleagues[49] compared the performance of SSFP, IM-weighted FSE, and SPGR sequences in assessing cartilage lesions at cadaver ankles and found the highest ROC values for the IM-weighted FSE sequences at 3.0 T, but IM-weighted FSE and SSFP sequences showed a similar performance at 1.5 T, and both showed better results than the SPGR sequence at 3.0 T and 1.5 T. To the author's knowledge, larger clinical studies have not yet been performed using this sequence. The previously described DESS sequence also is a steady-state sequence and thus has cartilage signal features similar to the SSFP sequences, but the parameters differ in some respects.

Recently 3D FSE sequences have been used for clinical imaging of the knee and ankle.[50,51] These sequences generate isotropic voxels and allow high-quality reformations in any plane. Thus it may be possible to obtain only one sequence dataset and get the additional planes as reformations (**Fig. 13**). This technique potentially would save acquisition time and shorten patient examinations substantially. Ristow and colleagues[50] compared the image quality and diagnostic performance in assessing abnormal findings of the knee of a fat-suppressed IM-weighted 3D FSE sequence and a standard 2D IM-weighted FSE sequence. They found that isotropic 3D IM-weighted FSE imaging enhanced standard knee MR imaging by better visualizing high-contrast lesions; however, 3D FSE image quality was lower, and there were limitations in diagnostic performance compared with standard 2D FSE imaging. Clearly this technique has potential, however, and with further improvements in the sequence design it may replace 2D IM-weighted FSE sequences.

MR Arthrography

Direct MR arthrography with use of T1-weighted pulse sequences following intra-articular injection of gadolinium chelates has been shown to be a reliable imaging technique for detecting surface lesions of articular cartilage, with sensitivity and specificity ranging from 85% to 100%.[52,53] The injected fluid produces high contrast between joint space, cartilage, and subchondral bone and at the same time distends the joint and thus

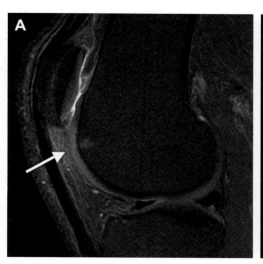 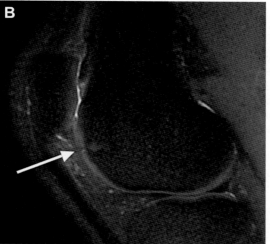

Fig. 13. (A) Sagittal 2D (4200/51 milliseconds) and (B) 3D (2500/38 milliseconds) FSE sequences of the knee show bone marrow edema pattern and a focal cartilage lesion. The cartilage fissure (arrow) is well depicted in (B) but is not well visualized in (A).

improves the separation of corresponding joint surfaces. Because of its invasive nature, however, this technique is of limited use for OA imaging.

A simple method for producing artificial arthrographic contrast in a T1-like FSE sequence using a driven equilibrium pulse (DRIVE) has been described recently. In contrast to the 3D DEFT sequence mentioned previously, this 2D technique provides bright signal intensity of joint fluid; signal intensities otherwise are the same as in a normal T1-weighted FSE sequence obtained at high spatial resolution and short scan times.[54] DRIVE also can be used to increase the contrast and/or spatial resolution of IM-weighted FSE images. This new technique and its value for cartilage imaging are still under clinical evaluation, however.

Quantitative Imaging of the Cartilage Matrix

In addition to assessing cartilage pathology, thickness, and volume, recent studies have shown the potential of MR imaging parameters to reflect changes in the biochemical composition of cartilage with early OA. These techniques include T2 quantification,[55] T1rho quantification,[13,56] and dGEMRIC.[57,58] These techniques allow characterization of the cartilage matrix and, potentially, quality before morphologic damage occurs.

T2 quantification

It has been shown that increased T2 relaxation time is proportional to the distribution of cartilage water and is sensitive to small changes in water content.[59] In an early study Dardzinski and colleagues[60] examined the spatial variation of in vivo cartilage T2 in young asymptomatic adults and found a reproducible pattern of increasing T2 that was proportional to the known spatial variation in cartilage water and that was inversely proportional to the distribution of proteoglycans. These authors postulated that the regional T2 differences were secondary to the restricted mobility of cartilage water within an anisotropic solid matrix. Thus measurement of the spatial distribution of the T2 reflecting areas of increased and decreased water content may be used to quantify cartilage degeneration before morphologic changes are appreciated.

In a preliminary study Mosher and colleagues[61] showed that aging is associated with an asymptomatic increase in T2 of the transitional zone of articular cartilage. The results of this study indicated that the diffuse increase in T2 relaxation time in senescent cartilage is different in appearance than the focally increased T2 observed in damaged articular cartilage.[61] Dunn and colleagues[55] analyzed 55 participants who were categorized radiographically as healthy (n = 7), as having mild OA (n = 20), or as having severe OA (n = 28). They found that healthy participants had mean T2 values of 32.1 to 35.0 milliseconds, whereas patients who had mild and severe OA had mean T2 values of 34.4 to 41.0 milliseconds. All cartilage compartments except the lateral tibia showed significant ($P < .05$) differences in T2 relaxation time between healthy and diseased knees. Correlation of T2 values with clinical symptoms and cartilage morphology was found predominantly in the medial compartments.

T1rho quantification

A different parameter that has been proposed for measuring cartilage composition is 3D T1rho relaxation mapping. T1rho describes the spin-lattice relaxation in the rotating frame, and changes in the extracellular matrix of cartilage (eg, the loss of glycosaminoglycans, GAG), may be reflected in measurements of T1rho because of the less restricted motion of water protons. Preliminary results demonstrated the in vivo feasibility of quantifying early biochemical changes in participants who had symptomatic OA using T1rho-weighted MR imaging on a 1.5-T clinical scanner.[13,56] In a study with a limited number of symptomatic participants, T1rho-weighted MR imaging provided a noninvasive marker for quantifying early degenerative changes in cartilage in vivo.[13] Li and colleagues[62] examined 10 healthy volunteers, and 9 patients who had OA at 3.0 T and found a significant difference ($P = .002$) in the average T1rho within patellar and femoral cartilage between controls (45.04 ± 2.59 milliseconds) and patients who had OA (53.06 ± 4.60 milliseconds). A significant correlation was found between T1rho and T2 relaxation measurements; however, the difference in T2 measurements between controls and patients who had OA was not significant. These initial results suggest that T1rho relaxation mapping may be a promising clinical tool for detecting OA and monitoring treatment. Stahl and colleagues[63] analyzed the diagnostic value of T2 and T1rho measurements in identifying asymptomatic physically active subjects with and without focal cartilage pathology. These investigators found that T1rho and T2 composition of cartilage differed in subjects with and without focal cartilage pathology and concluded that T1rho and T2 may be suitable parameters for identifying asymptomatic subjects at higher risk for developing cartilage degeneration (**Fig. 14**).

Further studies are underway in larger symptomatic populations to correlate T1rho

A   **B**

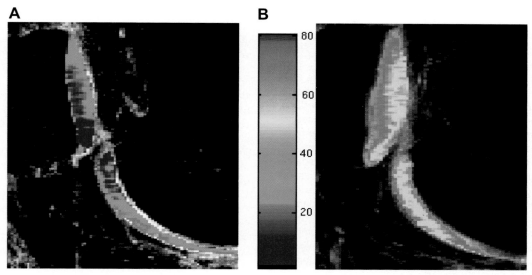

Fig. 14. Sagittal T1rho color maps [ms] of the patellofemoral cartilage. (*A*) An asymptomatic subject without focal cartilage pathology (low T1rho values). (*B*) An asymptomatic subject who has early, diffuse cartilage degeneration (high T1rho values) and focal cartilage defects (not shown). (*From* Stahl R, Luke A, Li X, et al. T1rho, T(2) and focal knee cartilage abnormalities in physically active and sedentary healthy subjects versus early OA patients—a 3.0-Tesla MRI study. Eur Radiol 2009;19:132–43.)

measurements with early OA with arthroscopy as a standard of reference. The advantage of T1rho and T2 measurements is that these techniques are noninvasive and do not require contrast injection.

Delayed gadolinium-enhanced MR imaging of cartilage

Cartilage consists of approximately 70% water, and the remainder is predominantly type II collagen fibers and GAG. The GAG macromolecules contain negative charges that attract sodium ions. One of the most commonly used MR imaging contrast agents, $Gd-DTPA^{2-}$ has a negative charge and therefore does not penetrate cartilage in areas where GAG concentrations are high. In fact, its distribution is concentrated in areas with lower GAG concentrations and thus pathologic cartilage composition. $Gd-DTPA^{2-}$ concentrations in cartilage can be quantified, and this technique has been defined as "delayed gadolinium-enhanced MR imaging of cartilage," dGEMRIC. Initial studies have shown that the dGEMRIC measurement of GAG corresponds to the true GAG concentration as measured with biochemistry and histology.[57,64] This technique has also been used in a number of clinical studies, and variations in this measurement have been shown in patients who have OA, in trials of autologous chondrocyte implants, and in comparisons between participants with a sedentary lifestyle and those who exercise regularly.[11,65–67]

Sequence protocols in relation to joint-specific requirements

MR imaging of OA currently concentrates mostly on the knee joint, but an increasing number of studies have focused on the hip joint.[68–72] There is a limited role for wrist and ankle MR imaging in OA.[73] The shoulder and elbow are rarely affected by OA, and thus MR imaging is not expected to have a significant role in assessing OA in these joints.

An optimal MR imaging protocol for knee OA would include morphologic IM-weighted FSE sequences in a coronal and sagittal orientation as well as quantitative sequences for volumetric and cartilage matrix assessment (SPGR/FLASH sequence as well as T1rho, T2, or dGEMRIC maps). Depending on clinical or research indications, axial IM-weighted sequences may be included for better assessment of the patella. Imaging of the hip would include coronal and sagittal IM-weighted FSE sequences. Oblique axial images are useful in measuring the alpha angle, which is required for assessment of femoroacetabular impingement and plays a major role in the evolution of accelerated OA.[74] Morphologic evaluation of cartilage and labrum at the hip joint without intra-articular contrast is limited. Initial studies have focused on quantitative MR imaging of the hip,[68,69,72,74] but segmentation of the femoral and acetabular cartilage layers at the hip is challenging, and frequently the two cartilage layers cannot be differentiated.

SUMMARY

To assess all tissues affected by OA, "whole-organ" MR imaging protocols are required. These protocols include morphologic sequences, such as IM-weighted FSE sequences, that are well suited to detect abnormalities of cartilage, menisci, bone marrow, ligaments, and tendons, and quantitative sequences that allow the assessment of cartilage volumes (SPGR, FLASH) and the analysis of cartilage biochemical composition (T2, T1rho, and dGEMRIC techniques). Dedicated surface coils are required for optimal visualization of joints affected by OA, in particular the knee joint, and multichannel phased-array coils with parallel imaging have been shown to improve image quality and/or shorten acquisition time. Image quality also benefits from increased field strength, and 3.0-T MR imaging is used increasingly for assessing joints with OA.

REFERENCES

1. Kladny B, Gluckert K, Swoboda B, et al. Comparison of low-field (0.2 Tesla) and high-field (1.5 Tesla) magnetic resonance imaging of the knee joint. Arch Orthop Trauma Surg 1995;114:281–6.

2. Rand T, Imhof H, Turetschek K, et al. Comparison of low field (0.2T) and high field (1.5T) MR imaging in the differentiation of torn from intact menisci. Eur J Radiol 1999;30:22–7.

3. Woertler K, Strothmann M, Tombach B, et al. Detection of articular cartilage lesions: experimental evaluation of low- and high-field-strength MR imaging at 0.18 and 1.0 T. J Magn Reson Imaging 2000;11: 678–85.

4. Ahn JM, Kwak SM, Kang HS, et al. Evaluation of patellar cartilage in cadavers with a low-field-strength extremity-only magnet: comparison of MR imaging sequences, with macroscopic findings as the standard. Radiology 1998;208:57–62.

5. Felson D, Chaisson C, Hill C, et al. The association of bone marrow lesions with pain in knee osteoarthritis. Ann Intern Med 2001;134:541–9.

6. Hunter DJ, Lo GH, Gale D, et al. The reliability of a new scoring system for knee osteoarthritis MRI and the validity of bone marrow lesion assessment: BLOKS (Boston Leeds Osteoarthritis Knee Score). Ann Rheum Dis 2008;67:206–11.

7. Link TM, Steinbach LS, Ghosh S, et al. Osteoarthritis: MR imaging findings in different stages of disease and correlation with clinical findings. Radiology 2003;226:373–81.

8. Phan CM, Link TM, Blumenkrantz G, et al. MR imaging findings in the follow-up of patients with different stages of knee osteoarthritis and the correlation with clinical symptoms. Eur Radiol 2006;16:608–18.

9. Eckstein F, Heudorfer L, Faber SC, et al. Long-term and resegmentation precision of quantitative cartilage MR imaging (qMRI). Osteoarthr Cartil 2002; 10:922–8.

10. Peterfy CG, Guermazi A, Zaim S, et al. Whole-Organ Magnetic Resonance Imaging Score (WORMS) of the knee in osteoarthritis. Osteoarthr Cartil 2004; 12:177–90.

11. Burstein D, Gray M. New MRI techniques for imaging cartilage. J Bone Joint Surg Am 2003; 85(Suppl 2):70–7.

12. Mosher TJ, Dardzinski BJ. Cartilage MRI T2 relaxation time mapping: overview and applications. Semin Musculoskelet Radiol 2004;8:355–68.

13. Regatte RR, Akella SV, Wheaton AJ, et al. 3D-T1rho-relaxation mapping of articular cartilage: in vivo assessment of early degenerative changes in symptomatic osteoarthritic subjects. Acad Radiol 2004; 11:741–9.

14. Barr C, Bauer JS, Malfair D, et al. MR imaging of the ankle at 3 Tesla and 1.5 Tesla: protocol optimization and application to cartilage, ligament and tendon pathology in cadaver specimens. Eur Radiol 2007; 17:1518–28.

15. Bauer JS, Barr C, Henning TD, et al. Magnetic resonance imaging of the ankle at 3.0 Tesla and 1.5 Tesla in human cadaver specimens with artificially created lesions of cartilage and ligaments. Invest Radiol 2008;43:604–11.

16. Bauer JS, Krause SJ, Ross CJ, et al. Volumetric cartilage measurements of porcine knee at 1.5-T and 3.0-T MR imaging: evaluation of precision and accuracy. Radiology 2006;241:399–406.

17. Kijowski R, Blankenbaker D, Davis K, et al. Comparison of 1.5T and 3T magnetic resonance imaging systems for evaluating the articular cartilage of the knee joint. Chicago: RSNA; 2007. p. 125.

18. Link TM, Sell CA, Masi JN, et al. 3.0 vs 1.5T MRI in the detection of focal cartilage pathology—ROC analysis in an experimental model. Osteoarthr Cartil 2005;14:63–70.

19. Masi JN, Sell CA, Phan C, et al. Cartilage MR imaging at 3.0 versus that at 1.5 T: preliminary results in a porcine model. Radiology 2005;236: 140–50.

20. Kijowski R, Blankenbaker DG, Davis KW, et al. Comparison of 1.5- and 3.0-T MR imaging for evaluating the articular cartilage of the knee joint. Radiology 2009;250:839–48.

21. Eckstein F, Charles HC, Buck RJ, et al. Accuracy and precision of quantitative assessment of cartilage morphology by magnetic resonance imaging at 3.0T. Arthritis Rheum 2005;52:3132–6.

22. Peterfy CG, Schneider E, Nevitt M. The osteoarthritis initiative: report on the design rationale for the

magnetic resonance imaging protocol for the knee. Osteoarthr Cartil 2008;16:1433–41.

23. Kraff O, Theysohn JM, Maderwald S, et al. MRI of the knee at 7.0 Tesla. Rofo 2007;179:1231–5.

24. Krug R, Carballido-Gamio J, Banerjee S, et al. In vivo bone and cartilage MRI using fully-balanced steady-state free-precession at 7 Tesla. Magn Reson Med 2007;58:1294–8.

25. Roemer FW, Guermazi A, Lynch JA, et al. Short tau inversion recovery and proton density-weighted fat suppressed sequences for the evaluation of osteoarthritis of the knee with a 1.0 T dedicated extremity MRI: development of a time-efficient sequence protocol. Eur Radiol 2005;15:978–87.

26. Yamamura M, Miki H, Nakamura N, et al. Open-configuration MRI study of femoro-acetabular impingement. J Orthop Res 2007;25:1582–8.

27. Hinterwimmer S, von Eisenhart-Rothe R, Siebert M, et al. Patella kinematics and patello-femoral contact areas in patients with genu varum and mild osteoarthritis. Clin Biomech (Bristol, Avon) 2004;19:704–10.

28. Nishii T, Kuroda K, Matsuoka Y, et al. Change in knee cartilage T2 in response to mechanical loading. J Magn Reson Imaging 2008;28:175–80.

29. Amin S, Guermazi A, Lavalley MP, et al. Complete anterior cruciate ligament tear and the risk for cartilage loss and progression of symptoms in men and women with knee osteoarthritis. Osteoarthr Cartil 2008;16:897–902.

30. Logan M, Dunstan E, Robinson J, et al. Tibiofemoral kinematics of the anterior cruciate ligament (ACL)-deficient weightbearing, living knee employing vertical access open "interventional" multiple resonance imaging. Am J Sports Med 2004;32:720–6.

31. Logan MC, Williams A, Lavelle J, et al. Tibiofemoral kinematics following successful anterior cruciate ligament reconstruction using dynamic multiple resonance imaging. Am J Sports Med 2004;32:984–92.

32. Lutterbey G, Behrends K, Falkenhausen MV, et al. Is the body-coil at 3 Tesla feasible for the MRI evaluation of the painful knee? A comparative study. Eur Radiol 2007;17:503–8.

33. Bauer JS, Banerjee S, Henning TD, et al. Fast high-spatial-resolution MRI of the ankle with parallel imaging using GRAPPA at 3 T. AJR Am J Roentgenol 2007;189:240–5.

34. Zuo J, Li X, Banerjee S, et al. Parallel imaging of knee cartilage at 3 Tesla. J Magn Reson Imaging 2007;26:1001–9.

35. Naraghi A, White L. MRI evaluation of the postoperative knee: special considerations and pitfalls. Clin Sports Med 2006;25:703–25.

36. Saadat E, Jobke B, Chu B, et al. Diagnostic performance of in vivo 3T fast spin echo MRI for articular cartilage abnormalities in human osteoarthritic knees using histology as standard of reference. Eur Radiol 2008;18:2292–302.

37. Kawahara Y, Uetani M, Nakahara N, et al. Fast spin-echo MR of the articular cartilage in the osteoarthrotic knee. Correlation of MR and arthroscopic findings. Acta Radiol 1998;39:120–5.

38. Link TM, Sell CA, Masi JN, et al. 3.0 vs 1.5 T MRI in the detection of focal cartilage pathology–ROC analysis in an experimental model. Osteoarthr Cartil 2006;14:63–70.

39. Potter HG, Linklater JM, Allen AA, et al. Magnetic resonance imaging of articular cartilage in the knee. An evaluation with use of fast-spin-echo imaging. J Bone Joint Surg Am 1998;80:1276–84.

40. Ramnath RR, Magee T, Wasudev N, et al. Accuracy of 3-T MRI using fast spin-echo technique to detect meniscal tears of the knee. AJR Am J Roentgenol 2006;187:221–5.

41. Bredella MA, Tirman PF, Peterfy CG, et al. Accuracy of T2-weighted fast spin-echo MR imaging with fat saturation in detecting cartilage defects in the knee: comparison with arthroscopy in 130 patients. AJR Am J Roentgenol 1999;172:1073–80.

42. Eckstein F, Burstein D, Link TM. Quantitative MRI of cartilage and bone: degenerative changes in osteoarthritis. NMR Biomed 2006;19:822–54.

43. Yoshioka H, Stevens K, Hargreaves BA, et al. Magnetic resonance imaging of articular cartilage of the knee: comparison between fat-suppressed three-dimensional SPGR imaging, fat-suppressed FSE imaging, and fat-suppressed three-dimensional DEFT imaging, and correlation with arthroscopy. J Magn Reson Imaging 2004;20:857–64.

44. Ruehm S, Zanetti M, Romero J, et al. MRI of patellar articular cartilage: evaluation of an optimized gradient echo sequence (3D-DESS). J Magn Reson Imaging 1998;8:1246–51.

45. Hargreaves BA, Gold GE, Lang PK, et al. MR imaging of articular cartilage using driven equilibrium. Magn Reson Med 1999;42:695–703.

46. Gold GE, Fuller SE, Hargreaves BA, et al. Driven equilibrium magnetic resonance imaging of articular cartilage: initial clinical experience. J Magn Reson Imaging 2005;21:476–81.

47. Hargreaves BA, Gold GE, Beaulieu CF, et al. Comparison of new sequences for high-resolution cartilage imaging. Magn Reson Med 2003;49:700–9.

48. Kornaat PR, Reeder SB, Koo S, et al. MR imaging of articular cartilage at 1.5T and 3.0T: comparison of SPGR and SSFP sequences. Osteoarthr Cartil 2005;13:338–44.

49. Bauer J, Barr C, Steinbach L, et al. Imaging of the articular cartilage of the ankle at 3.0 and 1.5 Tesla. Eur Radiol 2006;16(Suppl 1):238 [abstract].

50. Ristow O, Steinbach L, Sabo G, et al. Isotropic 3D fast spin-echo imaging versus standard 2D imaging

at 3.0 T of the knee-image quality and diagnostic performance. Eur Radiol 2009;19:1263–72.

51. Stevens KJ, Busse RF, Han E, et al. Ankle: isotropic MR imaging with 3D-FSE-cube—initial experience in healthy volunteers. Radiology 2008;249:1026–33.

52. Gagliardi JA, Chung EM, Chandnani VP, et al. Detection and staging of chondromalacia patellae: relative efficacies of conventional MR imaging, MR arthrography, and CT arthrography. AJR Am J Roentgenol 1994;163:629–36.

53. Kramer J, Recht MP, Imhof H, et al. Postcontrast MR arthrography in assessment of cartilage lesions. J Comput Assist Tomogr 1994;18:218–24.

54. Woertler K, Rummeny EJ, Settles M. A fast high-resolution multislice T1-weighted turbo spin-echo (TSE) sequence with a DRIVen equilibrium (DRIVE) pulse for native arthrographic contrast. AJR Am J Roentgenol 2005;185:1468–70.

55. Dunn TC, Lu Y, Jin H, et al. T2 relaxation time of cartilage at MR imaging: comparison with severity of knee osteoarthritis. Radiology 2004;232:592–8.

56. Regatte RR, Akella SV, Borthakur A, et al. In vivo proton MR three-dimensional T1rho mapping of human articular cartilage: initial experience. Radiology 2003;229:269–74.

57. Bashir A, Gray ML, Hartke J, et al. Nondestructive imaging of human cartilage glycosaminoglycan concentration by MRI. Magn Reson Med 1999;41:857–65.

58. Burstein D, Bashir A, Gray ML. MRI techniques in early stages of cartilage disease. Invest Radiol 2000;35:622–38.

59. Liess C, Lusse S, Karger N, et al. Detection of changes in cartilage water content using MRI T2-mapping in vivo. Osteoarthr Cartil 2002;10:907–13.

60. Dardzinski BJ, Mosher TJ, Li S, et al. Spatial variation of T2 in human articular cartilage. Radiology 1997;205:546–50.

61. Mosher TJ, Dardzinski BJ, Smith MB. Human articular cartilage: influence of aging and early symptomatic degeneration on the spatial variation of T2—preliminary findings at 3 T. Radiology 2000;214:259–66.

62. Li X, Han ET, Ma CB, et al. In vivo 3T spiral imaging based multi-slice T(1rho) mapping of knee cartilage in osteoarthritis. Magn Reson Med 2005;54:929–36.

63. Stahl R, Luke A, Li X, et al. T1rho, T(2) and focal knee cartilage abnormalities in physically active and sedentary healthy subjects versus early OA patients—a 3.0-Tesla MRI study. Eur Radiol 2009;19:132–43.

64. Trattnig S, Mlynarik V, Breitenseher M, et al. MRI visualization of proteoglycan depletion in articular cartilage via intravenous administration of Gd-DTPA. Magn Reson Imaging 1999;17:577–83.

65. Gillis A, Bashir A, McKeon B, et al. Magnetic resonance imaging of relative glycosaminoglycan distribution in patients with autologous chondrocyte transplants. Invest Radiol 2001;36:743–8.

66. Williams A, Gillis A, McKenzie C, et al. Glycosaminoglycan distribution in cartilage as determined by delayed gadolinium-enhanced MRI of cartilage (dGEMRIC): potential clinical applications. AJR Am J Roentgenol 2004;182:167–72.

67. Williams A, Sharma L, McKenzie CA, et al. Delayed gadolinium-enhanced magnetic resonance imaging of cartilage in knee osteoarthritis: findings at different radiographic stages of disease and relationship to malalignment. Arthritis Rheum 2005;52:3528–35.

68. Carballido-Gamio J, Link TM, Li X, et al. Feasibility and reproducibility of relaxometry, morphometric, and geometrical measurements of the hip joint with magnetic resonance imaging at 3T. J Magn Reson Imaging 2008;28:227–35.

69. Cheng Y, Wang S, Yamazaki T, et al. Hip cartilage thickness measurement accuracy improvement. Comput Med Imaging Graph 2007;31:643–55.

70. Kim YJ, Bixby S, Mamisch TC, et al. Imaging structural abnormalities in the hip joint: instability and impingement as a cause of osteoarthritis. Semin Musculoskelet Radiol 2008;12:334–45.

71. Taljanovic MS, Graham AR, Benjamin JB, et al. Bone marrow edema pattern in advanced hip osteoarthritis: quantitative assessment with magnetic resonance imaging and correlation with clinical examination, radiographic findings, and histopathology. Skeletal Radiol 2008;37:423–31.

72. Tiderius CJ, Jessel R, Kim YJ, et al. Hip dGEMRIC in asymptomatic volunteers and patients with early osteoarthritis: the influence of timing after contrast injection. Magn Reson Med 2007;57:803–5.

73. Eckstein F, Siedek V, Glaser C, et al. Correlation and sex differences between ankle and knee cartilage morphology determined by quantitative magnetic resonance imaging. Ann Rheum Dis 2004;63:1490–5.

74. Pfirrmann CW, Mengiardi B, Dora C, et al. Cam and pincer femoroacetabular impingement: characteristic MR arthrographic findings in 50 patients. Radiology 2006;240:778–85.

MRI of Hip Osteoarthritis and Implications for Surgery

Tallal C. Mamisch, MD[a,b,*], Christoph Zilkens, MD[c,d],
Klaus A. Siebenrock, MD, PhD[a], Bernd Bittersohl, MD[a,c],
Young-Jo Kim, MD, PhD[d], Stefan Werlen, MD[b]

KEYWORDS

- Osteoarthritis • Hip • Femoroacetabular impingement
- MRI • dGEMRIC • Surgery

Osteoarthritis (OA) of the hip is caused by a combination of intrinsic factors, such as joint anatomy, and extrinsic factors, such as body weight, injuries, diseases, and load.[1] Possible risk factors for OA are especially instability and impingement. Different surgical tequniques such as osteotomies of the pelvis and the femur,[2] surgical dislocation,[3] and hip arthroscopy[4,5] are being performed to delay or halt OA. Success of salvage hip procedures depends on the existing cartilage and joint damage prior to surgery; the likelihood of therapy failure rises with cases of advanced OA.[6–8]

For imaging of intra-articular pathology, MR imaging represents the best technique because of its ability to directly visualize cartilage, superior soft tissue contrast, and the prospect of multi-dimensional imaging. Opinions differ on the diagnostic efficacy of MR imaging and the question of which MR imaging technique is most appropriate. Many techniques showing similar promising data have been introduced for the knee.[9–12] Conditions within the hip are different, and the relatively thin hip cartilage and the spherical-shaped joint pose difficulties in the diagnosis of cartilage and labral injury. High MR imaging resolution and contrast-to-noise ratio between bone,

cartilage, synovium, and soft tissue such as labrum and capsule are required.

There is an ongoing investigation for the optimal MR imaging technique for imaging of the hip.[13–15] Currently, MR arthrography using intra-articular contrast material has been established as the standard method for imaging of labral lesions;[13,16–18] however, the diagnostic reliability of cartilage lesion remains moderate.[19,20] The diagnostic reliability of acetabular cartilage delamination by MR imaging is still challenenging.[21] The aim of this article is to discuss the current use of MR imaging in hip OA and its implications for surgery. As femoroacetabular impingement (FAI) becomes an increasingly important clinical diagnosis of the hip joint and is recognized as a precursor to the onset of hip OA, we will focus on this entity. Current standards, difficulties, and possible solutions using high-field MR imaging and future approaches are covered.

FEMOROACETABULAR IMPINGEMENT

During the past decade, FAI has gained increasing attentiveness as a possible trigger of hip OA. The incongruency of the hip (eg, after Perthes disease)

This article originally appeared in *Radiologic Clinics of North America* 2009;47(4):713–22.
[a] Department of Orthopedic Surgery, University of Bern, Freiburgstrasse, 3010 Bern, Switzerland
[b] Department of Radiology, Sonnenhof Clinics, 3010 Bern, Switzerland
[c] Department of Orthopedic Surgery, University of Düsseldorf, 41313 Düsseldorf, Germany
[d] Department of Orthopedic Surgery, Children's Hospital, Harvard Medical School, Boston, MA 02215, USA
* Corresponding author. Department of Orthopedic Surgery, University of Bern, Freiburgstrasse, 3010 Bern, Switzerland.
E-mail address: mamisch@bwh.harvard.edu (T.C. Mamisch).

Magn Reson Imaging Clin N Am 18 (2010) 111–120
doi:10.1016/j.mric.2009.09.008

mri.theclinics.com

might be denominated as static form of impinge-ment, whereas more subtle anatomic deformities, in which the incongruency of the hip joint exists only in certain positions during motion, are the dynamic form of impingement.[4,22,23] Depending on the anatomic abnormality, there are two types of FAI: cam and pincer. In cam FAI, the cause of impact is a nonspherical shape of the femoral head coming along with insufficient femoral head-neck offset. In cam FAI, shear forces lead to acetabular cartilage damage (**Fig. 1**), especially through forced flexion and internal rotation of the hip. In pincer FAI, the impact arises from acetab-ular overcoverage or other false configuration or shape of the acetabulum. The shape of the femoral head is spherical; however, the proximal femoral neck abuts frontally against the labrum and the acetabular rim. That way, the labrum is damaged primarily through recurrent trauma (**Fig. 2**) before a cartilage damage occurs.[24] Further causes for FAI are rotational anomalies with reduced femoral neck antetorsion and reduced acetabular version[25,26] or an overcorrection after periacetab-ular osteotomy (PAO), also called "Bernese disease."[27]

Untreated FAI can lead to premature OA of the hip.[28] To relieve symptoms such as limited range of motion and pain and further delay or halt the progression of OA, surgical treatment is neces-sary. Surgery includes reshaping of nonspherical femoral head in terms of cam, trimming the acetabular rim, or use of PAO in case of pincer FAI. The outcome of surgery depends on the quantity of pre-existing OA, with poor results occurring in patients with advanced degenerative changes. Follow-up examinations after open or arthroscopic FAI surgery showed favorable results, particularly in the subgroup of patients who did not have signs of advanced hip OA.[28] In patients who have FAI, it is important to identify early stages of cartilage degeneration to identify patients who could profit from osteo- or chondro-plastic types of surgery.

Diagnosis of Femoroacetabular Impingement

Diagnosis of FAI is based on clinical findings and radiographic analysis, including MR arthrogra-phy.[29] Clinical symptoms of FAI include a slow onset of inguinal pain, which is usually pronounced with physical activities or prolonged sitting.[30] During physical examination this can be reproduced by the "impingement test," which examines hip pain produced by passive flexion, internal rotation, and adduction.[31] A positive impingement test result can be corre-lated to acetabular labrum lesions.[24] Radio-graphic assessment by means of standard anteroposterior and lateral views[32] is used to asses late stages of hip OA[33] and abnormal femoral head morphology,[34,35] specifically the pistol grip deformity.[36] Plain radiographic anal-ysis is important in assessing acetabular version and coverage.

In cases of FAI, plain radiographs are often inad-equate in terms of femoral head-neck junction morphology assessment and assessment of early-stage OA.[37] Because of the importance of de-tecting these early hip joint lesions in FAI, MR imaging assessment is quickly becoming the stan-dard tool for diagnostic assessment.[16] It is becoming clear that standard coronal, axial, and sagittal MR imaging planes are less reliable than radially reconstructed planes perpendicular to the acetabular labrum in detecting early degenerative pathologies of the hip (**Fig. 3**).[16,38] For the

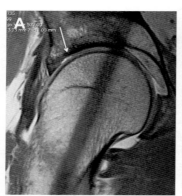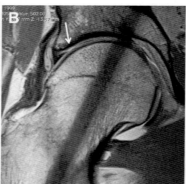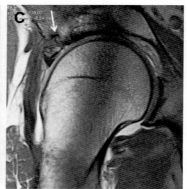

Fig. 1. (*A, B*) Radial turbo spin-echo proton density-weighted MR arthrography images at 3.0 T show cartilage damage (*arrow*) at the anterosuperior to superior portion of the acetabular rim caused by cam-type impinge-ment. (*C*) Severe cartilage degeneration is associated with intact labrum and cystic deformation (*arrow*) of the acetabular rim.

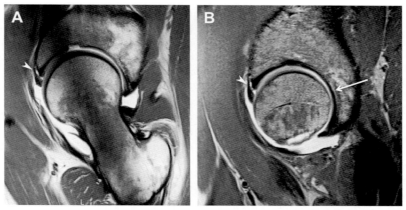

Fig. 2. (A) Radial and (B) sagittal turbo spin-echo proton density-weighted MR arthrography images at 3.0 T demonstrate labral tear in pincer-type impingement at the anterior position (*arrowhead*) and posterior femoroacetabular cartilage degeneration (*arrow*).

assessment of the femoral head-neck morphology, radial reconstructions along the femoral neck axis[35,39,40] improve the understanding of the FAI pathomechanism and correlate well with the prediction of FAI and intraoperative findings.[41] This imaging technique is increasingly recognized as an important tool for morphologic assessment

of FAI and an improved technique to detect early labral and chondral damage in the hip.[29]

Measurements in Femoroacetabular Impingement

Different MR imaging parameters are defined for assessment of FAI, such as alpha angle,

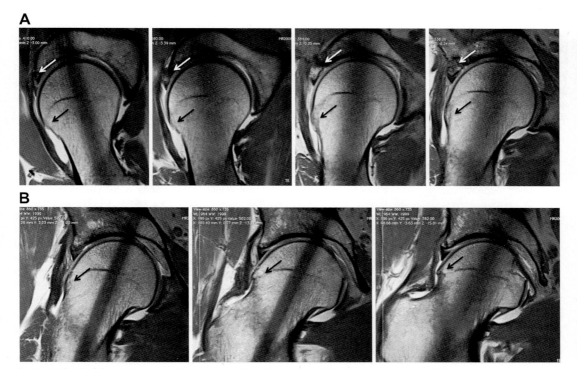

Fig. 3. Multiple (A) radial perpendicular reconstructions around the femoral neck and (B) coronal proton density-weighted MR imaging show loss of femoral head-neck offset from anterior to superior (*white arrows*). The radial reconstructions (A) also show a labral tear with exact anatomic localization at the anterosuperior position (*black arrows*).

head-neck-offset, acetabular depth, and acetabular version. According to Pfirrmann and colleagues,[21] the alpha angle can be measured between an axis parallel to the femoral neck passing through the narrowest portion of the femoral neck and an axis passing through the point at which the head contour passes into the metaphysis (**Fig. 4**). An angle of 55° or more is considered increased and pathologic. An interval of 30° among the radial reformats should be used to assess alpha angle. The offset can be determined based on the method described by Ito and colleagues.[39] It is the quotient of two lines defining the radius of the femoral head and the extension of the head-neck junction, which is defined by point at which the head contour passes into the metaphysis.

Offset is considered as reduced when it has a ratio of 1.2 or less. The acetabular coverage can be measured by assessing the acetabular depth within the axial reformat. The depth is expressed as distance between a line drawn among anterior and posterior acetabular horn and the center of the femoral head (**Fig. 5**). The acetabular version can be measured using two- or three-dimensional axial T1-weighted MR imaging through the acetabular roof as the anterior and posterior rims become apparent. The acetabular version is measured between the distance of the acetabular and posterior rim to the anterior and posterior axis of the pelvis, as shown in **Fig. 6**. **Fig. 7** shows examples of different acetabular versions in patients with cam-type impingement (anteversion), mixed-type impingement (no version), and pincer-type impingement (retroversion).

ASSESSMENT OF THE ACETABULAR LABRUM

For MR imaging assessment of the acetabular labrum, noncontrast techniques and arthrographic techniques are used. Based on comparison studies of different techniques in correlation to intraoperative findings, MR arthrography is more reliable in the diagnosis of acetabular labrum lesions. The contrast material, which is administered into the joint under fluoroscopic control, distends the capsule and allows better separation of the labrum and joint capsule. Labral tears may be better revealed through contrast filling into the clefts of the labrum. The diagnostic sensitivity of MR arthrography ranges from 90%[13] to 71%;[42] however, the interobserver reliability is only moderate.[20,42]

It is not possible to assess the thickness and orientation of the acetabular lesion when a two-dimensional MR imaging technique is used.[13,42] It is an invasive procedure that bears the risk of iatrogenic injury to adjacent neurovascular structures. Regarding staging and grading, most evaluation studies that have been described only determine location (anterosuperior, superolateral, and posterior) and whether a lesion is present.[42] The added grading classification of grades 1 to 3 used by Czerny and colleagues[43] depends on the degree of infiltration of the contrast agent into the acetabular labrum, a description of the tear, and changes of signal intensity, not yet correlated with structural changes of the acetabular labrum. In addition to staging there is still a lack of diagnosis for changes of the surface morphology, such as fibrillation, and changes on the junction between the acetabular cartilage and the acetabular labrum at 1.5 T.

ASSESSMENT OF ACETABULAR CARTILAGE

Compared to the well-established detection of osteonecrosis[44] and evaluation of the acetabular labrum, the role of cartilage lesion assessment is not well defined in the hip.[45] As in acetabular labrum diagnosis, noncontrast techniques and MR arthrography are used. Noncontrast techniques using two- and three-dimensional sequences analyze thickness measurement patterns for detection of the osteoarthritic changes.[46] Reported sensitivity for these measurements is 47% for grade 1 lesions and 49% for grade 2, which reveals low diagnostic efficiency and indicates that these measurements are more useful in follow-up studies.[46] Mintz and colleagues[47] tried to classify cartilage based on cartilage thickness and signal intensity changes according to the Outerbridge Score,[48] but the

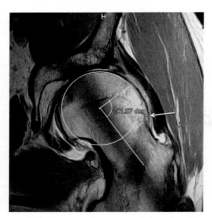

Fig. 4. Radial proton density-weighted reformatted MR imaging shows the assessment of increased alpha-angle (91°) at the anterosuperior position in a cam-type patient (*arrow*).

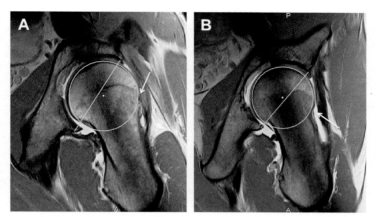

Fig. 5. Assessment of the acetabular depth according to Pfirrmann et al[21] in a radial position. Depth of the acetabulum was defined by the distance between the center of the femoral neck and the line that connects the anterior and posterior acetabular rim. Radial proton density-weighted reformatted MR imaging (A) shows the acetabulum is deeper the patient with pincer FAI and concave head-neck offset (*arrow*) (center of femoral head inside the acetabular fossa; acetabular depth negative) than in (B) the patient with cam FAI and loss of head-neck offset (*arrow*) (center of femoral head outside the acetabular fossa; acetabular depth positive).

results were unreliable. They compared only grades 1 to 3 lesions to no lesion (grade 0) for sensitivity and accuracy. The results are only comparable to thickness measurement studies with the same limitations. With the use of MR arthrography the detection of cartilage lesions could be improved,[20] but the classification within this study was done without staging or grading and the accuracy was only moderate (sensitivity of 47%). The analysis also was limited by low spatial resolution, particularly with regard to separated diagnosis of acetabular and femoral cartilage, restriction to two-dimensional imaging, and low signal-to-noise ratio caused by field strength of only 1.0 T or 1.5 T. High interobserver variability was reported.

Beaulé and colleagues[45] described cartilage delamination using MR arthrography and its correlation with intraoperative findings in four patients. Based on the subdivision of cartilage delamination by Beck and colleagues,[41] it was only possible to detect a cleavage (with a frayed edge). On the other hand, detection of debonding, in which the cartilage appears macroscopically sound but is mobile and simulates a carpet phenomenon that is observed intraoperatively anterosuperiorly in patients with FAI, was not possible. Overall, the cartilage diagnosis in the hip is limited so far, and no reliable staging and grading system has been established. The use of 3.0-T imaging in combination with MR arthrography in the future can overcome these limitations and improve cartilage diagnosis significantly (**Fig. 8**). Distinction of femoral and acetabular cartilage layer remains challenging because the cartilage of the femoroacetabular joint is thin and the

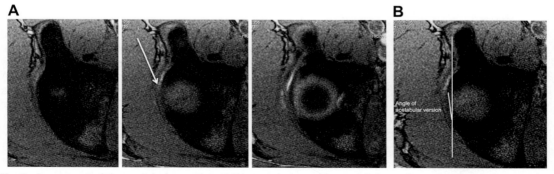

Fig. 6. Assessment of the acetabular version at the acetabular roof on axial three-dimensional, fat-suppressed, 2-mm slice thickness T1-weighted MR imaging shows (A, *left* to *right*) opening of the acetabulum (*arrow*) and (B) measurement of the acetabular version.

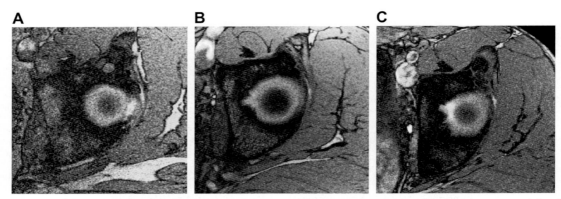

Fig. 7. Examples of acetabular version. Axial three-dimensional, fat-suppressed, 2-mm slice thickness T1-weighted MR imaging shows (*A*) cam-type hip with anteversion (12°), (*B*) mixed-type hip with neutral version (0°), and (*C*) pincer-type hip with retroversion (-9°).

cavity is circumferential, which makes it difficult to differentiate both cartilages from each other.

BIOCHEMICAL IMAGING

Articular cartilage is a highly structured tissue made up of chondrocytes and extracellular matrix composed of water, collagen fibers, negatively charged proteoglycan molecules, and glycosaminoglycans (GAG).[49,50] The collagen fibers network shows a specific arrangement. Fibers are oriented perpendicularly to the bone-cartilage interface within the radial zone (deepest zone); the orientation is oblique within the intermediate zone, and a parallel orientation is seen within the superficial zone. Not only does the orientation of collagen fibers differ between layers of cartilage but so

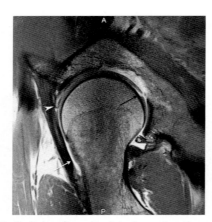

Fig. 8. Radial reformatted turbo spin-echo proton density-weighted MR imaging at 3.0 T in a patient with a cam-type impingement (*white arrow*) shows femoral cartilage lesion (*black arrow*) and intrasubstance lesion of the labrum (*white arrowhead*).

does the concentration of proteoglycans, which is superior within the intermediate zone, and the amount of water, which is greatest within the superficial zone.

During the progress of OA, cartilage constitution is altered (eg, in water content, collagen orientation, and proteoglycan/GAG content).[51] Biochemical MR imaging approaches, such as T1 mapping after gadolinium administration, T2 mapping, T2 magnetization transfer, and diffusion-weighted imaging sensitive for cartilage microstructure and biochemical content, may—in addition to morphologic evaluation—provide further insight into the progress of cartilage changing. One promising technique that was recently developed and applied to daily clinical routine is contrast-enhanced MR imaging, referred to as delayed gadolinium-enhanced MR imaging of cartilage (dGEMRIC). This technique is based on findings that GAG contributes a strong negative charge to the cartilage matrix. If a negatively charged contrast agent such as Gd(DTPA)$^{2-}$ is given time to distribute in the cartilage, it distributes in inverse proportion to the GAG content. By means of gadolinium-enhancement within cartilage and subsequent T1 quantification, T1 values can be used as an index for GAG concentration within cartilage. Because GAG seems to be lost early in cartilage degeneration, this technique may improve OA diagnosis at early stages.[12,52] dGEMRIC has been investigated in vitro,[53–55] in vivo,[56–60] and for follow-up of cartilage repair procedures.[61]

Kim and colleagues[52] investigated the applicability of dGEMRIC in hip dysplasia. In 68 hips (43 patients), the dGEMRIC index and joint space width were compared to radiographically and clinically relevant factors such as pain, severity of dysplasia, and age. The dGEMRIC index correlated significantly with pain (r = −0.50, P<.0001) and lateral center-edge angle as measure of severity of dysplasia (r = 0.52, P<.0001). In contrast, joint space width did not correlate with pain or severity of dysplasia. A statistically significant difference of the dGEMRIC index (P<.0001) among mild, moderate, and severe dysplasia could be observed. The average dGEMRIC index ranged from 570 ms (no dysplasia), to 550 ms (mild dysplasia), to 500 ms (moderate dysplasia), to 420 ms (severe dyplasia).

In another study, a cohort of 47 patients who underwent PAO for hip dysplasia was investigated prospectively.[62] In addition to patient age, radiographic severity of OA, and severity of dysplasia, the dGEMRIC index was evaluated. This study showed that PAO is an expedient tool to reduce pain and ameliorate joint function. Conversely, dGEMRIC was reported as the factor best applicable to identify possible failures of PAO preoperatively. The long-term follow-up of a cohort of patients after PAO with preoperatively low dGEMRIC index showed an increase of the dGEMRIC index postoperatively, which indicated that in defined and reversible stages of cartilage degeneration, OA might be reversible through disease-modifying procedures.[63]

Jessel and colleagues[64] used dGEMRIC to establish a prediction model in 96 hips (74 patients who had symptomatic dysplasia) and identified age, severity of dysplasia, and labral tear as factors associated with significant hip OA. They showed that dGEMRIC might be able to identify patients who would develop significant hip OA and potentially would profit from a salvage procedure such as PAO. This finding was consistent with the other preliminary studies. Concerning the FAI group, Jessel and colleagues described 30 symptomatic patients (37 hips) who were treated with open surgery and were assessed by dGEMRIC preoperatively.[64] The dGEMRIC index (487 ± 70 ms) was significantly lower than in the control group (570 ± 90 ms). A statistically significant correlation could be established between dGEMRIC index and alpha angle (P<.05), although there was no correlation between age or gender of patients. They concluded that dGEMRIC index qualifies as a measure for the severity of cartilage damage in patients with FAI and reflects the severity of anatomic deformity. The results in the group of FAI patients are less consistent than in the group of dysplasia patients, which might be because of the complex nature of the deformity in FAI.

To reduce acquisition time, a gradient-echo approach for T1 mapping instead of multi-spin-echo using a dual flip angle technique to obtain T1 values has been developed. This technique has shown promising results in phantom

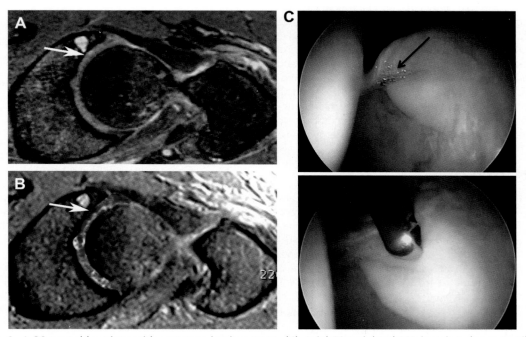

Fig. 9. A 36-year-old patient with cam-type impingement. (A) Axial T2-weighted MR imaging shows possible cartilage damage (arrow). (B) Axial dGEMRIC clearly shows an area of cartilage damage under the cyst (arrow). (C) Arthroscopic views demonstrate the cartilage lesion (arrow).

experiments and in vivo for the evaluation of reparative cartilage within the knee after matrix-associated autologous chondrocyte transplantation at 3.0 T.[61] Besides a significant reduction of scanning time, the great advantage is the possibility to create three-dimensional maps of the hip cartilage that allow for the assessment of the complex special structure of damage pattern in FAI (**Fig. 9**).

SUMMARY

MR imaging represents the best available noninvasive tool for hip evaluation in terms of indication and planning for surgical treatment in OA. It still has limitations in diagnosing cartilage, especially in the early OA stage. The relatively thin cartilage, the spherical joint shape, and narrowness of tissue structures pose logistical difficulties and demand high MR imaging technology standards. So far, MR arthrography using an intra-articular contrast material in combination with radial reconstructed planes is the method of choice for hip assessment in early OA.

FAI has been identified as a cause of early-onset OA in the hip. Therapeutic strategies do exist but only achieve good results in hips without degenerative changes at the early stage. This finding emphasizes the need for diagnostic concepts that enable the detection of early cartilage and labral degeneration. Recent developments in high-resolution isotropic imaging, cartilage-specific MR imaging sequences, local gradient and radio frequency coils, and high field MR systems have improved diagnostic capabilities in terms of signal-to-noise ratio, contrast-to-noise ratio, and shorter acquisition times. In addition to morphologic MR imaging, biochemical MR imaging approaches that characterize cartilage microstructure and biochemical content will contribute to a better understanding of cartilage degeneration.

REFERENCES

1. Felson DT. An update on the pathogenesis and epidemiology of osteoarthritis. Radiol Clin North Am 2004;42(1):1–9, v.
2. Jäger M, Wild A, Westhoff B, et al. Femoroacetabular impingement caused by a femoral osseous head-neck bump deformity: clinical, radiological, and experimental results. J Orthop Sci 2004;9(3):256–63 [in German].
3. Ganz R, Gill TJ, Gautier E, et al. Surgical dislocation of the adult hip a technique with full access to the femoral head and acetabulum without the risk of avascular necrosis. J Bone Joint Surg Br 2001;83(8):1119–24.
4. Ganz R, Parvizi J, Beck M, et al. Femoroacetabular impingement: a cause for osteoarthritis of the hip. Clin Orthop Relat Res 2003;417:112–20.
5. Guanche CA, Bare AA. Arthroscopic treatment of femoroacetabular impingement. Arthroscopy 2006;22(1):95–106.
6. Murphy S, Tannast M, Kim YJ, et al. Debridement of the adult hip for femoroacetabular impingement: indications and preliminary clinical results. Clin Orthop Relat Res 2004;429:178–81.
7. Trousdale RT, Ekkernkamp A, Ganz R, et al. Periacetabular and intertrochanteric osteotomy for the treatment of osteoarthrosis in dysplastic hips. J Bone Joint Surg Am 1995;77(1):73–85.
8. Trumble SJ, Mayo KA, Mast JW. The periacetabular osteotomy: minimum 2 year followup in more than 100 hips. Clin Orthop Relat Res 1999;363:54–63.
9. Eckstein F. Noninvasive study of human cartilage structure by MRI. Methods Mol Med 2004;101:191–217.
10. Eckstein F, Glaser C. Measuring cartilage morphology with quantitative magnetic resonance imaging. Semin Musculoskelet Radiol 2004;8(4):329–53.
11. Koo S, Gold GE, Andriacchi TP. Considerations in measuring cartilage thickness using MRI: factors influencing reproducibility and accuracy. Osteoarthr Cartil 2005;13(9):782–9.
12. Recht MP, Goodwin DW, Winalski CS, et al. MRI of articular cartilage: revisiting current status and future directions. AJR Am J Roentgenol 2005;185(4):899–914.
13. Czerny C, Hofmann S, Neuhold A, et al. Lesions of the acetabular labrum: accuracy of MR imaging and MR arthrography in detection and staging. Radiology 1996;200(1):225–30.
14. Balkissoon A. MR imaging of cartilage: evaluation and comparison of MR imaging techniques. Top Magn Reson Imaging 1996;8(1):57–67.
15. Plotz GM, Brossmann J, Schunke M, et al. Magnetic resonance arthrography of the acetabular labrum: macroscopic and histological correlation in 20 cadavers. J Bone Joint Surg Br 2000;82(3):426–32.
16. Locher S, Werlen S, Leunig M, et al. [MR-Arthrography with radial sequences for visualization of early hip pathology not visible on plain radiographs]. Z Orthop Ihre Grenzgeb 2002;140(1):52–7 [in German].
17. Petersilge CA, Haque MA, Petersilge WJ, et al. Acetabular labral tears: evaluation with MR arthrography. Radiology 1996;200(1):231–5.
18. Petersilge CA. MR arthrography for evaluation of the acetabular labrum. Skeletal Radiol 2001;30(8):423–30.
19. Knuesel PR, Pfirrmann CW, Noetzli HP, et al. MR arthrography of the hip: diagnostic performance of

a dedicated water-excitation 3D double-echo steady-state sequence to detect cartilage lesions. AJR Am J Roentgenol 2004;183(6):1729–35.

20. Schmid MR, Notzli HP, Zanetti M, et al. Cartilage lesions in the hip: diagnostic effectiveness of MR arthrography. Radiology 2003;226(2):382–6.

21. Pfirrmann CW, Mengiardi B, Dora C, et al. Cam and pincer femoroacetabular impingement: characteristic MR arthrographic findings in 50 patients. Radiology 2006;240(3):778–85.

22. Kim YJ, Bixby S, Mamisch TC, et al. Imaging structural abnormalities in the hip joint: instability and impingement as a cause of osteoarthritis. Semin Musculoskelet Radiol 2008;12(4):334–45.

23. Kim YJ. Nonarthroplasty hip surgery for early osteoarthritis. Rheum Dis Clin North Am 2008;34(3): 803–14.

24. Leunig M, Beck M, Dora C, et al. [Femoroacetabular impingement: trigger for the development of osteoarthritis]. Orthopade 2005;35(1):77–84 [in German].

25. Reynolds D, Lucas J, Klaue K. Retroversion of the acetabulum: a cause of hip pain. J Bone Joint Surg Br 1999;81(2):281–8.

26. Dora C, Zurbach J, Hersche O, et al. Pathomorphologic characteristics of posttraumatic acetabular dysplasia. J Orthop Trauma 2000;14(7): 483–9.

27. Dora C, Mascard E, Mladenov K, et al. Retroversion of the acetabular dome after Salter and triple pelvic osteotomy for congenital dislocation of the hip. J Pediatr Orthop B 2002;11(1):34–40.

28. Beck M, Kalhor M, Leunig M, et al. Hip morphology influences the pattern of damage to the acetabular cartilage: femoroacetabular impingement as a cause of early osteoarthritis of the hip. J Bone Joint Surg Br 2005;87(7):1012–8.

29. Kassarjian A, Yoon LS, Belzile E, et al. Triad of MR arthrographic findings in patients with cam-type femoroacetabular impingement. Radiology 2005; 236(2):588–92.

30. Leunig M, Ganz R. [Femoroacetabular impingement: a common cause of hip complaints leading to arthrosis]. Unfallchirurg 2005;108(1):9–17 [in German].

31. MacDonald S, Garbuz D, Ganz R. Clinical evaluation of the symptomatic young adult hip. Semin Arthroplasty 1997;8:3–9.

32. Siebenrock KA, Schoeniger R, Ganz R. Anterior femoro-acetabular impingement due to acetabular retroversion: treatment with periacetabular osteotomy. J Bone Joint Surg Am 2003;85(2):278–86.

33. Kellgren JH, Lawrence JS. Radiological assessment of osteo-arthrosis. Ann Rheum Dis 1957;16: 494–502.

34. Eijer H, Myers SR, Ganz R. Anterior femoroacetabular impingement after femoral neck fractures. J Orthop Trauma 2001;15(7):475–81.

35. Siebenrock KA, Wahab KH, Werlen S, et al. Abnormal extension of the femoral head epiphysis as a cause of cam impingement. Clin Orthop Relat Res 2004;418:54–60.

36. Stulberg SD, Cordell LD, Harris WH, et al. Unrecognized childhood hip disease: a major cause of idiopathic osteoarthritis of the hip. Proceedings of the Third Open Scientific Meeting of the Hip. St Louis (MO); 1975. p. 212–28.

37. Locher S, Werlen S, Leunig M, et al. [Inadequate detectability of early stages of coxarthrosis with conventional roentgen images]. Z Orthop Ihre Grenzgeb 2001;139(1):70–4 [in German].

38. Kubo T, Horii M, Harada Y, et al. Radial-sequence magnetic resonance imaging in evaluation of acetabular labrum. J Orthop Sci 1999;4(5):328–32.

39. Ito K, Minka MA II, Leunig M, et al. Femoroacetabular impingement and the cam-effect: a MRI-based quantitative anatomical study of the femoral head-neck offset. J Bone Joint Surg Br 2001;83(2): 171–6.

40. Leunig M, Werlen S, Ungersbock A, et al. Evaluation of the acetabular labrum by MR arthrography. J Bone Joint Surg Br 1997;79(2):230–4.

41. Beck M, Leunig M, Parvizi J, et al. Anterior femoroacetabular impingement: part II. Midterm results of surgical treatment. Clin Orthop Relat Res 2004; 418:67–73.

42. Keeney JA, Peelle MW, Jackson J, et al. Magnetic resonance arthrography versus arthroscopy in the evaluation of articular hip pathology. Clin Orthop Relat Res 2004;429:163–9.

43. Czerny C, Kramer J, Neuhold A, et al. [Magnetic resonance imaging and magnetic resonance arthrography of the acetabular labrum: comparison with surgical findings]. Rofo 2001;173(8):702–7 [in German].

44. Mont MA, Hungerford DS. Non-traumatic avascular necrosis of the femoral head. J Bone Joint Surg Am 1995;77(3):459–74.

45. Beaulé PE, Zaragoza E, Copelan N. Magnetic resonance imaging with gadolinium arthrography to assess acetabular cartilage delamination: a report of four cases. J Bone Joint Surg Am 2004;86(10): 2294–8.

46. Nishii T, Nakanishi K, Sugano N, et al. Articular cartilage evaluation in osteoarthritis of the hip with MR imaging under continuous leg traction. Magn Reson Imaging 1998;16(8):871–5.

47. Mintz DN, Hooper T, Connell D, et al. Magnetic resonance imaging of the hip: detection of labral and chondral abnormalities using noncontrast imaging. Arthroscopy 2005;21(4):385–93.

48. Outerbridge RE. The etiology of chondromalacia patellae. J Bone Joint Surg Br 1961;43:752–7.

49. Poole AR, Kojima T, Yasuda T, et al. Composition and structure of articular cartilage: a template for

tissue repair. Clin Orthop Relat Res 2001;(Suppl 391):S26–33.

50. Cova M, Toffanin R. MR microscopy of hyaline cartilage: current status. Eur Radiol 2002;12(4): 814–23.

51. Venn M, Maroudas A. Chemical composition and swelling of normal and osteoarthrotic femoral head cartilage. I. Chemical composition. Ann Rheum Dis 1977;36(2):121–9.

52. Kim YJ, Jaramillo D, Millis MB, et al. Assessment of early osteoarthritis in hip dysplasia with delayed gadolinium-enhanced magnetic resonance imaging of cartilage. J Bone Joint Surg Am 2003;85(10): 1987–92.

53. Woertler K, Buerger H, Moeller J, et al. Patellar articular cartilage lesions: in vitro MR imaging evaluation after placement in gadopentetate dimeglumine solution. Radiology 2004;230(3):768–73.

54. Mlynarik V, Trattnig S, Huber M, et al. The role of relaxation times in monitoring proteoglycan depletion in articular cartilage. J Magn Reson Imaging 1999;10(4):497–502.

55. Bashir A, Gray ML, Burstein D. Gd-DTPA2- as a measure of cartilage degradation. Magn Reson Med 1996;36(5):665–73.

56. Bashir A, Gray ML, Boutin RD, et al. Glycosaminoglycan in articular cartilage: in vivo assessment with delayed Gd(DTPA) (2-)-enhanced MR imaging. Radiology 1997;205(2):551–8.

57. Burstein D, Velyvis J, Scott KT, et al. Protocol issues for delayed Gd(DTPA) (2-)-enhanced MRI (dGEMRIC) for clinical evaluation of articular cartilage. Magn Reson Med 2001;45(1):36–41.

58. Tiderius C, Olsson L, de Verdier H, et al. Gd-DTPA2-enhanced MRI of femoral knee cartilage: a dose response study in healthy volunteers. Magn Reson Med 2001;46:1067–71.

59. Tiderius CJ, Olsson LE, Leander P, et al. Delayed gadolinium-enhanced MRI of cartilage (dGEMRIC) in early knee osteoarthritis. Magn Reson Med 2003;49(3):488–92.

60. Williams A, Gillis A, McKenzie C, et al. Glycosaminoglycan distribution in cartilage as determined by delayed gadolinium-enhanced MRI of cartilage (dGEMRIC): potential clinical applications. AJR Am J Roentgenol 2004;182(1):167–72.

61. Trattnig S, Marlovits S, Gebetsroither S, et al. Three-dimensional delayed gadolinium-enhanced MRI of cartilage (dGEMRIC) for in vivo evaluation of reparative cartilage after matrix-associated autologous chondrocyte transplantation at 3.0T: preliminary results. J Magn Reson Imaging 2007; 26(4):974–82.

62. Cunningham T, Jessel R, Zurakowski D, et al. Delayed gadolinium-enhanced magnetic resonance imaging of cartilage to predict early failure of Bernese periacetabular osteotomy for hip dysplasia. J Bone Joint Surg Am 2006;88(7):1540–8.

63. Jessel R, Zurakowski D, Zilkens C, et al. Radiographic and patient factors associated with pre-radiographic osteoarthritis in hip dysplasia. J Bone Joint Surg Am 2009;91(5):1120–9.

64. Jessel R, Zilkens C, Tiderius C, et al. Assessment of osteoarthritis in hips with femoroacetabular impingement using delayed gadolinium enhanced MRI of cartilage. JMRM, in press.

MRI in Dementia

Reinhold Schmidt, MD[a],[*], Daniel Havas, MSc[b],
Stefan Ropele, PhD[a], Christian Enzinger, MD[a],
Franz Fazekas, MD[a]

KEYWORDS

- MRI • Cognitive disorder • Alzheimer's disease
- Imaging • Dementia

The incidence of both cognitive disorders and dementing illnesses is rising in our ageing population. As a consequence, imaging modalities are becoming increasingly important for differential diagnosis and monitoring of disease progression in daily clinical practice and for use as surrogate markers in treatment trials. Such technologies as conventional CT, MRI, proton magnetic resonance spectroscopy (MRS), positron emission tomography (PET), and single photon emission CT are currently being applied for this purpose.

Additionally, diffusion-weighted imaging, diffusion tensor imaging (DTI), perfusion-weighted MRI, magnetic transfer imaging, and a combined visualization of different modalities (eg, MRI/PET) have been proposed for in vivo tracing of biomarkers. We provide a review of original papers as well as published review articles on the role of MRI in various cognitive disorders.

In general, every measurement method runs through different stages of development and validation before it can be used as a routine tool (**Fig. 1**). Along these lines, we will assess the usefulness of MRI for early diagnosis, for monitoring of disease progression, and for use as a surrogate marker for documenting drug efficacy in therapeutic clinical studies.

ALZHEIMER'S DISEASE

Conceptually, treatment of Alzheimer's disease should start early in the disease, ideally in a clinically presymptomatic stage, before widespread synaptic and neuronal loss has occurred. This approach would require tools that already pick up with high sensitivity subtle Alzheimer's disease–related brain changes.

Structural MRI

Methods to assess brain volume changes in Alzheimer's disease patients include voxel-based morphometry or the voxel-based specific regional analysis system for Alzheimer's disease involving transformation to a normalized brain,[1–5] cortical pattern matching,[6–8] and brain boundary shift integral measurements.[9] These techniques make it possible for clinicians to discriminate between the magnitude of progression of brain atrophy in normal ageing and the higher rates of volume loss observed in Alzheimer's disease. Brain boundary shift integral measurements might additionally be useful for assessing subtle regional volume changes. Such assessments have been helpful for demonstrating significant drug effects even in relatively small patient groups.[9]

Structural MRI has also been used in several studies to predict progression from mild cognitive impairment to Alzheimer's disease. Other MRI measurement techniques employed in the assessment of Alzheimer's disease are manual and semi-automated measurements of regional atrophy in specific regions of interest (**Fig. 2**). Studies using this approach have focused primarily on the hippocampus and the medial temporal lobes, yet the corpus callosum has also been shown to be vulnerable to Alzheimer's disease–related brain atrophy.[10] In this context, it is of note that hippocampal atrophy in MRI is strongly related to the histologic finding of neuronal loss[11] and to the

This article originally appeared in *Neurologic Clinics of North America* 2009;27(1):221–36.
[a] Department of Neurology, Medical University of Graz, Auenbruggerplatz 22, A-8036 Graz, Austria
[b] JSW CNS Research Graz, Parkring 12, 8074 Grambach, Austria
* Corresponding author.
E-mail address: reinhold.schmidt@meduni-graz.at (R. Schmidt).

Magn Reson Imaging Clin N Am 18 (2010) 121–132
doi:10.1016/j.mric.2009.09.009

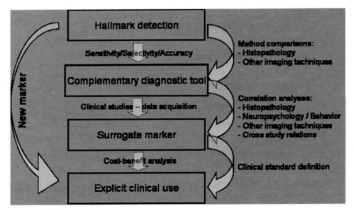

Fig. 1. Stages of a measurement method from detection of a disease hallmark to the explicit clinical use of the technique for diagnosis.

severity of Alzheimer's disease pathology,[12,13] and that hippocampal atrophy correlates with cognitive impairment.[14–16]

In even earlier disease stages, tracking shrinkage of the entorhinal cortex may also be useful for predicting Alzheimer's disease.[17–19] Atrophy rates have been reported to be larger in entorhinal cortex than in the hippocampus (~7% per year versus ~6% per year),[20] but difficulties in unambiguously defining this brain structure on the basis of landmarks make entorhinal cortex measurements highly variable.[21] In general, manual regions-of-interest measurements are both operator-dependent and labor-intensive.

Both regions-of-interest measurements and automated measurement approaches assessing hippocampal volume changes have already proven meaningful and feasible in clinical trials. However, a recent study suggested that whole brain atrophy measures might even be more closely related to clinical and cognitive scores (Mini-Mental State Examination, Dementia Rating Scale, Clinical Dementia Rating) than to the annual change in hippocampal and entorhinal cortex volume.[22]

MRI indices enable assessments of processes linked to disease progression with sensitivity far beyond what would be detectable on the basis of cognitive and clinical scores. Consequently, trials incorporating such MRI markers require fewer subjects, which in turn makes it easier to conduct proof-of-concept studies[9,22–24] (for a more detailed review on quantitative MRI of different brain regions see Ramani and colleagues[25]). As for potential applications of MRI in related clinical trials, a consensus report of the Alzheimer's Association[2] identified two main areas: (1) for supplementary exclusion and for more stringent stratification criteria to define a homogeneous study population, and (2) for strong correlation with clinical symptoms and neuropathology at earlier stages of the disease and the possibility to trace the progression of the disease.

Nonetheless, because of its lack in specificity, structural MRI cannot currently be considered an

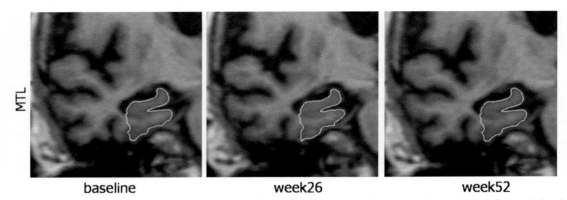

baseline   week26   week52

Fig. 2. Measurement of medial temporal lobe (MTL) atrophy using manual segmentation on coronal T1-weighted scans.

established diagnostic tool on an individual basis. Also, for research purposes, standardized acquisition schemes, procedures for regular checks on scanner quality, and standardized protocols for processing and analyzing MRI data in dementia need to be developed.[21]

Diffusion-Weighted Imaging and Diffusion-Tensor Imaging

Several studies have used the apparent diffusion coefficient or diffusion characteristics derived from DTI to gain information on demyelinization and axonal loss in the context of Alzheimer's disease. The apparent diffusion coefficient provides information on the overall mobility of tissue water while DTI provides additional directional information on this diffusion process.

White matter changes of the brain can be associated with a net loss of barriers restricting the motion of water molecules and tissue anisotropy of white matter.[25] Histopathology of Alzheimer's disease brains also shows partial loss of myelin, axons, and oligodendrial cells, and reactive gliosis in the white matter.[26] However, diminished fractional anisotropy in normal-appearing white matter may also be caused by other factors, such as membrane damage, edema, reduced axoplasmatic flow related to cytoskeletal dysfunction, and alterations of ion or fluid homeostasis.[27,28] Several studies set out to define in vivo estimates of Alzheimer's disease–related structural changes by using DTI techniques and measuring increased apparent diffusion coefficient and decreased fractional anisotropy in the temporal lobe white matter,[29] the hippocampus,[30] the posterior white matter,[31] and the corpus callosum of patients with mild to moderate Alzheimer's disease.[32] Another approach found a correlation between the lattice index and the Mini-Mental State Examination score in the splenium of the corpus callosum.[33] Together, these measures may reflect very early biophysical alterations linked to the progression of Alzheimer's disease, although an overlap between patients and groups of healthy controls also has been noted.[34]

Albeit not yet validated to the extent of structural MRI, both diffusion-weighted imaging and DTI appear as promising candidates with potential to support an imaging diagnosis of Alzheimer's disease.[21] A strong correlation between apparent diffusion coefficient and Mini-Mental State Examination scores underlines a possible role for clinical use.[32] However, some technical issues still must be resolved regarding the optimum diffusion time and the optimal strength of the diffusion gradients (b values). Generally, the use of higher b values has been shown to provide a better lesion-to–normal tissue contrast and a better contrast-to-noise ratio in Alzheimer's disease.[35] Magnetic resonance units with more powerful gradients should, therefore, be able to markedly improve the signal-to-noise ratio and thus allow higher spatial resolution with less susceptibility effects.[25] However, standardization and quality assurance procedures are still lacking, although endeavors to overcome these problems on different scanner systems have already been proposed.[36]

Magnetization Transfer Ratio

Magnetization transfer imaging can provide pathophysiological information on brain structure on a microscopic level. This notion is supported by magnetic resonance histopathological studies demonstrating a correlation between the magnetization transfer ratio (MTR) and the extent of histologically defined demyelinization and axon loss.[37,38]

MTR has rarely been used so far to assess Alzheimer's disease. Further studies are needed to determine the effectiveness of this technique for the clinical diagnosis of Alzheimer's disease and to assess its value for monitoring disease progression. However, preliminary studies suggest that MTR holds promise as a tool for early diagnosis of Alzheimer's disease with an even higher specificity for neurodegeneration compared with other surrogate markers. This notion is supported by the observation that MTR in the hippocampus was found to be decreased in Alzheimer's disease patients[39] and by the detection of MTR changes in gray and white matter in mild cognitive impairment subjects who did not yet show notable brain volume change.[40] MTR changes therefore might precede gross regional atrophy.[41]

An additional future application for magnetic transfer imaging could be the detection of microglia surrounding neuritic plaques in Alzheimer's disease, as suggested by a 3-T MRI study. Song and colleagues[42] were able to detect exogenously administered microglia noninvasively in rat brains using magnetic transfer imaging, and corroborated their findings by histopathology. Because modern Alzheimer's disease therapy also aims to affect immunoreactive processes, such as microglia activation in the brain, such a noninvasive way to monitor the potential effects of anti-inflammatory therapies in clinical trials could turn out to be particularly useful.

Magnetic Resonance Spectroscopy

MRS provides biochemical information on the metabolism of the brain. Using MRS, differences in N-acetyl aspartate (NAA) and myoinositol levels between Alzheimer's disease patients and normal ageing persons have been demonstrated. NAA is thought to represent the neuroal dysfunction and loss, whereas myoinositol is deemed a marker of gliosis (**Fig. 3**).[43]

The combination of volumetric and spectroscopic magnetic resonance appears superior in terms of sensitivity and specificity to either measure alone.[44] Longitudinal MRS revealed correlations between NAA, choline, and cognitive function in clinical trials on cholinergic agents.[45–47] This leads some to speculate that MRS might serve to connect traditional measures of brain structure with traditional measures of brain function.[48]

Functional MRI

Functional MRI allows clinicians to noninvasively study changes in neural activity associated after an experimental paradigm (eg, during the performance of a cognitive task in the scanner). Clinical applications of this method mostly rely on the measurement of the so-called "blood oxygenation level–dependent" (BOLD) response, thereby providing a composite surrogate signal of neural activity as defined by the neurovascular coupling hypothesis.[49]

Regarding functional measurements in the field of Alzheimer's disease, functional MRI conceptually offers the opportunity to study deviations from normal functional processes on a neural system level, ideally and—like other functional techniques, such as PET—even before morphologic changes related to the disease process become detectable by other methods. Such study might finally lead to a definition of "functional phenotypes" of Alzheimer's disease patients, with individually differential risks for conversion to overt clinical disease, defined by a differential capacity to neural plasticity involved in the partial limitation of the clinical expression of the disease process.

Indeed, in cases with a clinical diagnosis of probable Alzheimer's disease, functional MRI studies assessing the neural response to different memory tasks relatively consistently reported decreased hippocampal and parahippocampal activation compared with age-matched elderly normal controls.[50–53] However, other brain regions also have been implicated as relevant in this context. Furthermore, in general, the number of patients studied was small (usually fewer than 10 subjects per study) and different functional MRI tasks have been used (eg, divided attention, subtraction, picture or face encoding, watching novel versus previously learned scenes or items, visual search tasks).[51,54–58] Together with the variability in the BOLD response, this might explain some of the inconsistencies in the findings among different studies.

However, preliminary studies suggested that functional MRI might prove particularly useful in short-term, early proof of concept studies, given its potential to evaluate acute und subacute effects of medications on neural activity. This notion is supported by the observation that cholinergic enhancement with a single dose of rivastigmine led to an increase in functional MRI activity both in the fusiform face area during face encoding and in the prefrontal cortex during a working memory task in subjects with mild Alzheimer's disease.[51]

Functional MRI therefore holds great promise to elucidate mechanisms of functional cortical and

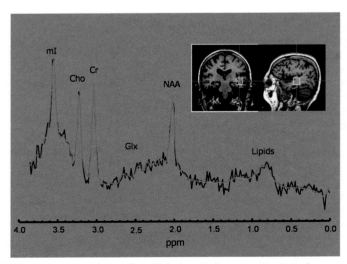

Fig. 3. Single voxel MRS in the temporal lobe of an Alzheimer's disease patient. An increased level of myoinositol (mI) concentration and a decreased NAA peak are noted. These two characteristics are thought to reflect gliosis and axonal dysfunction/loss. Cho, choline; Cr, creatine; Glx, glutamate; ppm, parts per million.

subcortical reorganization associated with the progression of the disease, as well as to allow clinicians to visualize how drugs modulate functional networks and potentially to define pharmacologic responders. However, using functional MRI in cohorts of demented or even more cognitively compromised subjects poses obvious challenges, especially regarding issues of reproducibility in longitudinal designs and, even more basically, concerning the applicability and feasibility of more complicated and refined functional MRI paradigms. To overcome some of these problems, resting state functional MRI has been proposed. This enables the study of functional default networks without the necessity for adhering to given tasks. However, the value of this approach in a clinical setting has yet to be determined.[59,60] Future functional MRI studies will certainly also need to address how much biochemical, (micro)-vascular, and morphologic changes associated with the disease process itself potentially affect or confound the surrogate signal under investigation.

Amyloid Imaging

Because Alzheimer's disease is characterized by aggregates of β-amyloid peptides forming senile plaques, in vivo imaging of these pathologic hallmarks would enable clinicians to monitor progression and effectiveness of amyloid-targeted therapies, such as vaccination, secretase inhibitors, or beta sheet breaker compounds.[61]

The first promising data about the use of such imaging came from studies with transgenic mice that harbor mutated forms of the human amyloid precursor protein as found in familial inherited Alzheimer's disease.[62–67] Both PET and MRI were used to assess the amyloid load noninvasively. The theoretic advantages of MRI over PET are its superior spatial resolution, its noninvasive nature, as well as the more widespread availability of MRI scanners compared with PET machines. Imaging strategies varied among the studies from ligand-based detection[64,66] to the use of the average MRI signal to gain information on the plaques.[63] The latter approach often has been combined with an optimized pulse sequence to be able to visualize individual plaques.[22] Using such an approach, the regional averaged MRI signal has been found to be different between transgenic and nontransgenic littermates[68] and refined pulse sequences have allowed measurements of signal changes corresponding spatially and quantitatively to individual plaques. However, concerns have been raised that these methods might be insensitive to plaques containing little or no iron. Furthermore, iron can be additionally

found not only in plaques but also in microhemorrhages, which also occur in Alzheimer's disease brains. Together, this furthered the renascence of ligand-based approaches, which are less likely to provide misleading findings.

The first ligands used in this context—gadolinium or iron nanoparticles binding to Aβ—necessitated the coadministration of mannitol to open the blood-brain barrier. Most recently, substances with potential to overcome this limitation have been proposed. Thus, ^{19}fluorine (^{19}F) has been shown to penetrate the brain after intravenous injection, at least in transgenic mice. While mannitol makes the application in humans difficult because of the reasons given, ^{19}fluorine does not inherit this intrinsic problem.

Skovronsky and colleagues[69] cross-correlated ^{19}F-containing (E,E)-1-fluoro-2,5-bis(3-hydroxy-carbonly-4-hydroxy)styrylbenzene (FSB) MRI maps with FSB binding in postmortem histologic slices, confirming this approach to be a reliable in vivo indicator of amyloid plaques and neurofibrillary tangles. Other researchers detected plaques in T2-weighted images and confirmed their results in Congo-red stained slices histopathologically.[67]

The main technical advances achieved over the last few years concerning MRI scanners were the increase of the magnetic field strength and the availability of high-performance gradient technology and array coils.[21] Together, these achievements in concert with further research efforts could finally result in the in vivo visualization of amyloid plaques in humans using MRI. Compared to other approaches, amyloid imaging will have the advantage of higher specificity because this pathology is typical in Alzheimer's disease dementia. Future studies should have three goals: (1) the identification of ligands to amyloid plaques safe for use in human studies, (2) exploration of approaches for detecting soluble Aβ species, and (3) determination of methods specific to the second hallmark of Alzheimer's disease, the neurofibrillary tangles.[70]

VASCULAR DEMENTIA

Vascular dementia is a heterogeneous disorder. Various subtypes can be defined clinically. These include poststroke dementia, multi-infarct dementia, dementia with strategically located infarctions, and, the most common type, subcortical ischemic vascular dementia, with white matter lesions and lacunes as hallmark lesions (**Fig. 4**). A first attempt to define imaging correlates has been provided in the NINDS-AIREN (National Institute of Neurological Disorders and Stroke–Association

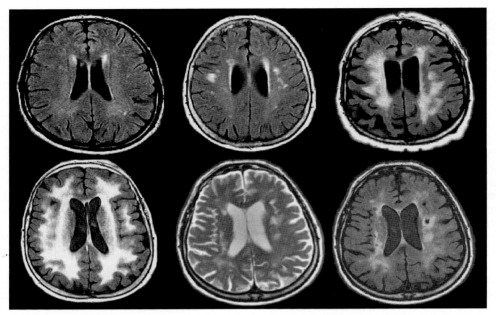

Fig. 4. The spectrum of small vessel disease–related brain changes in MRI: white matter lesions ranging from punctate foci (*upper left*) to extensive confluent abnormalities (*lower left*) and lacunar infarcts (*lower right*).

Internationale pour la Recherche et l'Enseignment en Neurosciences) criteria.[71] Yet, in a study on inter-rater reliability of these criteria, it became clear that they are very complex and not suited for use by inexperienced raters.[72]

The radiological criteria included in the NINDS-AIREN criteria for vascular dementia have suboptimal reproducibility. Use of operational criteria improves agreement to acceptable levels, but only in experienced readers. **Box 1** gives an overview of these operational criteria.

One of the most important findings in the context of vascular dementia during the last few years was the observation of a rapid progression of confluent white matter lesions, which several studies have consistently described.[72,73] These lesions were found to almost double in volume over an observational period of 6 years.[74] This has led to the hypothesis that progression of white matter lesions might be used as a surrogate marker in clinical trials of vascular cognitive impairment and vascular dementia.[75] This thinking follows the line of studies in multiple sclerosis where MRI also serves as a surrogate marker of disease progression and therapeutic efficacy.

The advent of new MRI techniques, including DTI, magnetization transfer imaging, advanced MRS, and functional imaging methods, such as functional MRI, single photon emission CT, or PET, promise further refinements in the characterization of brain lesions beyond that possible with conventional MRI.[76] These methods have the potential to demonstrate interruptions of white matter fiber tracks and to determine the severity of tissue destruction and axonal damage in the area of a given lesion but also in white matter that appears normal. These methods will likely allow the study of remote effects of lesions in different brain areas and the evaluation of brain plasticity compensating for lesion-related detrimental effects. The studies on DTI are most advanced and, in patients with cerebral autosomal dominant arteriopathy with subcortical infarcts and leukoencephalopathy (CADASIL), there exist correlations between changes of DTI histogram metrics and clinical measures over time. Therefore, it is speculated that DTI histograms may also be used as an adjunct outcome measure in future therapeutic trials.[72,77]

Several studies have demonstrated that the association between progression of white matter damage and cognitive decline is complex.[1] Measuring the increase of leukoaraiosis volume in isolation will probably not suffice to fully determine treatment response in trials on subcortical vascular dementia. It is likely that assessment of other morphologic expressions of the disease, including changes in brain volume and in normal-appearing white matter on standard MRI sequences, will be mandatory and will increase our pathophysiological understanding of this widely understudied disease.

Box 1
Operational criteria that increase reproducibility of NINDS-AIREN criteria for vascular dementia to an acceptable level in experienced readers

Topography

Large-vessel stroke: Large-vessel stroke is an infarction defined as a parenchymal defect in an arterial territory involving the cortical gray matter.

Anterior cerebral artery: Only bilateral anterior cerebral artery infarcts are sufficient to meet the NINDS-AIREN criteria.

Posterior cerebral artery: Infarcts in the posterior cerebral artery territory can be included only when they involve the following regions:

Paramedian thalamic infarction: The infarct includes the cortical gray matter of the temporal/occipital lobe and extends into the paramedian part (defined as extending to the third ventricle) of the thalamus; the extension may be limited to the gliotic rim of the infarct that surrounds the parenchymal defect.

Inferior medial temporal lobe lesions

Association areas: A middle cerebral artery infarction needs to involve the following regions:

Parietotemporal: The infarct involves both the parietal and temporal lobes (eg, angular gyrus).

Temporo-occipital: The infarct involves both the temporal and occipital lobes.

Watershed carotid territories: A watershed infarction is defined as an infarct in the watershed area between the middle cerebral artery and posterior cerebral artery or the middle cerebral artery and anterior cerebral artery in the following regions:

Superior frontal region

Parietal region

Small-vessel disease

Ischemic pathology resulting from occlusion of small perforating arteries may manifest itself as lacunes or white matter lesions. Lacune is defined as a lesion greater than 2 mm in diameter with cerebrospinal fluid–like intensity on all sequences on MRI (water density on CT) surrounded by white matter or subcortical gray matter. Care should be taken not to include Virchow-Robin spaces, which typically occur at the vertex and around the anterior commisure near the substantia perforata. Ischemic white matter lesions are defined as circumscribed abnormalities with high signal on T2-weighted images not following cerebrospinal fluid signal (mildly hypodense compared with surrounding tissue on CT) with a minimum diameter of 2 mm.

Multiple basal ganglia and frontal white matter lacunes: Criteria are met when at least two lacunes in the basal ganglia region (including thalamus and internal capsule) and at least two lacunes in the frontal white matter are present.

Extensive periventricular white matter lesions: Lesions in the white matter abutting the ventricles and extending irregularly into the deep white matter, or deep/subcortical white matter lesions. Smooth caps and bands by themselves are not sufficient. Gliotic areas surrounding large-vessel strokes should not be included here.

Bilateral thalamic lesions: To meet the criteria, at least one lesion in each thalamus should be present.

Severity

Large-vessel disease of the dominant hemisphere: If there is a large-vessel infarct as defined above, it has to be in the dominant hemisphere to meet the criteria. In the absence of clinical information, the left hemisphere is considered dominant.

Bilateral large-vessel hemispheric strokes: One of the infarcts should involve an area listed under topography but is in the nondominant hemisphere, while the infarct in the dominant hemisphere does not meet the topography criteria.

Leukoencephalopathy involving at least one fourth of the total white matter: Extensive white matter lesions are considered to involve one fourth of the total white matter when they are confluent (grade 3 in the Age-Related White-Matter Changes [ARWMC] scale) in at least two regions of the ARWMC scale and beginning confluent (grade 2 in the ARWMC scale) in two other regions. A lesion is considered confluent when greater than 20 mm in diameter, or consists of two or more smaller lesions fused by more than connecting bridges.

Fulfillment of radiological criteria for probable vascular dementia

Large-vessel disease: Both the topography and severity criteria should be met (a lesion must be scored in at least one subsection of both topography and severity).

Small-vessel disease: for white-matter lesions, both the topography and severity criteria should be met (a lesion must be scored in at least one subsection of both topography and severity); for multiple lacunes and bilateral thalamic lesions, the topography criterion alone is sufficient.

FRONTOTEMPORAL DEMENTIA

The clinical syndrome of frontotemporal dementia is often associated with tau- or ubiquitin-positive (TDP-43 variant) pathology, but distinctive histo-pathological hallmarks are lacking (dementia lacking distinctive histopathology [DLDH]). Patients develop behavioral as well as executive incompetence related to frontal lobe dysfunction. A specific treatment is not yet available.

Longitudinal structural MRI studies have revealed progressive frontal or temporal lobe atrophy.[78] Although some of these features, like peri-Sylvian atrophy, have been associated with phonologic and syntactic language components[79] affected in nonfluent aphasia, neither structural (MRI) nor functional (hexamethyly-propyleneamine–single photon emission CT) measures can currently be regarded as adequate surrogate markers.

Currently, the value of MRI in this setting lies in the differential diagnosis by detecting hallmarks more typical of other dementia types. Researchers still need to determine if high-field MRI and MRS have the power to identify the additional structural and metabolic changes that are more characteristic for frontotemporal dementia. For now, about the only identifiable hallmark considered typical of frontotemporal dementia is the so-called "knife-edged sign" (**Fig. 5**).

HUNTINGTON'S DISEASE

Huntington's disease represents a monogenic neurodegenerative disorder caused by an extended trinucleotide repeat (CAG), which is clinically characterized by progressive uncontrolled movements and by neuropsychiatric and cognitive disturbances. Both structural and functional MRI studies have been summarized in a recent review.[80]

Further work is needed to determine the precise relationship between cognitive and regional volume changes in Huntington's disease to define potential surrogate markers for the clinical onset of the disease and its progression. So far, functional MRI has been especially important in enhancing the pathophysiological understanding of Huntington's disease by emphasizing the specific functional role of the striatum and basal ganglia in the disease process. As caveats, Montoya and colleagues[80] listed differences in the design and analyses approaches used in these studies and also discussed the role of concomitant vascular changes in the interference with the metabolic response to neural activity assessed by functional neuroimaging techniques (functional MRI, PET).

To overcome these limitations, a combined application of several imaging techniques has been proposed[81] to provide parallel information on metabolic, functional, and neuroanatomical alterations as well as on the temporal changes in these parameters, and then to correlate these findings with histologic postmortem studies.[80] From such an approach, an improved understanding of cognitive dysfunction in Huntington's disease can be expected soon.

PSYCHIATRIC DISORDERS WITH COGNITIVE DISTURBANCES

Up to now, MRI has rarely been used in the investigation of psychiatric disorders, although a recent study in autistic patients provides an example for its general usefulness in this field.[82] Here, an atypically diffuse connectivity between the caudate nuclei and the cerebral cortex was interpreted as compatible with developmental differences in the subcortico-cortical and cortico-cortical connectivities between autistic and normal subjects. In addition, cortical thickness was found to be increased using structural MRI in autistic patients. However, these measures were not correlated to clinical autism scales. Nonetheless, such findings shed some light on possible structural correlates of autism, indicating that autism might be a developmental disorder of the central nervous system.

Further, a functional MRI study of emotional processing in mood disorders showed distinct differences in the patterns of response to emotional expressions in prefrontal and subcortical regions between patients diagnosed with major depression and those diagnosed with bipolar disorder.[83]

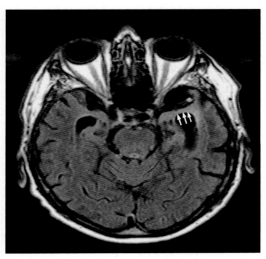

Fig. 5. The so-called "knife-edge sign" (*arrows*) as an imaging hallmark considered typical for the frontotemporal dementia type.

Researchers need to determine whether these findings could also assist in finding a correct diagnosis before the occurrence of a clinically manifest manic episode.[84]

AIDS DEMENTIA COMPLEX AND OTHER RARE DEMENTING DISORDERS OF THE CENTRAL NERVOUS SYSTEM

A general problem in rare forms of dementia is the lack of sufficient study data for the validation of MRI measures. However, using MRS, rather characteristic metabolite changes have been reported for HIV-positive patients,[85,86] These metabolic patterns, therefore, offer some potential to assist in the differential diagnosis and also appear to potentially be useful for monitoring the disease process in therapeutic trials.

SUMMARY

With increasing availability of MRI scanners and continuous development of more sophisticated magnetic resonance pulse sequences, better training of technical staff, and increasing experience of raters, as well as the availability of easily usable and more refined imaging software, MRI has been established as an important diagnostic and scientific tool for studying dementia over the last decades. Imaging at higher magnetic field strengths also has markedly improved the resolution of MRI, and combinations with functional techniques, such as PET, have offered additional insights into disease-related tissue changes and functional processes in the brain in vivo.

Similar to the evolution witnessed in the field of Alzheimer's disease, where MRI techniques have already become a valuable tool to monitor disease activity, MRI could similarly pave the way to improvements in diagnosing several other cognitive disorders and in the understanding of underlying pathophysiological changes of the brain. Defining clinical standards and precisely assuring quality will help to improve the quality of imaging data for future use in clinical multicenter trials. Such trials will ultimately form the foundation for the use of MRI measures of morphology and function as validated surrogate markers of disease progression, and will finally lead to tests to measure the effects of treatment.

REFERENCES

1. Ashburner J, Friston KJ. Voxel-based morphometry—the methods. Neuroimage 2000;11:805–21.
2. Goto M, Aoki S, Abe O, et al. [Examination of an imaging method in early Alzheimer disease diagnosis support system (VSRAD)]. Nippon Hoshasen Gijutsu Gakkai Zasshi 2006;62:1353–8.
3. Karas GB, Burton EJ, Rombouts SA, et al. A comprehensive study of gray matter loss in patients with Alzheimer's disease using optimized voxel-based morphometry. Neuroimage 2003;18(4):895–907.
4. Karas GB, Scheltens P, Rombouts SA, et al. Global and local gray matter loss in mild cognitive impairment and Alzheimer's disease. Neuroimage 2004; 23:708–16.
5. Thompson PM, Hayashi KM, de Zubicaray G, et al. Dynamics of gray matter loss in Alzheimer's disease. J Neurosci 2003;23:994–1005.
6. Csernansky JG, Wang L, Joshi S, et al. Early DAT is distinguished from aging by high-dimensional mapping of the hippocampus. Dementia of the Alzheimer type. Neurology 2000;55:1636–43.
7. Thompson PM, Mega MS, Woods RP, et al. Cortical change in Alzheimer's disease detected with a disease-specific population-based brain atlas. Cereb Cortex 2001;11:1–16.
8. Thompson PM, Moussai J, Zohoori S, et al. Cortical variability and asymmetry in normal aging and Alzheimer's disease. Cereb Cortex 1998;8:492–509.
9. Fox NC, Cousens S, Scahill R, et al. Using serial registered brain magnetic resonance imaging to measure disease progression in Alzheimer disease: power calculations and estimates of sample size to detect treatment effects. Arch Neurol 2000;57: 339–44.
10. Teipel SJ, Bayer W, Alexander GE, et al. Progression of corpus callosum atrophy in Alzheimer disease. Arch Neurol 2002;59:243–8.
11. Goncharova II, Dickerson BC, Stoub TR, et al. MRI of human entorhinal cortex: a reliable protocol for volumetric measurement. Neurobiol Aging 2001;22: 737–45.
12. Gosche KM, Mortimer JA, Smith CD, et al. Hippocampal volume as an index of Alzheimer neuropathology: findings from the Nun Study. Neurology 2002;58:1476–82.
13. Jack CR Jr, Dickson DW, Parisi JE, et al. Antemortem MRI findings correlate with hippocampal neuropathology in typical aging and dementia. Neurology 2002;58:750–7.
14. de Leon MJ, George AE, Golomb J, et al. Frequency of hippocampal formation atrophy in normal aging and Alzheimer's disease. Neurobiol Aging 1997;18: 1–11.
15. Toledo-Morrell L, Dickerson B, Sullivan MP, et al. Hemispheric differences in hippocampal volume predict verbal and spatial memory performance in patients with Alzheimer's disease. Hippocampus 2000;10:136–42.
16. Uotani C, Sugimori K, Kobayashi K. Association of minimal thickness of the medial temporal lobe with hippocampal volume, maximal and minimal

hippocampal length: volumetric approach with horizontal magnetic resonance imaging scans for evaluation of a diagnostic marker for neuroimaging of Alzheimer's disease. Psychiatry Clin Neurosci 2006;60:319–26.

17. Rose SE, McMahon KL, Janke AL, et al. Diffusion indices on magnetic resonance imaging and neuropsychological performance in amnestic mild cognitive impairment. J Neurol Neurosurg Psychiatry 2006;77:1122–8.

18. Stoub TR, Bulgakova M, Leurgans S, et al. MRI predictors of risk of incident Alzheimer disease: a longitudinal study. Neurology 2005;64:1520–4.

19. Stoub TR, deToledo-Morrell L, Stebbins GT, et al. Hippocampal disconnection contributes to memory dysfunction in individuals at risk for Alzheimer's disease. Proc Natl Acad Sci U S A 2006;103: 10041–5.

20. Du AT, Schuff N, Kramer JH, et al. Higher atrophy rate of entorhinal cortex than hippocampus in AD. Neurology 2004;62:422–7.

21. Coimbra A, Williams DS, Hostetler ED. The role of MRI and PET/SPECT in Alzheimer's disease. Curr Top Med Chem 2006;6:629–47.

22. Jack CR Jr, Shiung MM, Gunter JL, et al. Comparison of different MRI brain atrophy rate measures with clinical disease progression in AD. Neurology 2004;62:591–600.

23. Jack CR Jr, Slomkowski M, Gracon S, et al. MRI as a biomarker of disease progression in a therapeutic trial of milameline for AD. Neurology 2003;60: 253–60.

24. Mungas D, Harvey D, Reed BR, et al. Longitudinal volumetric MRI change and rate of cognitive decline. Neurology 2005;65:565–71.

25. Ramani A, Jensen JH, Helpern JA. Quantitative MR imaging in Alzheimer disease. Radiology 2006;241: 26–44.

26. Brun A, Englund E. A white matter disorder in dementia of the Alzheimer type: a pathoanatomical study. Ann Neurol 1986;19:253–62.

27. Mark RJ, Hensley K, Butterfield DA, et al. Amyloid beta-peptide impairs ion-motive ATPase activities: evidence for a role in loss of neuronal Ca2+ homeostasis and cell death. J Neurosci 1995;15: 6239–49.

28. Terry RD. The pathogenesis of Alzheimer disease: an alternative to the amyloid hypothesis. J Neuropathol Exp Neurol 1996;55:1023–5.

29. Hanyu H, Sakurai H, Iwamoto T, et al. Diffusion-weighted MR imaging of the hippocampus and temporal white matter in Alzheimer's disease. J Neurol Sci 1998;156:195–200.

30. Sandson TA, Felician O, Edelman RR, et al. Diffusion-weighted magnetic resonance imaging in Alzheimer's disease. Dement Geriatr Cogn Disord 1999;10:166–71.

31. Bozzao A, Floris R, Baviera ME, et al. Diffusion and perfusion MR imaging in cases of Alzheimer's disease: correlations with cortical atrophy and lesion load. AJNR Am J Neuroradiol 2001;22:1030–6.

32. Bozzali M, Falini A, Franceschi M, et al. White matter damage in Alzheimer's disease assessed in vivo using diffusion tensor magnetic resonance imaging. J Neurol Neurosurg Psychiatry 2002;72: 742–6.

33. Rose SE, Chen F, Chalk JB. Loss of connectivity in Alzheimer's disease: an evaluation of white matter tract integrity with colour coded MR diffusion tensor imaging. J Neurol Neurosurg Psychiatry 2000;69: 528–30.

34. Kantarci K, Jack CR Jr, Xu YC, et al. Mild cognitive impairment and Alzheimer disease: regional diffusivity of water. Radiology 2001;219:101–7.

35. Yoshiura T, Mihara F, Kuwabara Y, et al. MR relative cerebral blood flow mapping of Alzheimer disease: correlation with Tc-99m HMPAO SPECT. Acad Radiol 2002;9:1383–7.

36. Pfefferbaum A, Sullivan EV. Increased brain white matter diffusivity in normal adult aging: relationship to anisotropy and partial voluming. Magn Reson Med 2003;49:953–61.

37. Dousset V, Grossman RI, Ramer KN, et al. Experimental allergic encephalomyelitis and multiple sclerosis: lesion characterization with magnetization transfer imaging. Radiology 1992;182:483–91.

38. van Waesberghe JH, van Walderveen MA, Castelijns JA, et al. Patterns of lesion development in multiple sclerosis: longitudinal observations with T1-weighted spin-echo and magnetization transfer MR. AJNR Am J Neuroradiol 1998;19:675–83.

39. Hanyu H, Asano T, Sakurai H, et al. Magnetization transfer measurements of the hippocampus in the early diagnosis of Alzheimer's disease. J Neurol Sci 2001;188:79–84.

40. Chertkow H, Bergman H, Schipper HM, et al. Assessment of suspected dementia. Can J Neurol Sci 2001;(28 Suppl 1):S28–41.

41. Hyman BT, Van Hoesen GW, Damasio AR, et al. Alzheimer's disease: cell-specific pathology isolates the hippocampal formation. Science 1984;225: 1168–70.

42. Song Y, Morikawa S, Morita M, et al. Comparison of MR images and histochemical localization of intra-arterially administered microglia surrounding beta-amyloid deposits in the rat brain. Histol Histopathol 2006;21:705–11.

43. Kantarci K, Jack CR Jr, Xu YC, et al. Regional metabolic patterns in mild cognitive impairment and Alzheimer's disease: A 1H MRS study. Neurology 2000; 55:210–7.

44. Schuff N, Amend D, Ezekiel F, et al. Changes of hippocampal N-acetyl aspartate and volume in Alzheimer's disease. A proton MR spectroscopic

imaging and MRI study. Neurology 1997;49: 1513–21.

45. Frederick B, Satlin A, Wald LL, et al. Brain proton magnetic resonance spectroscopy in Alzheimer disease: changes after treatment with xanomeline. Am J Geriatr Psychiatry 2002;10:81–8.

46. Krishnan KR, Charles HC, Doraiswamy PM, et al. Randomized, placebo-controlled trial of the effects of donepezil on neuronal markers and hippocampal volumes in Alzheimer's disease. Am J Psychiatry 2003;160:2003–11.

47. Satlin A, Bodick N, Offen WW, et al. Brain proton magnetic resonance spectroscopy (1H-MRS) in Alzheimer's disease: changes after treatment with xanomeline, an M1 selective cholinergic agonist. Am J Psychiatry 1997;154:1459–61.

48. Dickerson BC, Sperling RA. Neuroimaging biomarkers for clinical trials of disease-modifying therapies in Alzheimer's disease. NeuroRx 2005;2: 348–60.

49. Logothetis NK, Pfeuffer J. On the nature of the BOLD fMRI contrast mechanism. Magn Reson Imaging 2004;22:1517–31.

50. Kato T, Knopman D, Liu H. Dissociation of regional activation in mild AD during visual encoding: a functional MRI study. Neurology 2001;57:812–6.

51. Rombouts SA, Barkhof F, Van Meel CS, et al. Alterations in brain activation during cholinergic enhancement with rivastigmine in Alzheimer's disease. J Neurol Neurosurg Psychiatry 2002;73: 665–71.

52. Small SA, Perera GM, DeLaPaz R, et al. Differential regional dysfunction of the hippocampal formation among elderly with memory decline and Alzheimer's disease. Ann Neurol 1999;45: 466–72.

53. Sperling RA, Bates JF, Chua EF, et al. fMRI studies of associative encoding in young and elderly controls and mild Alzheimer's disease. J Neurol Neurosurg Psychiatry 2003;74:44–50.

54. Bondi MW, Houston WS, Eyler LT, et al. fMRI evidence of compensatory mechanisms in older adults at genetic risk for Alzheimer disease. Neurology 2005;64:501–8.

55. Dannhauser TM, Walker Z, Stevens T, et al. The functional anatomy of divided attention in amnestic mild cognitive impairment. Brain 2005;128:1418–27.

56. Dickerson BC, Salat DH, Greve DN, et al. Increased hippocampal activation in mild cognitive impairment compared to normal aging and AD. Neurology 2005; 65:404–11.

57. Golby A, Silverberg G, Race E, et al. Memory encoding in Alzheimer's disease: an fMRI study of explicit and implicit memory. Brain 2005;128: 773–87.

58. Johnson SC, Schmitz TW, Moritz CH, et al. Activation of brain regions vulnerable to Alzheimer's disease: the effect of mild cognitive impairment. Neurobiol Aging 2006;27:1604–12.

59. De Luca M, Beckmann CF, De Stefano N, et al. fMRI resting state networks define distinct modes of long-distance interactions in the human brain. Neuroimage 2006;29:1359–67.

60. Liu Y, Wang K, Yu C, et al. Regional homogeneity, functional connectivity and imaging markers of Alzheimer's disease: a review of resting-state fMRI studies. Neuropsychologia 2008;46:1648–56.

61. Selkoe DJ. Imaging Alzheimer's amyloid. Nat Biotechnol 2000;18:823–4.

62. Dhenain M, Privat N, Duyckaerts C, et al. Senile plaques do not induce susceptibility effects in T2*-weighted MR microscopic images. NMR Biomed 2002;15:197–203.

63. Helpern JA, Lee SP, Falangola MF, et al. MRI assessment of neuropathology in a transgenic mouse model of Alzheimer's disease. Magn Reson Med 2004;51:794–8.

64. Higuchi M, Iwata N, Matsuba Y, et al. 19F and 1H MRI detection of amyloid beta plaques in vivo. Nat Neurosci 2005;8:527–33.

65. Vanhoutte G, Dewachter I, Borghgraef P, et al. Noninvasive in vivo MRI detection of neuritic plaques associated with iron in APP[V717I] transgenic mice, a model for Alzheimer's disease. Magn Reson Med 2005;53:607–13.

66. Wadghiri YZ, Sigurdsson EM, Sadowski M, et al. Detection of Alzheimer's amyloid in transgenic mice using magnetic resonance microimaging. Magn Reson Med 2003;50:293–302.

67. Zhang J, Yarowsky P, Gordon MN, et al. Detection of amyloid plaques in mouse models of Alzheimer's disease by magnetic resonance imaging. Magn Reson Med 2004;51:452–7.

68. Helpern JA. The promise of high-field-strength MR imaging. AJNR Am J Neuroradiol 2003;24: 1738–9.

69. Skovronsky DM, Zhang B, Kung MP, et al. In vivo detection of amyloid plaques in a mouse model of Alzheimer's disease. Proc Natl Acad Sci U S A 2000;97:7609–14.

70. Huddleston DE, Small SA. Technology insight: imaging amyloid plaques in the living brain with positron emission tomography and MRI. Nat Clin Pract Neurol 2005;1:96–105.

71. van Straaten EC, Scheltens P, Knol DL, et al. Operational definitions for the NINDS-AIREN criteria for vascular dementia: an interobserver study. Stroke 2003;34:1907–12.

72. vanStraaten ECW, Scheltens P, Barkhof F. MRI and CT in the diagnosis of vascular dementia. J Neurol Sci 2004;226(1–2):9–12.

73. Schmidt R, Petrovic K, Ropele S, et al. Progression of leukoaraiosis and cognition. Stroke 2007;38: 2619–25.

74. Schmidt R, Enzinger C, Ropele S, et al. Progression of cerebral white matter lesions: 6-year results of the Austrian stroke prevention study. Lancet 2003;361: 2046–8.

75. Schmidt R, Scheltens P, Erkinjuntti T, et al. White matter lesion progression: a surrogate endpoint for trials in cerebral small-vessel disease. Neurology 2004;63:139–44.

76. Fazekas F. RSBRKPSWSRSR: Novel imaging technologies in the assessment of cerebral ageing and vascular dementia. In: Jellinger K, Schmidt R, Windisch M, editors. Advances in dementia research. Wien, New York: Springer Medicine; 2000. p. 15–21.

77. Holtmannspotter M, Peters N, Opherk C, et al. Diffusion magnetic resonance histograms as a surrogate marker and predictor of disease progression in CADASIL: a two-year follow-up study. Stroke 2005;36: 2559–65.

78. Avants B, Grossman M, Gee JC. The correlation of cognitive decline with frontotemporal dementia induced annualized gray matter loss using diffeomorphic morphometry. Alzheimer Dis Assoc Disord 2005;(19 Suppl 1):S25–8.

79. Hodges JR. Frontotemporal dementia (Pick's disease): clinical features and assessment. Neurology 2001;56: S6–10.

80. Montoya A, Price BH, Menear M, et al. Brain imaging and cognitive dysfunctions in Huntington's disease. J Psychiatry Neurosci 2006;31: 21–9.

81. Rosas HD, Koroshetz WJ, Chen YI, et al. Evidence for more widespread cerebral pathology in early HD: an MRI-based morphometric analysis. Neurology 2003;60:1615–20.

82. Turner KC, Frost L, Linsenbardt D, et al. Atypically diffuse functional connectivity between caudate nuclei and cerebral cortex in autism. Behav Brain Funct 2006;2:34–46.

83. Lawrence NS, Williams AM, Surguladze S, et al. Subcortical and ventral prefrontal cortical neural responses to facial expressions distinguish patients with bipolar disorder and major depression. Biol Psychiatry 2004;55:578–87.

84. Abou-Saleh MT. Neuroimaging in psychiatry: an update. J Psychosom Res 2006;61:289–93.

85. Lin A, Grossman T, Shriner K, et al. Double blind trial of H^1 MRS monitoring antiretroviral therapy. Proc Int Soc Magn Reson Med 2000;8:1174.

86. Meyerhoff DJ, Bloomer C, Cardenas V, et al. Elevated subcortical choline metabolites in cognitively and clinically asymptomatic HIV+ patients. Neurology 1999;52:995–1003.

The Clinical Role of Fusion Imaging Using PET, CT, and MR Imaging

Habib Zaidi, PhD, PD[a],*, Marie-Louise Montandon, PhD[a],
Abass Alavi, MD, PhD (Hon), DSc (Hon)[b]

KEYWORDS

- Multimodality imaging • Image fusion • PET/CT
- PET/MRI • Quantification

Medical imaging has evolved rapidly during the last 2 decades, and we are now observing radical changes in the way medicine is practiced as a logical consequence of this growth. Nowadays, clinical diagnosis is rarely done without imaging, which makes molecular imaging an essential component of the clinical decision-making tree. Contemporary molecular imaging technologies now represent the leading component of any health care institution and have a pivotal role in the daily clinical management of patients.[1]

X-ray projection imaging, ultrasonography, CT, and MR imaging differentiate disease from normal tissue by revealing structural differences or differences in regional perfusion of the administered contrast media. The interpretation of the images can be complicated when normal perfusion patterns are disrupted by prior surgery or radiotherapy, which can lead to tissue damage or necrosis where contrast patterns can mimic those associated with neoplasia. This effect presents a significant challenge when imaging techniques are used to define the anatomic extent of disease, such as for planning highly conformal radiation treatment or highly targeted therapeutic regimens.[2]

In comparison with anatomic imaging techniques, functional imaging methods including planar scintigraphy, single-photon emission computed tomography (SPECT), positron emission tomography (PET), and MR spectroscopy assess regional differences in the biochemical status of tissues. In nuclear medicine, including SPECT and PET, this assessment is done by administering a biologically active molecule or pharmaceutical to the patient which is radiolabeled and accumulated in response to its biochemical attributes. The realization that the information provided by anatomic (CT and MR) and molecular (SPECT and PET) imaging modalities is complementarity spurred the development of various strategies for multimodality image registration and fusion. Correlative or fusion functional-anatomic imaging is now well established and its clinical value widely recognized.

Several investigators proposed and in most cases developed techniques to improve the correlation between the anatomic and physiologic information obtained using these anatomic and functional imaging studies. These methods include software-based image registration in which two or more sets of images from two or more different studies are fused following their separate acquisition on stand-alone imaging systems. Commonly, image registration techniques produce a single "fused" or "combined" image in which the functional SPECT or PET image is displayed in color over a gray-scale CT or MR image of the same anatomic region. Alternatively, hardware-based, dual-modality imaging systems including SPECT/CT, PET/CT, and, in the future,

---

This article originally appeared in *PET Clinics* 2008;3(3);275–91.
This work was supported by grant SNSF 3100A0-116547 from the Swiss National Foundation.
[a] Division of Nuclear Medicine, Geneva University Hospital, CH-1211 Geneva, Switzerland
[b] Division of Nuclear Medicine, Hospital of the University of Pennsylvania, 3400 Spruce Street, Philadelphia, PA 19104, USA
* Corresponding author.
E-mail address: habib.zaidi@hcuge.ch (H. Zaidi).

Magn Reson Imaging Clin N Am 18 (2010) 133–149
doi:10.1016/j.mric.2009.09.010

PET/MR imaging, more successfully achieve this goal, which underlies their wider clinical acceptance by the medical imaging community.

This article discusses recent advances in clinical multimodality imaging and the role of correlative fusion imaging in the clinical setting. Future opportunities and challenges facing the adoption of multimodality imaging are also addressed.

SOFTWARE-BASED IMAGE REGISTRATION AND FUSION

Software image fusion can be challenging to perform on a routine basis in the clinical setting because it requires exceptional digital communication in medicine (DICOM) connectivity, compatibility between the scanning protocols used by various imaging modalities, and outstanding collaboration between various clinical departments. These challenges may be overcome by the use of combined PET/CT systems described in the following section, although software-based coregistration offers greater flexibility and might in some cases offer some complementary advantages to hardware-based approaches.[3,4]

Achieving a high degree of accuracy for a spatial transformation between image sets can be complicated. Physical factors such as noise, limited spatial resolution, attenuation, scatter, and partial volume effect (PVE) and biologic factors such as persistent activity in the blood pool and nonspecific uptake may decrease the contrast and blur the images; therefore, it can be difficult to locate consistent landmarks. The coregistration problem in the brain is different from the situation in whole-body imaging. Furthermore, diagnostic CT images are usually taken using breath-holding techniques, whereas PET data are acquired during a relatively long time period with the resultant reconstructed image set being an average of all phases of respiration.[5] PET/CT investigations involving imaging of the thorax, abdomen, or pelvis, where organ motion exists, result in inconsistent image sets. This inconsistency can cause complications, for example, if the body boundaries of the CT data and the PET can be registered but the internal structures still differ significantly. Various PET/CT scanning protocols performed for a short period but with a similar breathing pattern have been designed to avoid the breath-holding problem.[6] The CT data acquired allow for both attenuation correction and registration of PET/CT data for accurate localization of metabolic abnormalities. Despite their difficulties, many semi- or fully automated registration methods have been developed and used with various degrees of success in research and clinical

settings. An in-depth overview of software-based registration techniques and algorithms is beyond the scope of this review. For a detailed survey of the algorithms developed so far, the reader is referred to recent comprehensive reviews.[7–10]

Two main strategies have emerged in the literature to perform so-called "rigid registration," such as brain PET-MR imaging registration of images of the same patient. The first strategy is based on the identification of similar structures in both images and subsequent minimization of a "distance measure" between them. The second strategy uses a voxel-per-voxel similarity measure of the full three-dimensional data set as a matching criterion (where *voxel* stands for a *volume element*, ie, a three-dimensional image point). The criterion that drives the registration algorithm is known as the "similarity measure." The most popular similarity measures find their origin in information theoretic approaches. These approaches include minimization of histogram dispersion,[11] maximization of mutual information,[12] or maximization of the correlation ratio.[13] The most widely used criterion is mutual information, an intensity-based similarity measure, and many variants to this approach (eg, normalized mutual information) have subsequently been proposed in the literature. Nonrigid registration approaches are usually required to correlate images of the thorax and abdomen. These approaches are usually combined with linear registration techniques to correct for changes in body configuration, differences in breathing patterns, or internal organ motion and associated displacements. Within the context of the assessment of response to treatment in which intrapatient registration of pre- and post-treatment whole-body PET images may be required to automate the analysis of lesion size and uptake,[14,15] nonrigid registration with position-dependent rigidity approaches have been suggested. These techniques assign a high degree of rigidity to some regions (eg, lesions, brain) that will remain unchanged following the registration process.[16]

HARDWARE-BASED MULTIMODALITY IMAGING
Combined PET/CT Instrumentation

The historical development of multimodality imaging is marked by various significant technical and scientific accomplishments driven by an unprecedented collaboration between multidisciplinary groups of investigators. Even though the introduction of commercial PET/CT units in a clinical setting is a recent feature, the prospective benefits of correlative multimodality imaging have been well established since the early years of medical imaging. Many pioneering radiologic scientists and physicians recognized that the capabilities of a radionuclide imaging system could be improved by adding an external source to allow acquisition of transmission data for anatomic correlation of the emission image.[2] Interestingly, the derived theoretical concepts that were occasionally patented[17,18] never materialized in practice until the late Dr Bruce Hasegawa and colleagues at the University of California, San Francisco[19,20] pioneered in the 1990s the development of dedicated SPECT/CT. Dr Hasegawa is the person to credit for the conception and design of the first combined SPECT/CT unit, which now stands as a wonderful tribute to his memory.[21] Later, Dr Townsend and coworkers at the University of Pittsburgh[22,23] pioneered in 1998 the development of combined PET/CT imaging systems, which have the capability to record both PET emission and x-ray transmission data for correlated functional/structural imaging. More compact and cost-effective designs of dual-modality systems have been explored more recently. One such

approach uses a rail-with-sliding-bed design in which a sliding CT bed is placed on a track in the floor and linked to a flexible SPECT camera.[24] A variety of rail-based, docking, and click-over concepts for correlating functional and anatomic images are also being considered with the goal of offering a more economic approach to multimodality imaging for institutions with limited resources.[25]

Among the many advantages offered by PET/CT is a reduction in the overall scanning time, allowing one to increase patient throughput by approximately 30%[26] owing to the use of fast CT-based attenuation correction when compared with lengthy procedures involving the use of external transmission rod sources. **Fig. 1** illustrates the timeline for various stand-alone PET and combined PET/CT scanning protocols following tracer injection and the typical 1-hour waiting time for ^{18}F-fluorodeoxyglucose (FDG). The patient is prepared for imaging by administering the radiopharmaceutical, typically 370 to 555 MBq (10 to 15 mCi) of ^{18}F-FDG in adults. A pre-injection transmission scan is usually performed

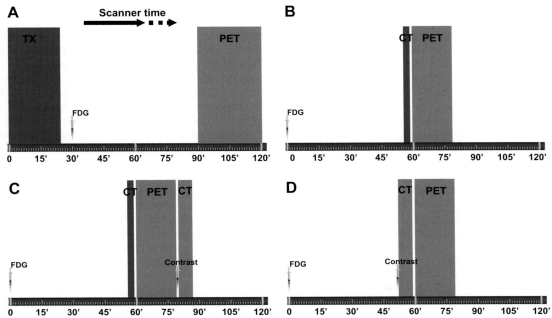

Fig. 1. Timeline for various stand-alone PET and PET/CT scanning protocols following tracer injection and typical 1 hour waiting time for ^{18}F-FDG. (*A*) The pre-injection transmission scan required on conventional stand-alone PET scanners (approximately 3 minutes per bed position on full-ring systems) is usually acquired before tracer injection. On contemporary combined PET/CT scanners equipped with fast detectors, the acquisition time is practically half the time required on conventional detectors. A low-dose CT for attenuation correction (*B*) or a study combined with a diagnostic quality contrast-enhanced CT (*C*) is usually performed depending on the clinical indication. The latter can also be used for attenuation correction but might result in artifacts in some cases by overcorrecting for attenuation in regions containing contrast medium (*D*). PET/CT allows one to reduce the overall scanning time, thus increasing patient throughput.

on stand-alone PET scanners before tracer injection to reduce spillover of emission data into the transmission energy window, although post-injection transmission scanning protocols have been successfully used in the clinic with the use of contemporary PET scanners.[27] When using combined PET/CT units, the patient is asked to remove all metal objects that could introduce artifacts in the CT scan and is then positioned on the table of the dual-modality imaging system. The patient undergoes an "overview" or "scout" scan during which x-ray projection data are obtained from the patient to identify the axial extent of the CT and PET study. The patient then undergoes a low-dose spiral CT acquisition followed by the PET study starting approximately 1 hour after FDG administration. The CT and PET data are reconstructed and registered, with the CT data used for attenuation correction of the reconstructed PET images. Depending on institutions and agreements between clinical departments and clinical requirements,[28–30] the images might be interpreted in tandem by a radiologist and nuclear medicine physician who can view the CT scan, the PET images, and the fused PET/CT data, followed by preparation of the associated clinical report. Some clinical indications commonly require administration with contrast media to acquire a relatively high-dose diagnostic quality CT scan.[31] The latter scan can be performed either before or following the PET study. In the former case, the contrast-enhanced CT is also used to correct the PET data for photon attenuation, and the low-dose CT scan is no longer needed. Care should be taken to avoid hot-spot artifacts in the attenuation-corrected PET images that might be caused by overcorrection of radio-dense oral and intravenous contrast agents. As a rule of thumb, examination of the uncorrected images is recommended to distinguish technical artifacts from physiologic/pathologic hypermetabolism. Alternatively, post-processing correction methods have been proposed in the literature.[32,33]

Combined PET/MR Imaging Instrumentation

The interest in PET scanning within strong magnetic fields was first motivated by the need to reduce the distance positrons travel before annihilation (positron range) through magnetic confinement of the emitted positrons.[34–36] Indeed, Monte Carlo simulation studies predicted improvements in spatial resolution for high-energy positron emitters ranging between 18.5% (2.73 mm instead of 3.35 mm) for ^{68}Ga and 26.8% (2.68 mm instead of 3.66 mm) for [82]Rb for a magnetic field strength of 7 T.[36] These improvements are in agreement with the results obtained using another Monte Carlo code in which a 27% improvement in spatial resolution for a PET scanner incorporating a 10 T magnetic field was reported.[37]

The history of combined PET/MR imaging dates back to the mid-1990s even before the advent of PET/CT.[35,37,38] Early attempts to design MR-compatible PET units relied on slight modification of PET detector blocks of a preclinical PET scanner to keep the photomultiplier tubes (PMTs) at a reasonable distance from the strong magnetic field of a clinical MR imaging unit.[39–43] The detectors were coupled to long optical fibers (4–5 m), leading the weak scintillation light outside the fringe magnetic field to position-sensitive PMTs. Despite the limitations of this design, similar approaches were adopted by other investigators.[44–47] Other related design concepts based on conventional PMT-based PET detectors rely on more complex magnet designs, including a split magnet[48] or field-cycled MR imaging.[49]

Other investigators have developed PET/MR imaging systems configured with suitable solid-state detectors that can be operated within a magnetic field for PET imaging. These systems include avalanche photodiodes (APDs)[50] and Geiger-mode avalanche photodiodes (G-APDs).[51,52] APD-based readout has already been implemented on a commercial preclinical PET system, the LabPET scanner,[53] 10 years after the development of the first prototype based on this technology.[54] Various MR-compatible preclinical PET prototypes have been designed using both APD-based[55–60] and G-APD based[61,62] technologies. Other promising technologies that might be used for the design of future generation PET/MR imaging systems include amorphous selenium avalanche photodetectors, which have an excellent quantum efficiency, a large avalanche gain, and a rapid response time.[63,64]

Most of these systems have been tested within a high field (up to 9.7 T) and have produced PET and MR images that appear to be free of distortion, consolidating the hypothesis that there is no significant interference between the two systems, and that each modality is virtually invisible to the other.

The promising results obtained on preclinical systems have encouraged one of the major industrial players (Siemens Medical Solutions, Knoxville, TN) to develop the first clinical PET/MR imaging prototype (BrainPET), dedicated for simultaneous brain imaging, in collaboration with the University of Tuebingen in Germany.[65] **Fig. 2** illustrates the conceptual design and a photograph of the integrated MR/PET scanner, showing isocentric layering of the MR head coil, PET detector ring, and MR

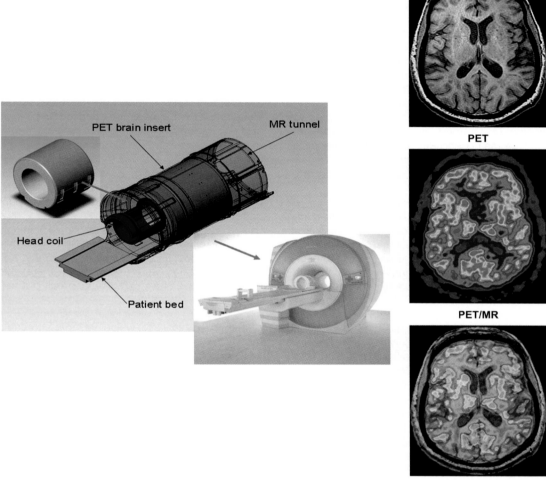

MRI

PET

PET/MR

Fig. 2. Drawing and photograph of integrated PET/MR imaging design showing isocentric layering of MR head coil, PET detector ring, and MR magnet tunnel (*left*). Simultaneously acquired MR images, PET, and fused combined PET/MR images of 66-year-old man after intravenous injection of 370 MBq of FDG are shown. Tracer distribution was recorded for 20 minutes at steady state after 120 minutes. (*Adapted from* Schlemmer HP, Pichler BJ, Schmand M, et al. Simultaneous MR/PET imaging of the human brain: feasibility study. Radiology 2008; 248:1030; with permission.)

magnet tunnel together with concurrently acquired clinical MR, PET, and fused MR/PET images. The system is being assessed in a clinical setting by exploiting the full potential of anatomic MR imaging in terms of high soft-tissue contrast sensitivity in addition to the many other possibilities offered by this modality, including blood oxygenation level dependant (BOLD) imaging, functional MR imaging, diffusion-weighted imaging, perfusion-weighted imaging, and diffusion tensor imaging.[66] The prospective applications of a hypothetical whole-body PET/MR imaging system are being explored in the literature.[67–70] Such a system

would allow one to exploit, in addition to the previously discussed applications, the power of MR spectroscopy to measure the regional biochemical content and to assess the metabolic status or the presence of neoplasia and other diseases in specific tissue areas.[71]

CLINICAL ROLE OF CORRELATIVE FUSION IMAGING

The clinical role of correlative imaging encompasses a wide variety of applications. It is now performed routinely with commercially available radiopharmaceuticals to answer important clinical questions in oncology,[72] cardiology,[73] neurology, and psychiatry.[74,75] As discussed previously, much of the early image registration effort was restricted to intrasubject brain applications, where the confinement of compact brain tissues within the skull renders a rigid-body model a satisfactory approximation.[76,77] Correlative fusion imaging techniques were introduced in the clinic, mostly for neuroimaging applications, well before the advent of hardware-based, dual-modality imaging. Multimodality imaging had a pivotal role in the assessment of central nervous system disorders such as seizures, Alzheimer's and Parkinson's disease, head injury, and inoperable brain tumors.[78–80]

Brain SPECT imaging using ^{99m}Tc-labeled perfusion ligands shows a sharp increase during an epileptic seizure (ictal scan) at the position of the epileptogenic focus, whereas most epileptic foci show a diminished perfusion on the interictal scan. By means of ictal/interictal subtraction studies, with subsequent coregistration onto MR imaging (Subtraction *I*ctal SPECT *Co*registered to *M*R imaging [SISCOM]), a predictive value up to 97% for the correct localization of an epileptic focus has been reported,[81] which is higher than any other competing modality. Fig. 3 shows an example of a ^{99m}Tc-labelled ethylene cysteine dimer (ECD) perfusion SPECT and FDG-PET studies of the same patient coregistered to an anatomic T1-weighted MR imaging study for the evaluation of epilepsy. The two ^{99m}Tc-ECD scans were performed during seizure (ictal) and when the patient was seizure free (interictal) the following day. Both SPECT studies and a three-dimensional, T1-weighted MR imaging study were coregistered using the normalized mutual information criterion, which is similar to mutual information but usually more robust and efficient in finding the correct fitting transform.[82] The differences between the ictal and interictal SPECT studies were overlaid on transaxial slices of the MR imaging study to permit accurate localization of the focus of the epilepsy. A coregistered FDG-PET study superimposed on the MR imaging study is also shown. This type of image registration and fusion technique has been a standard component of many clinical practices for the last 2 decades and is used routinely in the authors' institution. Corresponding techniques for other regions of the body have not achieved the same widespread clinical use.

Another example from the neuro-oncology field shows a patient with a glioblastoma (WHO IV) in the left temporal and frontal areas (Fig. 4).

A similar registration approach as for Fig. 3 was used for coregistration of an ^{18}F-fluoro-ethyl-tyrosine (^{18}F-FET) brain PET scan and gadolinium-enhanced, T2-weighted MR imaging. This study showed that PET frequently detected tumors that were not visible on MR imaging. Moreover, substantial differences in terms of gross tumor volume delineation were reported when compared with MR imaging–guided treatment planning.[83]

A plethora of novel tracers are used routinely for assessing tumor metabolism and other biologic and physiologic parameters associated with many diseases.[84,85] These tracers have clearly demonstrated the enormous potential of PET/CT as an emerging modality in the field of molecular imaging. Multiple studies have demonstrated unequivocally the role of PET/CT, especially for oncologic applications.[72,86] Nevertheless, the limited role of PET/CT in some clinical indications, including central nervous system disorders, orthopedic infections, and inflammatory disorders, and in the evaluation and follow-up of metastatic disease has been advocated as a serious concern against the decision of vendors to stop manufacturing less expensive stand-alone PET systems for clinical use, which are more affordable for economically depressed nations.[87,88]

Molecular imaging in its broad definition represents methodologies and probes that allow visualization of events at the cellular and molecular levels.[89] The intended targets for this purpose include cells surface receptors, transporters, intracellular enzymes, or messenger RNA. The source of the signal detected by these techniques could originate directly from the molecule or its surrogates. In both clinical and research studies involving control subjects or volunteers, an accurate estimate of the tracer biodistribution and its pharmacokinetics is frequently a goal to understand the biochemical behavior of the probe and its suitability for the task at hand. This assessment also allows radiation dosimetry estimates to be performed to assess potential radiation risks associated with novel tracers before their administration to patients. Fig. 5 shows typical biodistributions of ^{18}F-choline and ^{11}C-acetate probes in a subject. The CT scan can be used for attenuation correction of the PET data and for anatomic localization of tracer uptake and organ/tissue volumetric estimation, which is also required for dosimetry calculations. FDG-PET has limited impact in many malignancies presenting with low FDG avidity (eg, prostate cancer, hepatic metastases, and associated lymph nodes), where more specific tracers should be used. Fig. 6 shows a clinical PET/CT study illustrating the limitations of ^{18}F-FDG for the detection of hepatic metastases and lymph node involvement which are clearly visible on the ^{18}F-FDopa study. In addition, the high sensitivity and specificity of FDG-PET for lymph node involvement and the capacity to better discriminate between tumor extent and atelectasis may substantially alter the delineation of target volumes in radiotherapy.[86,90–94] **Fig. 7** shows an example where PET allowed excluding associated atelectasis that was impossible to differentiate using CT alone.[94]

ADVANCES IN ANATOMICALLY GUIDED QUANTIFICATION OF PET DATA

The primary motivation for multimodality imaging has been image fusion of functional and anatomic data to facilitate anatomic localization of functional abnormalities and to assist region-of-interest (ROI) definition for quantitative analysis. The anatomic information also can be useful for many other tasks, including attenuation compensation, transmission-based scatter modeling, motion detection, and correction, introducing a priori anatomic information into reconstruction of the PET emission data and partial volume correction.[95]

Anatomically Guided PET Attenuation and Scatter Compensation

The use of CT-based[96,97] and, more recently, MR imaging–guided[98,99] attenuation compensation has received a great deal of attention in the scientific literature. As discussed earlier, the former has many advantages when compared with conventional transmission-based scanning, which is now considered obsolete following the advent of hybrid systems.[100] Nevertheless, CT-based attenuation correction has many drawbacks that need to be addressed through research, including polychromaticity of x-ray photons and the beam-hardening effect, misregistration between CT and PET images resulting from respiratory motion, truncation artifacts, the presence of oral and intravenous contrast medium, metallic implants, x-ray scatter in CT images, and other CT artifacts from any source.[97] MR imaging–guided attenuation correction is in its infancy and remains challenging for whole-body imaging.[98,99] This very active research topic will certainly impact the future of hybrid PET/MR imaging technology.

Traditionally, approximate scatter compensation techniques in PET have been applied in which the scatter component is estimated from measurements using additional energy windows placed adjacent to the photopeak window used to acquire the primary PET emission data. The expanding diagnostic and therapeutic applications of quantitative PET imaging have motivated the development of scatter correction techniques, which incorporate patient-specific attenuation maps derived from either transmission scans or CT imaging and the physics of interaction and detection of emitted photons to estimate the scatter magnitude and distribution accurately.[101] Transmission-based scatter correction methods use an attenuation map to define the inhomogeneous properties of the scattering object and derive a distribution of scattered events using line integrals calculated as part of the attenuation correction method. Algorithms belonging to this class of model-based methods have been successfully applied in a clinical setting.[102–105] Although computationally intensive, more refined algorithms that use a patient-specific attenuation map, an estimate of the emission image, and Monte Carlo–based radiation transport calculations to estimate the magnitude and spatial distribution of Compton scattered events that would be detected have also been considered.[106–108]

Anatomically Guided PET Image Reconstruction

An undesirable property of the statistical iterative reconstruction techniques including the popular maximum likelihood–expectation maximization (ML-EM) algorithm is that large numbers of iterations increase the noise content of the reconstructed PET images.[109] The noise characteristics can be controlled by incorporating a prior distribution to describe the statistical properties of the unknown image and thus produce a posteriori probability distributions from the image conditioned upon the data. Bayesian reconstruction methods form a powerful extension of the ML-EM algorithm. Maximization of the a posteriori (MAP) probability over the set of possible images results in the MAP estimate.[110] This approach has many advantages because the various components of the prior, such as the pseudo-Poisson nature of statistics, non-negativity of the solution, local voxel correlations (local smoothness), or known existence of anatomic boundaries, may be added one by one into the estimation process, assessed individually, and used to guarantee a fast working implementation of preliminary versions of the algorithms. A Bayesian model also can incorporate prior anatomic information derived from a registered CT[111] or MR[112,113] image in the reconstruction of PET data with the aim of avoiding resolution loss due to the regularization, exploiting the superior resolution of the anatomic images.

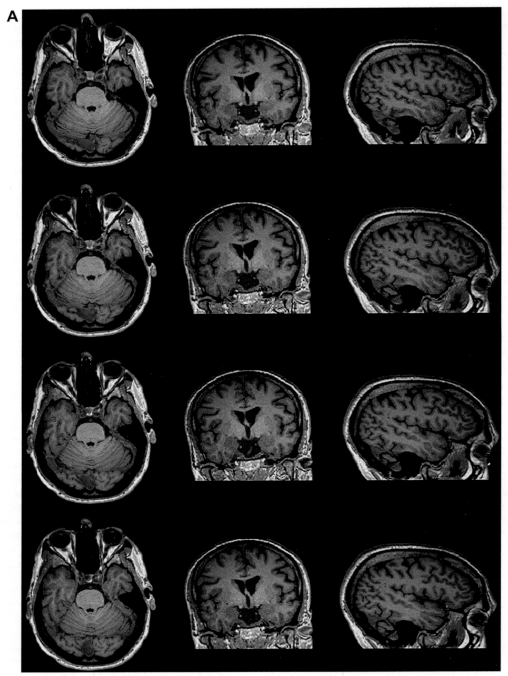

Fig. 3. Representative slices of a patient showing an example of SPECT/PET and MR imaging registration and fusion for the evaluation of epilepsy. Two ^{99m}Tc-ECD scans performed during seizure (ictal) and when the patient was seizure free (interictal) the following day are shown. Both SPECT studies and a three-dimensional, T1-weighted MR imaging study were coregistered using the normalized mutual information criterion. (*A*) The differences between the ictal and interictal SPECT studies are overlaid on transaxial slices of the MR imaging study to permit accurate localization of the focus of the epilepsy. (*B*) A coregistered FDG-PET study superimposed on the MR imaging study is also shown.

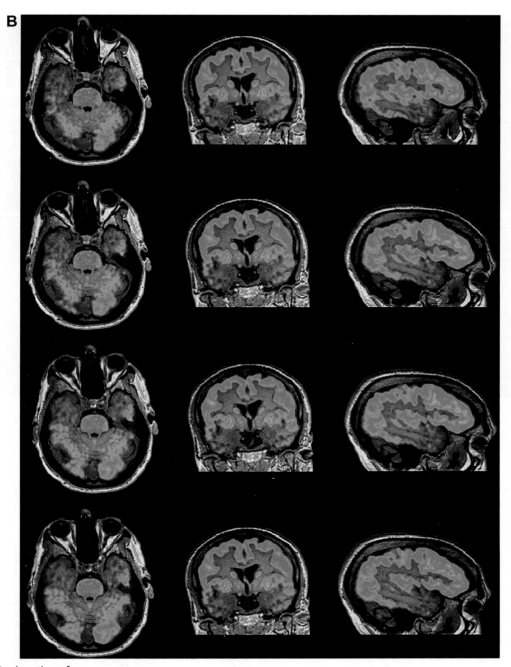

Fig. 3. (*continued*)

This class of algorithms incorporates a coupling term in the reconstruction procedure that favors the formation of edges in the PET data that are associated with the location of noteworthy anatomic edges from the anatomic images. A Gibbs prior distribution is usually used to encourage the piece-wise smoothness of reconstructed PET images. A Gibbs prior of piece-wise smoothness can also be incorporated in the bayesian model. Some groups have published preliminary promising results with segmentation-free anatomic priors based on measures similar to mutual information, but further investigation is required. In this way, the development of dual-modality imaging systems producing accurately registered anatomic and functional image

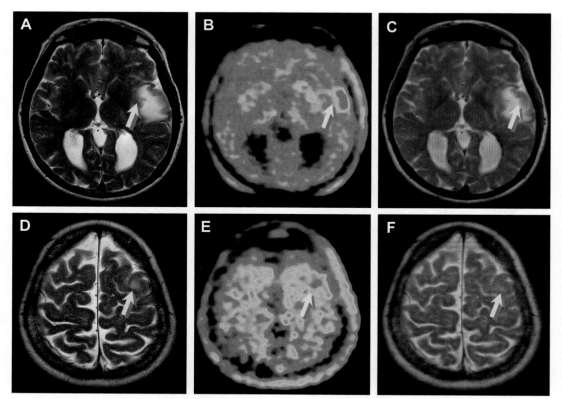

Fig. 4. Example of a patient with a glioblastoma (WHO IV) (*arrows*) in the left temporal and frontal areas. The images shown on the top row (temporal area) correspond to gadolinium-enhanced, T2-weighted MR imaging (*A*), coregistered ^{18}F-FET (*B*), and fused PET/MR imaging (*C*) of the first study. The same images are shown in the bottom row for the frontal area (*D*, *E*, and *F*). The ^{18}F-FET PET study revealed an additional lesion missed on MR imaging. In addition, the T2-weighted MR image and the ^{18}F-FET PET show substantially different gross tumor volume extension for radiotherapy treatment planning.

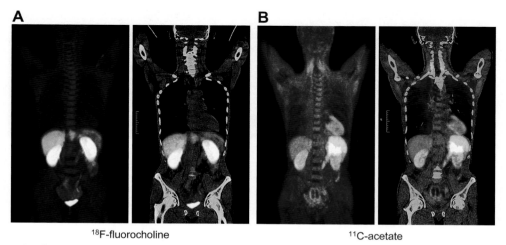

^{18}F-fluorocholine ^{11}C-acetate

Fig. 5. Role of PET/CT in novel tracer biodistribution studies showing typical biodistributions for ^{18}F-fluorocholine (*A*) and ^{11}C-acetate (*B*) in the same subject. The CT scan is used for attenuation correction of the PET data and for anatomic localization of tracer uptake and organ/tissue volumetric estimation which is required for dosimetry calculations.

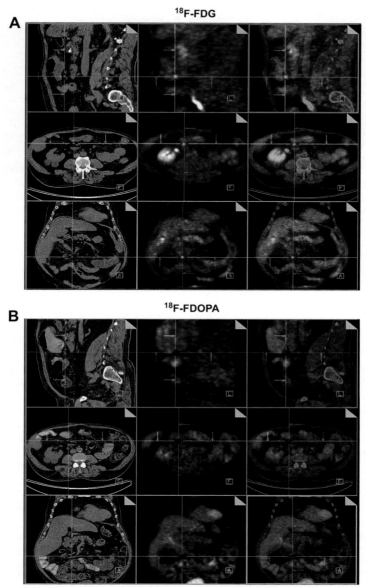

Fig. 6. Illustration of a clinical PET/CT study showing the limitations of ^{18}F-FDG for the detection of hepatic metastases and lymph node involvement, which are clearly visible on the ^{18}F-FDopa study.

data[23,114] is motivating the further investigation of the potential of bayesian MAP reconstruction techniques.

Anatomically Guided Partial Volume Correction in PET

The quantitative accuracy of PET is hampered by the low spatial resolution capability of currently available clinical scanners. The well-accepted criterion is that one can accurately quantify the activity concentration for sources having dimensions equal to or larger than twice the system's spatial resolution measured in terms of its full-width-at-half-maximum (FWHM). Sources of smaller size only partly occupy this characteristic volume, and, as such, the counts are spread over a larger volume than the physical size of the object owing to the limited spatial resolution of the imaging system. The total number of counts is conserved in the corresponding PET images. In this case, the resulting PET images reflect the

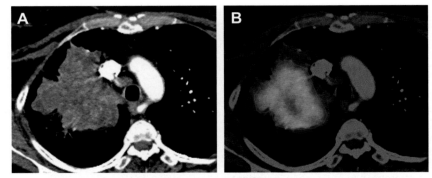

Fig. 7. Transaxial CT (*A*) and FDG-PET (*B*) images of a clinical PET/CT study of a patient with non-small cell lung cancer of the right upper lobe. PET/CT allowed excluding associated atelectasis that was impossible using a diagnostic quality CT alone, modifying the gross tumor volume delineated for radiotherapy treatment planning.

total amount of the activity within the object but not the actual activity concentration. This phenomenon is referred to as the PVE and can be corrected using one of the various strategies developed for this purpose.[115,116] The simplest technique uses recovery coefficients determined in a calibration measurement for objects of simple geometric shape.[117] This technique works relatively well for objects that can be approximated by simple geometric shapes (eg, tumors of spherical shape).[118] More sophisticated anatomy-based, post-reconstruction approaches have also been developed to correct for this effect knowing the size and shape of corresponding structures as assessed by structural imaging (MR imaging or CT).[119,120]

Fig. 8 shows the principle of the MR imaging–guided partial volume correction approach in functional brain PET imaging. The procedure used follows the approach described by Matsuda and colleagues,[121] which involves realigning the PET and MR image volumes followed by segmenting

the MR image into white and gray matter using the statistical parametric mapping (SPM5) segmentation toolbox.[122] The next step of this correction method consists in convolving the segmented white and gray matter images by the PET scanner's spatial resolution modeled by a gaussian response function. The gray matter PET image is then obtained by subtraction of the convolved PET white matter image from the original PET image. The PVE corrected gray matter PET image is then obtained by dividing the gray matter PET image by the convolved gray matter MR image. A binary mask for gray matter is finally applied. The accuracy of MR imaging–guided PVE correction in PET largely depends on the accuracy achieved by the PET–MR imaging coregistration procedure and MR imaging segmentation algorithm. The impact of image misregistration and segmentation errors has been assessed by some investigators.[119,123–127]

More recent techniques using multi-resolution synergetic approaches that combine functional

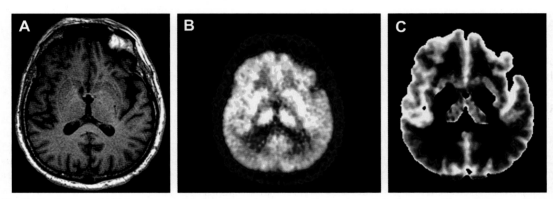

Fig. 8. Illustration of MR imaging–guided partial volume correction approach in functional brain PET showing the original T1-weighted MR image (*A*) and PET image before (*B*) and after (*C*) voxel-by-voxel PVE correction.

and anatomic information from various sources appear promising and should be investigated further in a clinical setting.[128] The corrections for the PVE can also be applied during the reconstruction process by incorporating a mathematical model for PVE along with other physical perturbations (photon attenuation, scattered radiation, and other physical effects) directly into the reconstruction algorithm.[129]

SUMMARY AND FUTURE PROSPECTS

This article has attempted to summarize important themes of ongoing advancements by providing an overview of current state-of-the art developments in software- and hardware-based multimodality imaging combining PET with other structural imaging modalities (PET/CT and PET/MR imaging). Clearly, multimodality imaging has changed drastically over the last 2 decades. The pace of change has accelerated rapidly in the last decade driven by the introduction and widespread acceptance of combined PET/CT units in the clinic and the likely deployment of compact PET/MR imaging systems in the near future. Navigating beyond the sixth dimension is now becoming possible with recent progress in multidimensional and multiparametric multimodality imaging combining the latest advances in sophisticated software to make use of existing advanced hardware.[130] A controversy arose recently regarding the future role of SPECT in the era of PET.[131–134] Time will determine whether these predictions are wrong or will come true. Given that the role of any molecular imaging technology is established with respect to the benefits conveyed to patients, dual-modality imaging systems using PET as the key component are here to stay and will definitely maintain an exclusive standing in clinical diagnosis, the assessment of response to treatment, and the delivery of personalized treatments and targeted therapies.

ACKNOWLEDGMENTS

The authors would like to thank Dr C. Steiner for providing some of the clinical illustrations used in this manuscript.

REFERENCES

1. Webb S. Combating cancer in the third millennium: the contribution of medical physics. Phys Med 2008;24:42–8.
2. Hasegawa B, Zaidi H. Dual-modality imaging: more than the sum of its components. In: Zaidi H, editor. Quantitative analysis in nuclear medicine imaging. New York: Springer; 2006. p. 35–81.
3. Pietrzyk U. Does PET/CT render software fusion obsolete? Nuklearmedizin 2005;44:S13–7.
4. Weigert M, Pietrzyk U, Muller S, et al. Whole-body PET/CT imaging: combining software- and hardware-based co-registration. Z Med Phys 2008;18:59–66.
5. Nehmeh SA, Erdi YE. Respiratory motion in positron emission tomography/computed tomography: a review. Semin Nucl Med 2008;38:167–76.
6. Slomka PJ, Dey D, Przetak C, et al. Automated 3-dimensional registration of stand-alone (18)F-FDG whole-body PET with CT. J Nucl Med 2003;44:1156–67.
7. Hill DL, Batchelor PG, Holden M, et al. Medical image registration. Phys Med Biol 2001;46:R1–45.
8. Hutton BF, Braun M. Software for image registration: algorithms, accuracy, efficacy. Semin Nucl Med 2003;33:180–92.
9. Maes F, Vandermeulen D, Suetens P. Medical image registration using mutual information. Proceedings of the IEEE 2003;91:1699–722.
10. Slomka PJ. Software approach to merging molecular with anatomic information. J Nucl Med 2004;45(Suppl 1):36S–45S.
11. Hill DLG, Studholme C, Hawkes DJ. Voxel similarity measures for automated image registration. In: Robb R, editor. Visualization in biomedical computing, vol 2359. Bellingham (DC): SPIE Press; 1994. p. 205–16.
12. Maes F, Collignon A, Vandermeulen D, et al. Multimodality image registration by maximization of mutual information. IEEE Trans Med Imaging 1997;16:187–98.
13. Lau YH, Braun M, Hutton BF. Non-rigid image registration using a median-filtered coarse-to-fine displacement field and a symmetric correlation ratio. Phys Med Biol 2001;46:1297–319.
14. Juweid ME, Cheson BD. Positron-emission tomography and assessment of cancer therapy. N Engl J Med 2006;354:496–507.
15. Weber WA, Figlin R. Monitoring cancer treatment with PET/CT: does it make a difference? J Nucl Med 2007;48:36S–44S.
16. De Moor K, Nuyts J, Plessers L, et al. Non-rigid registration with position dependent rigidity for whole body PET follow-up studies. Proceedings of the Nuclear Science Symposium and Medical Imaging Conference. San Diego, CA; 2006. p. 3502–6.
17. Mirshanov DM. Transmission-emission computer tomograph. USSR Patent No. 621.386:616–073 20.01.87-SU-181935, 1987.
18. Kaplan CH. Transmission/emission registered image (TERI) computed tomography scanners. International Patent No. PCT/US90/03722, 1989.
19. Hasegawa BH, Gingold EL, Reilly SM, et al. Description of a simultaneous emission-

transmission CT system. Proc Soc Photo Instrum Eng 1990;1231:50–60.

20. Hasegawa BH, Iwata K, Wong KH, et al. Dual-modality imaging of function and physiology. Acad Radiol 2002;9:1305–21.

21. Jones EF, Gould RG, VanBrocklin HF. Bruce H. Hasegawa, PhD, 1951–2008. J Nucl Med 2008; 49:37N–8N.

22. Beyer T, Townsend D, Brun T, et al. A combined PET/CT scanner for clinical oncology. J Nucl Med 2000;41:1369–79.

23. Townsend DW. Multimodality imaging of structure and function. Phys Med Biol 2008;53:R1–39.

24. Bailey D, Roach P, Bailey E, et al. Development of a cost-effective modular SPECT/CT scanner. Eur J Nucl Med Mol Imaging 2007;34:1415–26.

25. Beekman F, Hutton B. Multi-modality imaging on track. Eur J Nucl Med Mol Imaging 2007;34: 1410–4.

26. Steinert HC, von Schulthess GK. Initial clinical experience using a new integrated in-line PET/CT system. Br J Radiol 2002;73:S36–8.

27. Luk WR, Digby WD, Jones WF, et al. An analysis of correction methods for emission contamination in PET postinjection transmission measurement. IEEE Trans Nucl Sci 1995;42:2303–8.

28. Coleman RE, Delbeke D, Guiberteau MJ, et al. Concurrent PET/CT with an integrated imaging system: intersociety dialogue from the joint working group of the American College of Radiology, the Society of Nuclear Medicine, and the Society of Computed Body Tomography and Magnetic Resonance. J Nucl Med 2005;46: 1225–39.

29. Bischof Delaloye A, Carrio I, Cuocolo A, et al. White paper of the European Association of Nuclear Medicine (EANM) and the European Society of Radiology (ESR) on multimodality imaging. Eur J Nucl Med Mol Imaging 2007;34:1147–51.

30. Stegger L, Schäfers M, Weckesser M, et al. EANM-ESR white paper on multimodality imaging. Eur J Nucl Med Mol Imaging 2008;35:677–80.

31. Antoch G, Freudenberg LS, Beyer T, et al. To enhance or not to enhance? 18F-FDG and CT contrast agents in dual-modality 18F-FDG PET/CT. J Nucl Med 2004;45(Suppl 1):56S–65S.

32. Mawlawi O, Erasmus JJ, Munden RF, et al. Quantifying the effect of IV contrast media on integrated PET/CT: clinical evaluation. AJR Am J Roentgenol 2006;186:308–19.

33. Ahmadian A, Ay MR, Bidgoli JH, et al. Correction of oral contrast artifacts in CT-based attenuation correction of PET images using an automated segmentation algorithm. Eur J Nucl Med Mol Imaging 2008;35:1812–23.

34. Rickey D, Gordon R, Huda W. On lifting the inherent limitations of positron emission tomography by using magnetic fields (MagPET). Automedica 1992;14:355–69.

35. Hammer BE, Christensen NL, Heil BG. Use of a magnetic field to increase the spatial resolution of positron emission tomography. Med Phys 1994; 21:1917–20.

36. Wirrwar A, Vosberg H, Herzog H, et al. Muller-Gartner H-W 4.5 Tesla magnetic field reduces range of high-energy positrons: potential implications for positron emission tomography. IEEE Trans Nucl Sci 1997;44:184–9.

37. Raylman RR, Hammer BE, Christensen NL. Combined MRI-PET scanner: a Monte-Carlo evaluation of the improvements in PET resolution due to the effects of a static homogeneous magnetic field. IEEE Trans Nucl Sci 1996;43:2406–12.

38. Christensen NL, Hammer BE, Heil BG, et al. Positron emission tomography within a magnetic field using photomultiplier tubes and light guides. Phys Med Biol 1995;40:691–7.

39. Shao Y, Cherry SR, Farahani K, et al. Simultaneous PET and MR imaging. Phys Med Biol 1997;42: 1965–70.

40. Shao Y, Cherry SR, Farahani K, et al. Development of a PET detector system compatible with MRI/NMR systems. IEEE Trans Nucl Sci 1997;44: 1167–71.

41. Slates R, Cherry SR, Boutefnouchet A, et al. Design of a small animal MR compatible PET scanner. IEEE Trans Nucl Sci 1999;46:565–70.

42. Slates R, Farahani K, Shao Y, et al. A study of artifacts in simultaneous PET and MR imaging using a prototype MR compatible PET scanner. Phys Med Biol 1999;44:2015–27.

43. Marsden PK, Strul D, Keevil SF, et al. Simultaneous PET and NMR. Br J Radiol 2002;75:S53–9.

44. Mackewn JE, Strul D, Hallett WA, et al. Design and development of an MR-compatible PET scanner for imaging small animals. IEEE Trans Nucl Sci 2005; 52:1376–80.

45. Yamamoto S, Takamatsu S, Murayama H, et al. A block detector for a multislice, depth-of-interaction MR-compatible PET. IEEE Trans Nucl Sci 2005;52:33–7.

46. Raylman RR, Majewski S, Lemieux SK, et al. Simultaneous MRI and PET imaging of a rat brain. Phys Med Biol 2006;51:6371–9.

47. Raylman RR, Majewski S, Velan SS, et al. Simultaneous acquisition of magnetic resonance spectroscopy (MRS) data and positron emission tomography (PET) images with a prototype MR-compatible, small animal PET imager. J Magn Reson 2007;186:305–10.

48. Lucas AJ, Hawkes RC, Ansorge RE, et al. Development of a combined micro-PET-MR system. Technol Cancer Res Treat 2006;5: 337–41.

49. Handler WB, Gilbert KM, Peng H, et al. Simulation of scattering and attenuation of 511 keV photons in a combined PET/field-cycled MRI system. Phys Med Biol 2006;51:2479–91.

50. Renker D. Properties of avalanche photodiodes for applications in high energy physics, astrophysics and medical imaging. Nucl Instr Meth A 2002;486:164–9.

51. Renker D. Geiger-mode avalanche photodiodes, history, properties and problems. Nucl Instr Meth A 2006;567:48–56.

52. Llosa G, Battiston R, Belcari N, et al. Novel silicon photomultipliers for PET applications. IEEE Trans Nucl Sci 2008;55:877–81.

53. Pepin CM, St-Pierre C, Forgues J-C, et al. Physical characterization of the LabPET, LGSO, and LYSO scintillators. Nuclear Science Symposium Conference Record 2007;3:2292–5.

54. Lecomte R, Cadorette J, Rodrigue S, et al. Initial results from the Sherbrooke avalanche photodiode positron tomograph. IEEE Trans Nucl Sci 1996;43:1952–7.

55. Pichler BJ, Judenhofer MS, Catana C, et al. Performance test of an LSO-APD detector in a 7-T MRI scanner for simultaneous PET/MRI. J Nucl Med 2006;47:639–47.

56. Catana C, Wu Y, Judenhofer MS, et al. Simultaneous acquisition of multislice PET and MR images: initial results with a MR-compatible PET scanner. J Nucl Med 2006;47:1968–76.

57. Catana C, Procissi D, Wu Y, et al. Simultaneous in vivo positron emission tomography and magnetic resonance imaging. Proc Natl Acad Sci U S A 2008;105:3705–10.

58. Woody C, Schlyer D, Vaska P, et al. Preliminary studies of a simultaneous PET/MRI scanner based on the RatCAP small animal tomograph. Nucl Instr Meth A 2007;571:102–5.

59. Judenhofer MS, Catana C, Swann BK, et al. Simultaneous PET/MR images, acquired with a compact MRI compatible PET detector in a 7 Tesla magnet. Radiology 2007;244:807–14.

60. Judenhofer MS, Wehrl HF, Newport DF, et al. Simultaneous PET-MRI: a new approach for functional and morphological imaging. Nat Med 2008;14:459–65.

61. Moehrs S, Del Guerra A, Herbert DJ, et al. A detector head design for small-animal PET with silicon photomultipliers (SiPM). Phys Med Biol 2006;51:1113–27.

62. Hong SJ, Song IC, Ito M, et al. An investigation into the use of Geiger-mode solid-state photomultipliers for simultaneous PET and MRI acquisition. IEEE Trans Nucl Sci 2008;55:882–8.

63. Reznik A, Lui BJ, Rowlands JA. An amorphous selenium based positron emission mammography camera with avalanche gain. Technol Cancer Res Treat 2005;4:61–7.

64. Reznik A, Baranovskii SD, Rubel O, et al. Avalanche multiplication in amorphous selenium and its utilization in imaging. Journal of Non-Crystalline Solids 2008;354:2691–6.

65. Schlemmer HP, Pichler BJ, Schmand M, et al. Simultaneous MR/PET imaging of the human brain: feasibility study. Radiology 2008;248:1028–35.

66. Holdsworth SJ, Bammer R. Magnetic resonance imaging techniques: fMRI, DWI, and PWI. Semin Neurol 2008;28:395–406.

67. Gaa J, Rummeny EJ, Seemann MD. Whole-body imaging with PET/MRI. Eur J Med Res 2004;30:309–12.

68. Seemann MD. Whole-body PET/MRI: the future in oncological imaging. Technol Cancer Res Treat 2005;4:577–82.

69. Schlemmer HP, Pichler BJ, Krieg R, et al. An integrated MR/PET system: prospective applications. Abdom Imaging, in press.

70. Hicks RJ, Lau EW. PET/MRI: a different spin from under the rim. Eur J Nucl Med Mol Imaging 2009;36:10–4.

71. Payne GS, Leach MO. Applications of magnetic resonance spectroscopy in radiotherapy treatment planning. Br J Radiol 2006;79:S16–26 (Spec No 1).

72. Czernin J, Allen-Auerbach M, Schelbert HR. Improvements in cancer staging with PET/CT: literature-based evidence as of September 2006. J Nucl Med 2007;48:78S–88S.

73. Di Carli MF, Dorbala S, Meserve J, et al. Clinical myocardial perfusion PET/CT. J Nucl Med 2007;48:783–93.

74. Costa DC, Pilowsky LS, Ell PJ. Nuclear medicine in neurology and psychiatry. Lancet 1999;354:1107–11.

75. Tatsch K, Ell PJ. PET and SPECT in common neuropsychiatric disease. Clin Med 2006;6:259–62.

76. Pelizzari CA, Chen GT, Spelbring DR, et al. Accurate three-dimensional registration of CT, PET, and/or MR images of the brain. J Comput Assist Tomogr 1989;13:20–6.

77. Woods RP, Mazziotta JC, Cherry SR. MRI-PET registration with automated algorithm. J Comput Assist Tomogr 1993;17:536–46.

78. Gilman S. Imaging the brain. N Engl J Med 1998;338:812–20.

79. Viergever MA, Maintz JB, Niessen WJ, et al. Registration, segmentation, and visualization of multimodal brain images. Comput Med Imaging Graph 2001;25:147–51.

80. Muzik O, Chugani DC, Zou G, et al. Multimodality data integration in epilepsy. Int J Biomed Imaging 2007;2007:13963.

81. O'Brien TJ, Miles K, Ware R, et al. The cost-effective use of 18F-FDG PET in the presurgical

evaluation of medically refractory focal epilepsy. J Nucl Med 2008;49:931–7.

82. Studholme C, Hill DLG, Hawkes DJ. An overlap invariant entropy measure of 3D medical image alignment. Pattern Recognit 1999;32:71–86.

83. Vees H, Senthamizhchelvan S, Miralbell R, et al. Assessment of various strategies for 18F-FET PET-guided delineation of target volumes in high-grade glioma patients. Eur J Nucl Med Mol Imaging 2009;36:182–93.

84. Antoni G, Langstrom B. Radiopharmaceuticals: molecular imaging using positron emission tomography. Handb Exp Pharmacol 2008;185: 177–201.

85. Kumar R, Dhanpathi H, Basu S, et al. Oncologic PET tracers beyond [(18)F]FDG and the novel quantitative approaches in PET imaging. Q J Nucl Med Mol Imaging 2008;52:50–65.

86. Lardinois D, Weder W, Hany TF, et al. Staging of non-small-cell lung cancer with integrated positron-emission tomography and computed tomography. N Engl J Med 2003;348:2500–7.

87. Zaidi H. The quest for the ideal anato-molecular imaging fusion tool. Biomed Imaging Interv J 2006;2:e47.

88. Alavi A, Mavi A, Basu S, et al. Is PET-CT the only option? Eur J Nucl Med Mol Imaging 2007;34: 819–21.

89. Weissleder R, Mahmood U. Molecular imaging. Radiology 2001;219:316–33.

90. De Ruysscher D, Wanders S, Minken A, et al. Effects of radiotherapy planning with a dedicated combined PET-CT-simulator of patients with non-small cell lung cancer on dose limiting normal tissues and radiation dose-escalation: a planning study. Radiother Oncol 2005;77:5–10.

91. Nestle U, Walter K, Schmidt S, et al. 18F-deoxyglucose positron emission tomography (FDG-PET) for the planning of radiotherapy in lung cancer: high impact in patients with atelectasis. Int J Radiat Oncol Biol Phys 1999;44:593–7.

92. Messa C, Ceresoli GL, Rizzo G, et al. Feasibility of [18F]FDG-PET and coregistered CT on clinical target volume definition of advanced non-small cell lung cancer. Q J Nucl Med Mol Imaging 2005;49:259–66.

93. Luketich JD, Friedman DM, Meltzer CC, et al. The role of positron emission tomography in evaluating mediastinal lymph node metastases in non-small-cell lung cancer. Clin Lung Cancer 2001;2:229–33.

94. Zaidi H, Vees H, Wissmeyer M. Molecular PET/CT imaging-guided radiation therapy treatment planning. Acad Radiol 2009;16:1108–33.

95. Basu S, Zaidi H, Houseni M, et al. Novel quantitative techniques for assessing regional and global function and structure based on modern imaging modalities: implications for normal variation, aging

and diseased states. Semin Nucl Med 2007;37: 223–39.

96. Kinahan PE, Hasegawa BH, Beyer T. X-ray–based attenuation correction for positron emission tomography/computed tomography scanners. Semin Nucl Med 2003;33:166–79.

97. Zaidi H, Montandon M-L, Alavi A. Advances in attenuation correction techniques in PET. PET Clinics 2007;2:191–217.

98. Zaidi H. Is MRI-guided attenuation correction a viable option for dual-modality PET/MR imaging? Radiology 2007;244:639–42.

99. Hofmann M, Pichler B, Scholkopf B, et al. Towards quantitative PET/MRI: a review of MR-based attenuation correction techniques. Eur J Nucl Med Mol Imaging 2009;36:93–104.

100. Zaidi H. Is radionuclide transmission scanning obsolete for dual-modality PET/CT systems? Eur J Nucl Med Mol Imaging 2007;34:815–8.

101. Zaidi H, Montandon M-L. Scatter compensation techniques in PET. PET Clinics 2007;2:219–34.

102. Watson CC. New, faster, image-based scatter correction for 3D PET. IEEE Trans Nucl Sci 2000; 47:1587–94.

103. Watson CC, Casey ME, Michel C, et al. Advances in scatter correction for 3D PET/CT. Nuclear Science Symposium Conference Record, 19–22 October 2004, Rome, Italy 5:3008–12.

104. Wollenweber SD. Parameterization of a model-based 3-D PET scatter correction. IEEE Trans Nucl Sci 2002;49:722–7.

105. Accorsi R, Adam L-E, Werner ME, et al. Optimization of a fully 3D single scatter simulation algorithm for 3D PET. Phys Med Biol 2004;49: 2577–98.

106. Levin CS, Dahlbom M, Hoffman EJ. A Monte Carlo correction for the effect of Compton scattering in 3-D PET brain imaging. IEEE Trans Nucl Sci 1995;42:1181–8.

107. Zaidi H. Comparative evaluation of scatter correction techniques in 3D positron emission tomography. Eur J Nucl Med 2000;27:1813–26.

108. Holdsworth CH, Levin CS, Janecek M, et al. Performance analysis of an improved 3-D PET Monte Carlo simulation and scatter correction. IEEE Trans Nucl Sci 2002;49:83–9.

109. Reader AJ, Zaidi H. Advances in PET image reconstruction. PET Clinics 2007;2:173–90.

110. Green PJ. Bayesian reconstructions from emission tomography data using a modified EM algorithm. IEEE Trans Med Imaging 1990;9:84–93.

111. Comtat C, Kinahan PE, Fessler JA, et al. Clinically feasible reconstruction of 3D whole-body PET/CT data using blurred anatomical labels. Phys Med Biol 2002;47:1–20.

112. Gindi G, Lee M, Rangarajan A, et al. Bayesian reconstruction of functional images using

anatomical information as priors. IEEE Trans Med Imaging 1993;12:670–80.

113. Baete K, Nuyts J, Van Paesschen W, et al. Anatomical-based FDG-PET reconstruction for the detection of hypo-metabolic regions in epilepsy. IEEE Trans Med Imaging 2004;23:510–9.

114. Pichler BJ, Wehrl HF, Kolb A, et al. Positron emission tomography/magnetic resonance imaging: the next generation of multimodality imaging? Semin Nucl Med 2008;38:199–208.

115. Rousset O, Rahmim A, Alavi A, et al. Partial volume correction strategies in PET. PET Clinics 2007;2: 235–49.

116. Soret M, Bacharach SL, Buvat I. Partial-volume effect in PET tumor imaging. J Nucl Med 2007;48: 932–45.

117. Kessler RM, Ellis JR, Eden M. Analysis of emission tomographic scan data: limitations imposed by resolution and background. J Comput Assist Tomogr 1984;8:514–22.

118. Geworski L, Knoop BO, de Cabrejas ML, et al. Recovery correction for quantitation in emission tomography: a feasibility study. Eur J Nucl Med 2000;27:161–9.

119. Quarantelli M, Berkouk K, Prinster A, et al. Integrated software for the analysis of brain PET/SPECT studies with partial-volume-effect correction. J Nucl Med 2004;45:192–201.

120. Da Silva AJ, Tang HR, Wong KH, et al. Absolute quantification of regional myocardial uptake of 99mTc-sestamibi with SPECT: experimental validation in a porcine model. J Nucl Med 2001;42:772–9.

121. Matsuda H, Ohnishi T, Asada T, et al. Correction for partial-volume effects on brain perfusion SPECT in healthy men. J Nucl Med 2003;44:1243–52.

122. Ashburner J, Friston KJ. Unified segmentation. Neuroimage 2005;26:839–51.

123. Rousset OG, Collins DL, Rahmim A, et al. Design and implementation of an automated partial volume correction in PET: application to dopamine receptor quantification in the normal human striatum. J Nucl Med 2008;49:1097–106.

124. Meltzer CC, Kinahan PE, Greer PJ, et al. Comparative evaluation of MR-based partial-volume correction schemes for PET. J Nucl Med 1999;40: 2053–65.

125. Frouin V, Comtat C, Reilhac A, et al. Correction of partial volume effect for PET striatal imaging: fast implementation and study of robustness. J Nucl Med 2002;43:1715–26.

126. Zaidi H, Ruest T, Schoenahl F, et al. Comparative evaluation of statistical brain MR image segmentation algorithms and their impact on partial volume effect correction in PET. Neuroimage 2006;32: 1591–607.

127. Rousset O, Zaidi H. Correction of partial volume effects in emission tomography. In: Zaidi H, editor. Quantitative analysis of nuclear medicine images. New York: Springer; 2006. p. 236–71.

128. Shidahara M, Tsoumpas C, Hammers A, et al. Functional and structural synergy for resolution recovery and partial volume correction in brain PET. Neuroimage 2009;44:340–8.

129. Baete K, Nuyts J, Laere KV, et al. Evaluation of anatomy based reconstruction for partial volume correction in brain FDG-PET. Neuroimage 2004; 23:305–17.

130. Zaidi H. Navigating beyond the 6th dimension: a challenge in the era of multi-parametric molecular imaging. Eur J Nucl Med Mol Imaging, in press.

131. Rahmim A, Zaidi H. PET versus SPECT: strengths, limitations and challenges. Nucl Med Commun 2008;29:193–207.

132. Alavi A, Basu S. Planar and SPECT imaging in the era of PET and PET–CT: can it survive the test of time? Eur J Nucl Med Mol Imaging 2008;35: 1554–9.

133. Mariani G, Bruselli L, Duatti A. Is PET always an advantage versus planar and SPECT imaging? Eur J Nucl Med Mol Imaging 2008;35:1560–5.

134. Seret A. Will high-resolution/high-sensitivity SPECT ensure that PET is not the only survivor in nuclear medicine during the next decade? Eur J Nucl Med Mol Imaging 2009;36:533–5.

Index

Note: Page numbers of article titles are in **boldface** type.

A

Acetabular cartilage, MR imaging assessment of, 114–116
Acetabular labrum, MR imaging assessment of, 114
Advanced Multimodality Image Guided Operative (AMIGO) suite, 6–7, 8
AIDS, musculoskeletal lymphoma and, 84–85
AIDS dementia complex, 129
Alzheimer's disease, amyloid imaging in, 125
    diffusion-weighted imaging diffusion-tensor imaging in, 121–123
    functional MRI in, 124–125
    magnetic resonance spectroscopy in, 123–124
    magnetization transfer ratio in, 123
    structural MRI in, 121–123
Amyloid imaging, in Alzheimer's disease, 125
Angiography, MR, contrast-enhanced, in Takayasu arteritis, 52–53
        of aorta, 45–46
        of aortic aneurysm, 46, 47
        of aortic dissection, 49, 50
Aorta, contrast-enhanced MR angiography of, 45–46
    MR imaging of, **43–55**
        basic technical considerations in, 43–46
        black-blood vascular, 44
        bright-blood vascular, 44–45
        compared to CT imaging, 43
Aortic aneurysm, contrast-enhanced MR angiography of, 46, 47
    infected, MR imaging of, 46, 48
    inflammatory, MR imaging of, 46, 49
    spin echo MR imaging of, 46, 47, 48
Aortic disease, MR imaging in, 46–53
Aortic dissection, contrast-enhanced MR angiography of, 49, 50
    MR imaging of, 47–49, 50
Arterial curve, analysis of, gadolinium systemic model and, 35–36
Arthrography, MR, in osteoarthritis, 105–106
Atherosclerotic ulcer, penetrating, 51, 52

B

Blood flow, renal, single-kidney, calculation of, 35
Bone, chemotherapy and radiation of, complications of, 89, 90, 91
    lymphoma of. See *Lymphoma, of bone.*
Bone marrow, evaluation of, with FDG-positron emission tomography, 88–91
Bone scintigraphy, in lymphoma of bone, 77, 79

Brachytherapy, future of, 19
    MR imaging-guided, for prostate cancer, 16–19
        outcomes of, 19
        patient selection for, 17
        procedure for, 17–19
"Brain shift," 1, 2
Breast, contralateral, breast MR imaging in staging examination of, 65
Breast cancer, neoadjuvant chemotherapy response in, 66–67
    occult primary, 68
    patients at high risk for, screening of, 68
    residual disease in, assessment in, 67
    tumor recurrence in, at lumpectomy site, 67–68
Breast conservation therapy, breast MR imaging and, contraindications to, 63
Breast MR imaging, and breast conservation therapy, contraindications to, 63
    background of, 62
    diagnostic, current status and future directions in, **57–74**
        recent guidelines and recommendations for, 57–59
    for preoperative staging in, 62–66
    hormonal-related enhancement of, 69–71
    image acquisition for, 71
    in cancer staging, controversies in use of, 64–65
        issues to consider in, 65
    in inconclusive mammography, 68–69
    in recurrence of breast disease, 63
    new developments in technology of, 72
    of contralateral breast, in staging examination, 65
    of positive surgical margins, 64
    overuse/over-reliance on, pitfalls of, 69
    preoperative, identification of patients for, 65–88
    sensitivity and specificity issues in, 59–62

C

Cartilage matrix, quantitative imaging of, in osteoarthritis, 106–107
Central nervous system, dementing disorders of, 129
Chemotherapy, and radiation of, causing complications of bone, 89, 90, 91
Cognitive disturbances, MRI in, 128–129
Correlative fusion imaging, clinical role of, 137–140, 141, 142, 143, 144
Cryotherapy, for uterine fibroids, 14–15
    percutaneous, MR imaging-guided, of renal tumors, 21–22, 23

mri.theclinics.com

CT, and MR imaging of aorta, compared, 43
  in lymphoma of bone, 77–78, 79, 80
  in lymphoma of muscles, 81–82, 85
Cutaneous and subcutaneous tissue, lymphoma of, 83–84, 86

D

Dementia, frontotemporal, MRI in, 128
  MRI in, **121–132**
  vascular, MRI in, 125–127
    NINDS-AIREN criteria, 125–126, 127

F

FDG-Positron emission tomography, and MR imaging, monitoring treatment response of lymphoma with, 85–86, 87
  bone marrow evaluation using, 88–91
Femoroacetabular impingement, as trigger of hip osteoarthritis, 111–112, 113
  diagnosis of, 112–113
  measurements in, 113–114, 115, 116
Frontotemporal dementia, MRI in, 128
Fusion imaging, clinical role of, using PET, CT, and MR imaging, **133–149**
  correlative, clinical role of, 137–140, 141, 142, 143, 144
  future prospects for, 145

G

Gadlolinium-enhanced renal perfusion-distribution imaging, 33
Gadolinium-enhanced MR imaging, of cartilage, 107
Gadolinium kidney model, analysis of kidney curve and, 36–37
Gadolinium systemic model, analysis of arterial curve and, 35–36
Genital tract, female, 11
  male, 15
Genitourinary tract, MR imaging-guided interventions in, **11–28**
Glomerular filtration rate, single-kidney, calculation of, 35–37

H

Hardware-based multimodality imaging, 134–137
Hematoma, intramural, spin echo MR imaging of, 49–52
Hip, articular cartilage of, biochemical imaging of, 116–118
  osteoarthritis of, MRI in, and implications for surgery, **111–120**
    risk factors for, 111
Huntington's disease, MRI in, 128

I

Image registration, software-based, and fusion, 134
IMRIS iMRI, 5, 6

K

Kidney, MR imaging-guided radiofrequency ablation in, 21
  normal, 29, 30
  transplanted, diagnostic imaging of, 38, 40
Kidney curve, analysis of, gadolinium kidney model and, 36–37

L

Lymphoma, musculoskeletal, and AIDS, 84–85
  of bone, bone scintigraphy in, 77, 78
    clinical features of, 76
    CT in, 77–78, 79, 80
    imaging of, 76
    incidence of, 75
    MR imaging in, 78–80, 82, 83
    radiography of, 76–77, 78, 79
  of cutaneous and subcutaneous tissue, 83–84, 86
  of muscles, CT in, 81–82, 85
    differential diagnosis of, 82–83
    imaging of, 81
    incidence of, 80–81
    MR imaging of, 81, 84
    ultrasound in, 82, 85
  of musculoskeletal system, imaging of, **75–93**
    imaging modalities in, 75
  treatment of, response to, and treatment-related changes, 85–91

M

Magnetic resonance-guided focused ultrasound surgery, clinical trials in, 12–14
  equipment for fibroid treatment, 12
  for treating uterine fibroids, 11–14
  fundamentals, 12
  patient selection for, 12
  treatment planning for, 12
Magnetic resonance nephrourography, **29–42**
  image analysis in, 33–35
  in congenital anomalies and obstruction, 37–38, 39
  limitatitons of, 38–41
  renal function and, 3–33, 341
  structure of kidneys and, 29–31
Magnetic resonance spectroscopy, in Alzheimer's disease, 123–124
Magnetic Resonance Therapy (MRT) unit, 1–2, 3
MR angiography, contrast-enhanced, in Takayasu arteritis, 52–53

of aorta, 45–46
  of aortic aneurysm, 46, 47
  of aortic dissection, 49, 50
MR arthrography, in osteoarthritis, 105–106
MR imaging. See also *MRI*.
  and FDG-positron emission tomography,
    monitoring treatment response of lymphoma
    with, 85–86, 87
  black-blood vascular, of aorta, 44
  bright-blood vascular, of aorta, 44–45
  extremity-only, in osteoarthritis, 98–99
  gadolinium-enhanced, of cartilage, 107
  in lymphoma of bone, 78–80, 82, 83
  in lymphoma of muscles, 81, 84
  in osteoarthritis, field strength for, 95–98
    hardware, coils, and sequences, **95–110**
    sequence protocols for, 101–105
    three-dimensional gradient-echo and fast-low
      sequences for, 102–103, 104
  of aorta, **43–55**
    basic technical considerations in, 43–46
    compared to CT imaging, 43
  of breast. See *Breast MR imaging*.
  open, in osteoarthritis, 98–99
  recent developments in, 22–23
  surface coils for, in osteoarthritis, 99–101
  weight-bearing, in osteoarthritis, 99, 100
MR imaging-guided brachytherapy. See
  Brachytherapy, MR imaging-guided.
MR imaging-guided catheter-based ultrasound
  thermal therapy, of prostate, 20–21
MR imaging-guided interventions, in genitourinary
  tract, **11–28**
MR imaging-guided percutaneous cryotherapy, of
  renal tumors, 21–22, 23
MR imaging-guided prostate biopsy, 15–16
  future of, 16
  technique of, 16
MR imaging-guided radiofrequency ablation, in
  kidney, 21
MRI, closed-configuration intraoperative, origins of,
  4–5
  functional, in Alzheimer's disease, 124–125
  in dementia, **121–132**
  in frontotemporal dementia, 128
  in Huntington's disease, 128
  in psychiatric disorders and cognitive
    disturbances, 128–129
  in vascular dementia, 125–127
  intraoperative, future horizons of, 5–6
    origins of, **1–10**
      0.5T open-configuration prototype, 1–4
  of hip osteoarthritis, and implications for surgery,
    111–120
  open-configuration intraoperative, expanding
    scope of, 4–5
MRI robotics, intraoperative, 5, 7

MRI suites, intraoperative, future, 5–6
Multimodality imaging, hardware-based, 134–137
Muscles, lymphoma of. See *Lymphoma, of muscles*.
Musculoskeletal lymphoma, and AIDS, 84–85
Musculoskeletal system, lymphoma of, imaging of,
  75–93

N

Nephrourography, magnetic resonance, image
  analysis in, 33–35
    in congenital anomalies and obstruction,
      37–38, 39
    limitations of, 38–41
    renal function and, 31–33, 34
    structure of kidneys and, 29–31
NeuroArm MRI-compatible neurosurgical robot, 6, 7
Neurosurgical robot, NeuroArm MRI-compatible, 6, 7

O

Osteoarthritis, extremity and open MR imaging in,
  98–99
  MR arthrography in, 105–106
  MR imaging in, field strength for, 95–98
    hardware, coils, and sequences, **95–110**
    intermediate- and T1-weighted fast spin-echo
      sequences for, 102, 103
    sequence protocols for, 101–105
    surface coils for, 99–101
    three-dimensional gradient-echo and fast-low
      sequences for, 102–103, 104
  of hip, biochemical imaging of articular cartilage
    in, 116–118
    MRI in, and implications for surgery, **111–120**
  quantitative imaging of cartilage matrix in,
    106–107
  weight-bearing MR imaging in, 99, 100

P

PET/CT instrumentation, combined, 134–137
  advantages of, 135–136
  history of, 134–135
  instrumentation for, 136–137
PET imaging, anatomically guided attenuation, and
  scatter compensation, 141–142
  anatomically guided partial volume correction in,
    143–145
  anatomically guided reconstruction, 142–143
  data from, anatomically guided quantification of,
    advances in, 140–145
PoleStar iMRI, 5
Prostate, focused ultrasound surgery in, 19–20
  MR imaging-guided catheter-based ultrasound
    thermal therapy of, 20–21
Prostate biopsy, MR imaging-guided, 15–16

Prostate (*continued*)
  future of, 16
  technique of, 16
Prostate cancer, MR imaging-guided brachytherapy
  for, 16–19
    outcomes of, 19
    patient selection for, 17
    procedure for, 17–19
Psychiatric disorders, MRI in, 128–129

R

Radiation, and chemotherapy, causing complications
  of bone, 89, 90, 91
Radiofrequency ablation, MR imaging-guided, in
  kidney, 21
Radiography, in lymphoma of bone, 76–77, 78, 79
Renal artery, imaging techniques for, 33
Renal blood flow, single-kidney, calculation of, 35
Renal cell carcinoma, treatment of, 20
Renal tumors, MR imaging-guided percutaneous
  cryotherapy of, 21–22, 23

S

Software-based image registration, and fusion, 134

Spectroscopy, MR, in Alzheimer's disease, 123–124
Spin echo MR imaging, of aortic aneurysm, 46, 47, 48
  of intramural hematoma, 49–52

T

Takayasu arteritis, contrast-enhanced MR
  angiography in, 52–53

U

Ultrasound, in lymphoma of muscles, 82, 85
Ultrasound surgery, focused, in prostate, 19–20
Urinary tract, 20
Uterine fibroids, cryotherapy for, 14–15
  magnetic resonance-guided focused ultrasound
    surgery in, 11–14
  prevalence of, 11
  treatment options in, 11–12

V

Vascular dementia, MRI in, 125–127
  NINDS-AIREN criteria, 125–126, 127

Moving?

Make sure your subscription moves with you!

To notify us of your new address, find your **Clinics Account Number** (located on your mailing label above your name), and contact customer service at:

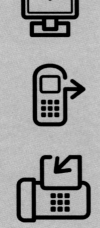

Email: journalscustomerservice-usa@elsevier.com

800-654-2452 (subscribers in the U.S. & Canada)
314-447-8871 (subscribers outside of the U.S. & Canada)

Fax number: 314-447-8029

Elsevier Health Sciences Division
Subscription Customer Service
3251 Riverport Lane
Maryland Heights, MO 63043

*To ensure uninterrupted delivery of your subscription, please notify us at least 4 weeks in advance of move.

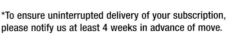